Allergen Immunotherapy

Guest Editor

LINDA COX, MD

IMMUNOLOGY AND ALLERGY CLINICS OF NORTH AMERICA

www.immunology.theclinics.com

Consulting Editor
RAFEUL ALAM, MD, PhD

May 2011 • Volume 31 • Number 2

SAUNDERS an imprint of ELSEVIER, Inc.

W.B. SAUNDERS COMPANY

A Division of Elsevier Inc.

1600 John F. Kennedy Blvd., ● Suite 1800 ● Philadelphia, PA 19103-2899.

http://www.theclinics.com

IMMUNOLOGY AND ALLERGY CLINICS OF NORTH AMERICA Volume 31, Number 2

May 2011 ISSN 0889–8561, ISBN-13: 978-1-4557-1148-2

Editor: Rachel Glover

Developmental Editor: Donald Mumford

Immunology and Allergy Clinics of North America (ISSN 0889–8561) is published quarterly by Elsevier Inc., 360 Park Avenue South, New York, NY 10010-1710. Months of issue are February, May, August, and November. Periodicals postage paid at New York, NY and additional mailing offices. Subscription prices are $272.00 per year for US individuals, $392.00 per year for US institutions, $129.00 per year for US students and residents, $334.00 per year for Canadian individuals, $187.00 per year for Canadian students, $486.00 per year for Canadian institutions, $379.00 per year for international individuals, $486.00 per year for international institutions, $187.00 per year for international students. To receive student/resident rate, orders must be accompanied by name of affiliated institution, date of term, and the *signature* of program/residency coordinator on institution letterhead. Orders will be billed at individual rate until proof of status is received. Foreign air speed delivery is included in all *Clinics* subscription prices. All prices are subject to change without notice. **POSTMASTER:** Send address changes to *Immunology and Allergy Clinics of North America,* Elsevier Health Sciences Division, Subscription Customer Service, 3251 Riverport Lane, Maryland Heights, MO 63043. **Customer Service: 1-800-654-2452 (U.S. and Canada); 314-447-8871 (outside U.S. and Canada). Fax: 314-447-8029. E-mail: journalscustomerservice-usa@elsevier.com(for print support);journalsonlinesupport-usa@elsevier. com(for online support).**

Reprints. For copies of 100 or more, of articles in this publication, please contact the Commercial Reprints Department, Elsevier Inc., 360 Park Avenue South, New York, New York 10010-1710. Tel. (212) 633-3812, Fax: (212) 462-1935, e-mail: reprints@elsevier.com.

Immunology and Allergy Clinics of North America is covered in MEDLINE/PubMed (Index Medicus), Current Contents/Life Sciences, Science Citation Index, ISI/BIOMED, Chemical Abstracts, and EMBASE/Excerpta Medica.

Printed and bound by CPI Group (UK) Ltd, Croydon, CR0 4YY

Transferred to Digital Print 2011

Contributors

CONSULTING EDITOR

RAFEUL ALAM, MD, PhD
Veda and Chauncey Ritter Chair in Immunology, Professor, and Director, Division of Immunology and Allergy, National Jewish Health; and University of Colorado Health Sciences Center, Denver, Colorado

GUEST EDITOR

LINDA COX, MD
Associate Clinical Professional of Medicine, Nova Southeastern University, Fort Lauderdale, Florida

AUTHORS

CEZMI A. AKDIS, MD
Professor; Director, Department of Dermatology, Swiss Institute of Allergy and Asthma Research (SIAF), University of Zurich, Davos, Switzerland

MUBECCEL AKDIS, MD, PhD
Privat Dozent, Department of Dermatology, Swiss Institute of Allergy and Asthma Research (SIAF), University of Zurich, Davos, Switzerland

DAVID I. BERNSTEIN, MD
Professor of Medicine and Environmental Health, Division of Immunology, Allergy and Rheumatology, University of Cincinnati College of Medicine, Cincinnati, Ohio

VÉRONIQUE BODO, PhD
Research and Development, Stallergènes, Antony, France

ROBERT J. BOYLE, MD, PhD
Clinical Senior Lecturer in Paediatric Allergy, Department of Paediatrics, Imperial College, St Mary's Hospital, London, United Kingdom

AMY BRONSTONE, PhD
Director of Medical Writing, BioMedEcon, LLC, Moss Beach, California

A. WESLEY BURKS, MD
Professor of Pediatrics and Division Chief, Division of Pediatric Allergy and Immunology, Duke University Medical Center, Durham, North Carolina

CHRISTOPHER W. CALABRIA, MD
ENTAA Care, PA, Glen Burnie, Maryland

MOISÉS A. CALDERÓN, MD, PhD
Honorary Clinical Senior Lecturer in Allergy; Head of Clinical Trials Unit, Department of Allergy and Respiratory Medicine, Imperial College, National Heart and Lung Institute, Royal Brompton and Harefield Trust, London, United Kingdom

GIORGIO WALTER CANONICA, MD
Allergy and Respiratory Diseases, Department of Internal Medicine, University of Genoa, Genoa, Italy

THOMAS B. CASALE, MD
Professor of Medicine, Department of Medicine; Chief, Division of Allergy and Immunology, Creighton University School of Medicine, Omaha, Nebraska

ENRICO COMPALATI, MD
Allergy and Respiratory Diseases, Department of Internal Medicine, University of Genoa, Genoa, Italy

LINDA COX, MD
Associate Clinical Professional of Medicine, Nova Southeastern University, Fort Lauderdale, Florida

STEPHEN R. DURHAM, MD
Professor and Head, Department of Allergy and Clinical Immunology, Imperial College; Professor, Allergy Department, Royal Brompton Hospital, London, United Kingdom

TOLLY EPSTEIN, MD, MS
Assistant Professor of Medicine, Division of Immunology, Allergy and Rheumatology, University of Cincinnati College of Medicine, Cincinnati, Ohio

ROBERT E. ESCH, PhD
Research and Development, Greer Laboratories, Inc, Lenoir, North Carolina

DAVID J. FITZHUGH, MD
Division of Allergy and Immunology, Department of Internal Medicine, University of South Florida College of Medicine; James A. Haley Veterans' Administration Hospital Medical Center, Tampa, Florida

THOMAS J. GRIER, PhD
Research and Development, Greer Laboratories, Inc, Lenoir, North Carolina

CHERYL S. HANKIN, PhD
President and Chief Scientific Officer, BioMedEcon, LLC, Moss Beach, California

K. HÖRMANN, Prof.MD
Department of Otorhinolaryngology–Head and Neck Surgery, University Hospital Mannheim, Wiesbaden, Germany

LOUISA K. JAMES, PhD
Allergy and Clinical Immunology Section, National Heart and Lung Institute, Medical Research Council and Asthma UK Centre for Allergic Mechanisms of Asthma, Imperial College London, London, United Kingdom

EDWIN H. KIM, MD
Fellow, Division of Pediatric Allergy and Immunology, Duke University Medical Center, Durham, North Carolina

J. KLEINE-TEBBE, MD
Outpatient Clinic and Associated Research Center Hanf, Herold & Kleine-Tebbe, Allergy and Asthma Center Westend, Berlin, Germany

L. KLIMEK, Prof.MD
Center for Rhinology and Allergology Wiesbaden, Department of Otorhinolaryngology, Head and Neck Surgery, University Hospital Mannheim, Wiesbaden, Germany

THOMAS M. KÜNDIG, MD
Department of Dermatology, University Hospital Zurich, Zurich, Switzerland

MICHAEL H. LAND, MD
Assistant Professor of Pediatrics, Division of Pediatric Allergy and Immunology, Duke University Medical Center, Durham, North Carolina

MARK LARCHÉ, PhD
Canada Research Chair in Allergy and Immune Tolerance; McMaster University/GSK Chair in Lung Immunology at St Joseph's Healthcare; Department of Medicine, Firestone Institute for Respiratory Health, McMaster University, Hamilton, Ontario, Canada

RICHARD F. LOCKEY, MD
Division of Allergy and Immunology, Department of Internal Medicine, University of South Florida College of Medicine; James A. Haley Veterans' Administration Hospital Medical Center, Tampa, Florida

VINCENT LOMBARDI, PhD
Research and Development, Stallergènes, Antony, France

LAURENT MASCARELL, PhD
Research and Development, Stallergènes, Antony, France

PHILIPPE MOINGEON, PhD
Research and Development, Stallergènes, Antony, France

HAROLD S. NELSON, MD
Professor of Medicine, Department of Medicine, National Jewish Health; and University of Colorado Health Sciences Center, Denver, Colorado

TRAN-HOAI T. NGUYEN, MD
Clinical Fellow, Department of Medicine, Division of Allergy and Immunology, Creighton University School of Medicine, Omaha, Nebraska

GIOVANNI PASSALACQUA, MD
Allergy and Respiratory Diseases, Department of Internal Medicine, University of Genoa, Genoa, Italy

MARTIN PENAGOS, MD, MSc
Academic Visitor, Department of Paediatric Allergy, St Thomas' Hospital, London, United Kingdom

O. PFAAR, MD
Center for Rhinology and Allergology Wiesbaden, Department of Otorhinolaryngology, Head and Neck Surgery, University Hospital Mannheim, Wiesbaden, Germany

NATHALIE SAINT-LU, PhD
Research and Development, Stallergènes, Antony, France

GUY SCADDING, MRCP
Registrar, Department of Allergy and Clinical Immunology, Imperial College; Allergy Department, Royal Brompton Hospital, London, United Kingdom

GABRIELA SENTI, MD
Clinical Trials Center, Center for Clinical Research, University and University Hospital Zurich, Zurich, Switzerland

MOHAMED H. SHAMJI, MSc, PhD
Faculty of Medicine, Allergy and Clinical Immunology Section, National Heart and Lung Institute, Medical Research Council and Asthma UK Centre for Allergic Mechanisms of Asthma, Imperial College London, London, United Kingdom

AZIZ SHEIKH, MD, FRCP, FRCGP
Professor of Primary Care Research and Development, Allergy and Respiratory Research Group, Centre for Population Health Sciences, The University of Edinburgh Medical School, Edinburgh, United Kingdom

OZGE U. SOYER, MD
Department of Pediatric Allergy, Ankara Education and Research Hospital, Ministry of Health, Ankara, Turkey

JEFFREY R. STOKES, MD
Associate Professor of Medicine, Department of Medicine, Division of Allergy and Immunology, Creighton University School of Medicine, Omaha, Nebraska

SOPHIE TOURDOT, PhD
Research and Development, Stallergènes, Antony, France

SERAINA VON MOOS, Med. Pract.
Clinical Trials Center, Center for Clinical Research, University and University Hospital Zurich, Zurich, Switzerland

Contents

Allergen-specific immunotherapy (SIT) defines and distinguishes the modern practice of clinical allergy and immunology as the 100th anniversary of this pioneering technique is celebrated. Despite the tremendous advancements made in therapeutics, pharmacology, and the basic science of allergy, SIT remains the only treatment modality that offers a potential cure for atopic diseases rather than simply an amelioration of symptoms. A historical perspective not only offers an opportunity to tell some of the fascinating stories that led to the conception of SIT but also gives an occasion to recognize, remember, and honor those individuals who have contributed to its development.

Meta-analysis is a powerful tool for evaluating the efficacy of a therapeutic intervention, and has clearly demonstrated that specific allergen immunotherapy (SIT) is effective for treating allergic rhinitis and asthma. Future research needs to focus on specifying the most effective forms of SIT for specific populations and allergens, using validated clinical outcomes, studying long-term outcomes (particularly the potential disease-modifying effect of immunotherapy), and assessing outcomes regarding health economics. The safety profile of SIT should be evaluated using international guidelines and terminology, and needs to include high-quality surveillance data.

IMMUNOLOGY

Allergen-specific immunotherapy (SIT) is the only curative approach in the treatment of allergic diseases defined up-to-date. Peripheral T-cell tolerance to allergens, the goal of successful allergen-SIT, is the primary mechanism in healthy immune responses to allergens. By repeated administration of increased doses of the causative allergen, allergen-SIT induces a state of immune tolerance to allergens through the constitution of T regulatory (Treg) cells, including allergen-specific interleukin (IL)-10–secreting Treg type 1 cells and $CD4^+CD25^+$Treg cells; induction of suppressive cytokines, such as IL-10 and transforming growth factor β; suppression of allergen-specific IgE and induction of IgG4 and IgA; and suppression of mast cells, basophils, eosinophils, and inflammatory dendritic cells. This review summarizes the current knowledge on the mechanisms of allergen-SIT with emphasis on the roles of Treg cells in allergen-SIT.

symptoms of both seasonal allergic rhinitis and asthma due to aeroaller-gens. However, clinical benefits of SCIT are tempered by risks of injec-tion-related systemic reactions and life-threatening anaphylaxis. This article reviews data derived from retrospective surveys conducted to define the incidence, prevalence, and factors contributing to injection-related fatal anaphylactic and near-fatal systemic reactions, as well as recently initiated longitudinal surveillance studies of SCIT reactions.

Accelerated Immunotherapy Schedules and Premedication   251

Christopher W. Calabria and Linda Cox

Subcutaneous immunotherapy is divided into a buildup and a maintenance phase. Accelerated immunotherapy has the advantage of a reduced num-ber of office visits. Rush and cluster immunotherapy schedules are the most common accelerated schedules used in the United States. A cluster immunotherapy schedule involves the patient receiving several allergen injections sequentially in a single day of treatment on nonconsecutive days. The maintenance dose is reached in 4 to 8 weeks. In rush immuno-therapy protocols, higher doses are administered at intervals of 15 to 60 minutes in a period of 1 to 3 days until the maintenance dose is achieved.

SUBLINGUAL IMMUNOTHERAPY

Sublingual Immunotherapy for Allergic Respiratory Diseases: Efficacy and Safety   265

Giovanni Passalacqua and Giorgio Walter Canonica

Subcutaneous immunotherapy (SCIT) is effective and safe when properly prescribed and administered. However, a certain risk of severe side effects exists, even when the reaction is managed correctly. These poten-tial adverse effects stimulated the search for new administration routes (nasal, bronchial, oral, sublingual), which were expected to be safer. Not all of these alternative routes provided an improved benefit–safety profile compared with SCIT. The sublingual route (SLIT) seemed to be a good candidate for the clinical practice because of its satisfactory safety profile and is now considered an acceptable alternative to SCIT in adults and children.

Sublingual Immunotherapy: Other Indications   279

Giovanni Passalacqua, Enrico Compalati, and Giorgio Walter Canonica

Sublingual immunotherapy (SLIT) represents a significant advance and it seems particularly suitable in pediatric patients. There are favorable results for food allergy in controlled trials. For latex allergy, the results of several trials are encouraging. For atopic dermatitis, previous experience with subcutaneous immunotherapy and some earlier trials suggest the possible application of SLIT in children with mild to moderate dermatitis and sensi-tization to dust mite, but this recommendation is considered insufficiently evidence based. In hymenoptera allergy, the only trial available is a proof-of-concept study in large local reactions that needs to be confirmed in well-controlled studies.

although most have failed to translate into successful human clinical trials. These results have helped to elucidate the pleotropic roles of cytokines as well as the diverse phenotypes of allergic diseases, particularly asthma. The goals of these therapies are to improve patient symptoms and quality of life, to prevent and favorably alter disease course, and to maintain a good risk/benefit ratio along with a cost-effective profile.

Food allergy has become an increasingly prevalent international health problem. Allergic reactions can result in life-threatening anaphylaxis in a short period of time, so the current standard of care dictates strict avoidance of suspected trigger foods and accessibility to injectable epinephrine. Intervention at the time of exposure is considered a rescue therapy rather than a disease-modifying treatment. Investigators have been studying allergen immunotherapy to promote induction of oral tolerance. This article examines the mechanisms of oral tolerance and the breakdown that leads to food allergy, as well as the history and current state of oral and sublingual immunotherapy development.

Because of the need to standardize allergen immunotherapy and the desire to reduce allergic adverse events during therapy, a transition to recombinant/synthetic hypoallergenic approaches is inevitable. Evidence supports the notion that effective therapy can be delivered using a limited panel of allergens or even epitopes, weakening the argument that all allergens must be present for optimal efficacy. Moreover, standardized products will allow direct comparisons between studies and, for the first time, immunotherapy studies will be truly blinded, allowing an accurate assessment of the actual treatment effect that can be achieved with this form of intervention.

For the past century, subcutaneous allergen-specific immunotherapy has been the state-of-the-art treatment for IgE-mediated allergic disease. Current research on allergen-specific immunotherapy is focused on enhancing its efficacy, safety, and patient convenience with the goal of offering a broadly accepted treatment option. There is a growing interest in intralymphatic allergen-specific immunotherapy because it is a highly efficacious and safe treatment route that requires only 3 injections. Concurrently, epicutaneous allergen-specific immunotherapy is attracting increasing attention because of its capacity to offer a safe, needle-free, and potentially self-administrable treatment option for IgE-mediated allergic diseases. In this article, we discuss the principles and immunologic rationale of these unconventional routes of allergen-specific immunotherapy while highlighting their developmental process and clinical relevance.

Allergen-specific immunotherapy represents a curative treatment of type I allergies. Subcutaneous immunotherapy is conducted with allergens adsorbed on aluminum hydroxide or calcium phosphate particles, whereas sublingual immunotherapy relies on high doses of soluble allergen without any immunopotentiator. There is a potential benefit of adjuvants enhancing regulatory and Th1 CD4+T cell responses during specific immunotherapy. Molecules affecting dendritic cells favor the induction of T regulatory cell and Th1 responses and represent valid candidate adjuvants for allergy vaccines. Furthermore, the interest in viruslike particles and mucoadhesive particulate vector systems, which may better address the allergen(s) to tolerogenic antigen-presenting cells, is documented.

RELATED INTEREST

Otolaryngologic Clinics of North America (Volume 44, Issue 3, June 2011)
Diagnosis and Treatment of Allergies for Otolaryngologists
Berrylin Ferguson, MD and Suman Golla, MD, *Guest Editors*

THE CLINICS ARE NOW AVAILABLE ONLINE!

Access your subscription at:
www.theclinics.com

Foreword

Allergen Immunotherapy

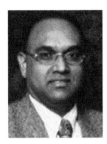

Rafeul Alam, MD, PhD
Consulting Editor

This year is the 100th anniversary of the first scientific publication on allergen immunotherapy. Leonard Noon, the father of allergen immunotherapy, called it "prophylactic inoculation against hay fever."[1] In his pioneering article, he acknowledged that Dunbar in Hamburg, Germany, through his animal experiments, provided the initial scientific understanding for sensitivity to pollens. Alexandre Besredka in Paris was the first to successfully perform allergen hyposensitization in animals.[2] The foregoing scientific works formed the foundation for "prophylactic inoculation" against hay fever. However, the concept of prophylactic inoculation, ie, vaccination, was introduced to the Western medicine more than 100 years earlier in 1798 by Edward Jenner.[3] Therefore, it is likely that Leonard Noon applied the principle and method of vaccination to hay fever. Vaccination is arguably the biggest discovery in modern medicine. It is important to note that Sir Edward Jenner was not the first to apply smallpox vaccination in humans. The earliest English language record of vaccination/inoculation comes from 1715. Dr P. Kennedy on his return from Constantinople (Istanbul) described how ingrafting of smallpox on two sisters successfully protected them from the epidemic disease. In his book entitled, *An essay on External Remedies* (Wellcome Trust Medical Library), he reveals how the ingrafting of smallpox was already in practice in Turkey, part of Persia at that time. The history of vaccination actually dates back much earlier. In 1767 the British surgeon, Dr J.Z. Holwell, FRS, wrote to the Royal College of Physicians in London about his observation on smallpox inoculation in Bengal, India.[4] He wrote about how the Brahmins of Bengal went from door to door to inoculate villagers against smallpox. He described how small wounds were made on the outside of the arm, between the elbow and the shoulder, and a piece of dry calico cloth with 'infected pustules' was rubbed onto the wound. Holwell described the method of inoculating with dried matter from other inoculated pustules from a previous year, dissolved in water from the Ganges; this would result in a weakened and contaminated virus. Dr Holwell went on to say that "When the before recited treatment is strictly followed, it comes to a miracle to hear that one in a million fails of receiving the infection."

Supported by NIH grants R56AI077535, PPG HL 36577, and N01 HHSN272200700048C.

Immunol Allergy Clin N Am 31 (2011) xv–xvi
doi:10.1016/j.iac.2011.03.009
0889-8561/11/$ – see front matter

The earliest record of the concept of inoculation is thought to be found in a book from the 7th century India, when Madhavacharaya wrote *Madhava Nidana* (an Ayurvedic system of pathology), a 79-chapter book that lists diseases along with their causes, symptoms, and complications. According to Donald R. Hopkins, Madhavacharya included a special chapter on smallpox (*masūrikā*) and described the method of inoculation to protect against smallpox.[5]

This idea of protection from smallpox by inoculation was picked up by Lady Mary Wortley Montague, the wife of a British ambassador, while living in Constantinople. She inoculated her own children for smallpox in 1718 and then tried to popularize this technique in England. She was indeed successful in her effort as her 3-year-old daughter survived the 1721 smallpox epidemic. This layperson's heroic effort took place nearly 80 years earlier than the famous publication of Sir Edward Jenner on vaccination in 1798. It is interesting that almost all the credit for the discovery of vaccination is now given to Dr Jenner but not to the old Indian tradition or Lady Montague.

With this brief history of prophylactic inoculation, I would like to present to the readership this latest issue of *Immunology and Allergy Clinics*. It illustrates the latest scientific progress on allergen immunotherapy under the excellent editorship of Dr Linda Cox. We invited leaders in the field to present the latest basic and translational innovations in the field of allergen immunotherapy.

Rafeul Alam, MD, PhD
Division of Allergy and Immunology
National Jewish Health and
University of Colorado
Denver Health Sciences Center
1400 Jackson Street
Denver, CO 80206, USA

E-mail address:
alamr@njc.org

REFERENCES

1. Noon L. Prophylactic inoculation against hay fever. Lancet 1911;1:1572–3.
2. Besredka A. Du mecanisme de l'anaphylaxie vis-a-visde serum de cheval. C R Soc Biol 1907;59:294–6.
3. Jenner E. An inquiry into the causes and effects of the variolae vaccinae. A disease discovered in some of the western counties of England, particularly Gloucestershire, and known by the name of the cow pox. London: Low; 1798. Available at: /wiki/Special:BookSources/0226351688. Accessed March 16, 2011. ISBN: 0226351688.
4. Holwell JZ. An account of the manner of inoculating for the smallpox in the East Indies. London: 1767. Available at: /wiki/Online_Computer_Library_Center; http://www.worldcat.org/oclc/181708667. Accessed March 16, 2011.
5. Hopkins DR. The greatest killer: smallpox in history. University of Chicago Press; 2002.

Preface

Allergen Immunotherapy: The First Centenary and Beyond

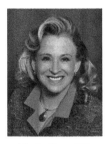

Linda Cox, MD
Guest Editor

One hundred years have elapsed since specific allergen immunotherapy (SIT) was first employed and found to be effective in the treatment of allergic respiratory diseases and 4 years since an edition of *Immunology and Allergy Clinics of North America* was dedicated to this topic. This publication offers a comprehensive review of this disease-modifying treatment, exploring its history, current status, and potential future.

The issue begins with a journey through thousands of years in Fitzhugh and Lockey's historical perspective that traces the roots of SIT back to early antiquity with Thucydides' (c. 460-400 BC) observation that plagues victims were often protected against subsequent plague outbreaks (ie, the plague infection-induced immunity). Nearly 600 years later, the observations that tolerance to snake venom toxicity could be induced by oral ingestion of snake venom likely influenced the snake charmers of that era to swim in snake-infested waters. Their perspective goes on to recount landmark events and discoveries, such as Dr Mary Loveless' discovery of "blocking antibodies" and the lack of efficacy of whole body insect immunotherapy versus purified venom extracts and Dr Ishizako's discovery of immunoglobulin E. Their article, also, describes early scientific experiments that laid the groundwork for future allergy/immunology advancements, such as the ryegrass nasal challenges, which Charles Blackey performed upon himself, which confirmed the causative effect of pollen on what was called *Cattarrhus aestivus* or "summer flow." Nasal and other organ challenges are tools that continue to be used in clinical trials to confirm clinical allergy and assess treatment outcome response.

This informative historical review is followed by Calderón and colleagues' critical evaluation of the published systematic reviews and meta-analyses on SIT. In addition to an analysis and critique of the specific systematic reviews and meta-analyses on subcutaneous (SCIT) and sublingual immunotherapy (SLIT), this article provides a cogent explanation of the methodologies used in performing these analyses.

Immunol Allergy Clin N Am 31 (2011) xvii–xix
doi:10.1016/j.iac.2011.03.006   **immunology.theclinics.com**
0889-8561/11/$ – see front matter © 2011 Elsevier Inc. All rights reserved.

A detailed discussion of the purported mechanisms and immunological changes associated with SCIT and SLIT is provided in Soyer and coworkers' and Scadding and Durham's articles, respectively.

A section dedicated to SCIT begins with Nelson's comprehensive review of the SCIT basics: indications, efficacy requirements (eg, allergen dose), efficacy of different individual allergens (eg, grass-pollen, cockroach, etc), and single versus polyallergen immunotherapy. The duration of SCIT efficacy and preventive effect is also reviewed in this article. Allergen extract preparation and stability are covered in Esch's article, which reviews many key issues germane to allergen extract preparations, such as the compatibility of different extract combinations in terms of proteolytic enzymes and the effect of different diluents, temperature storage, and other factors on extract stability. Different aspects of SCIT safety is reviewed in two articles. Bernstein and Epstein present the findings of the recent AAAAI/ACAAI 3-year collaborative immunotherapy safety survey, which was designed to collect data on SIT systemic reactions, including fatal and near-fatal reactions. Fortunately, no fatalities were reported in the approximately 18 million injections administered during the first 2 years of the survey, which is now in its final year. The authors speculated that this favorable safety trend may be in part due to the implementation of risk management strategies suggested by the Allergen Immunotherapy Practice Parameters (eg, 30-minute observation period). Calabria and Cox provide a different perspective on SCIT safety with a review of premedication and accelerated schedules, such as rush and cluster.

SLIT is a noninjection of immunotherapy prescribed nearly as frequently as SCIT worldwide. In parts of Europe, it represents the majority of new immunotherapy prescriptions (80%-90% in France and Italy). However, only a small percentage of US allergists (~6%) prescribe SLIT, likely because there is currently no Federal Drug Administration-approved SLIT formulation. Passalacqua and colleagues review the safety and efficacy of SLIT based on published clinical trials, meta-analyses, and postmarketing surveillance studies. In another article, they review novel indications for SLIT, such as recurrent large local reactions to venom stings and latex food allergy.

Monitoring SIT outcomes is reviewed from three different perspectives in the immunotherapy outcomes section: clinical, immunologic, and economics. Pfaar and coworkers provide a thorough balanced review of virtually all methods used to assess SIT response. The review discusses, in detail, the advantages and drawbacks of each assessment tool, such as symptom/medication scores, validated quality of life questionnaires, and allergen-provocation challenge, but concludes that SIT primary outcome parameters should include a measure of symptoms and concomitant medication usage, ideally as a combined score with weighted balance.

Changes in immunological parameters as a means to monitor SIT efficacy is discussed in Shamji and Durham's article, which focuses on the IgE-facilitated allergen-binding assay, routinely used in SIT clinical trials that may, in the future, be used in clinical practice as a surrogate marker to demonstrate and/or confirm SIT efficacy. This section concludes with Hankins' complete analysis of the cost-effectiveness of SIT, which includes a review of essentially all published data on SIT economics, including "real-life" studies of the Florida Medicaid population that have demonstrated up to 50% reduction in total health care costs.

The issue concludes with a series of articles that highlight future forms of SIT entitled novel approaches and formulations. It begins Nguyen and colleagues' excellent review of future forms of SIT formulations, which covers Toll-like receptor agonist adjuvants, cytokine blockers, transcription factor inhibitors, synthesis inhibitors, anti-IgE monoclonal antibodies, receptor antagonists, and other receptor modulators. Promising treatment for food allergies, a disease currently only managed with strict food avoidance, is discussed in Land and coworkers' review of the history and current state of oral and sublingual immunotherapy in which they examine—the mechanisms of oral tolerance and the breakdown that leads to food allergy.

A number of approaches to decrease the allergenicity (ie, safety), while maintaining immunogenicity (ie, efficacy) of allergen vaccines, have been explored. Some formulations/approaches are in the very early stages of development or have not yet been studied in humans, but demonstrated promise in these early studies or mouse models. Larché reviews peptide and recombinant allergens, which have been investigated for some years, as a means to provide more effective and consistent allergen extracts. von Moos and coworkers' article discusses promising and interesting alternative routes for administering SIT: epicutaneous and intralymphatic. In one open comparative study, three intralymphatic injections of allergen produced clinical benefits of 3 years of SCIT with conventional extracts. This issue concludes with Moingeon and colleagues' article discussing the potential role of adjuvants and mucoadhesives in enhancing SIT efficacy and safety.

In closing, this edition of *Immunology and Allergy Clinics of North America* celebrating the hundredth anniversary of specific allergen immunotherapy provides a wide-ranging review that includes the history, current status, and future approaches of SIT. It should be a "must-read" and bookshelf "staple" for all clinicians who provide and/or are interested in specific allergen immunotherapy.

Linda Cox, MD
5333 North Dixie Highway, Suite 210
Fort Lauderdale, FL 33334, USA

E-mail address:
lindaswolfcox@msn.com

History of Immunotherapy: The First 100 Years

David J. Fitzhugh, MD[a,b,*], Richard F. Lockey, MD[a,b]

KEYWORDS

- Allergen-specific immunotherapy • Allergic rhinitis
- Subcutaneous immunotherapy • Hypersensitivity

Allergen-specific immunotherapy (SIT) both defines and distinguishes the modern practice of clinical allergy and immunology as the 100th anniversary of this pioneering technique is celebrated. The ingenuity, resolve, and insight of the many forebears have led to this landmark achievement, and the progress that has been made after the original description of SIT in 1911 by Leonard Noon and John Freeman is remarkable. Despite the tremendous advancements made in therapeutics, pharmacology, and the basic science of allergy, SIT remains the only treatment modality that offers a potential cure for atopic diseases rather than simply an amelioration of symptoms. A historical perspective not only offers an opportunity to tell some of the fascinating stories that led to the conception of SIT but perhaps, more importantly, gives an occasion to recognize, remember, and honor those individuals who have contributed to its development (**Table 1**).

Although 1911 represents the beginning of the modern era of SIT, evidence supporting an understanding of the immune system and attempts to prevent or alter disease for the welfare of the patient dates to antiquity. Thucydides (circa 460–400 BC), an ancient Greek historian, observed that those patients fortunate enough to survive the plague were often protected against subsequent outbreaks, one of the first descriptions of immunity.[1] Mithadrates VI (circa 132–63 BC), king of Pontus and Armenia Minor, was so concerned about the possibility of poisoning that he developed a technique to protect against this danger in what may be considered the first example of oral tolerance, as recorded by Pliny the Elder: "By his unaided efforts he thought out the plan of drinking poison daily ... in order that sheer custom might render it

a Division of Allergy and Immunology, Department of Internal Medicine, University of South Florida College of Medicine, 12908 USF Health Drive, Tampa, FL 33612, USA
b James A. Haley Veterans' Administration Hospital Medical Center, 13000 Bruce B. Downs Boulevard, Tampa, FL 33612, USA
* Corresponding author. Division of Allergy and Immunology, Department of Internal Medicine, University of South Florida College of Medicine, 12908 USF Health Drive, Tampa, FL 33612.
E-mail address: dfitzhug@health.usf.edu

Immunol Allergy Clin N Am 31 (2011) 149–157
doi:10.1016/j.iac.2011.03.003 immunology.theclinics.com
0889-8561/11/$ – see front matter © 2011 Elsevier Inc. All rights reserved.

Table 1
Landmark achievements in the history of allergen-SIT

Jenner[1]	First demonstration of vaccine principles	1798
Blackley[2]	First attempt at SIT via pollen application to abraded skin	1880
Richet and Portier[3]	Experimental description of anaphylaxis	1902
Noon and Freeman[4]	First successful pollen SIT trial	1911
Cooke[3,5]	Discovery of house dust as ubiquitous antigen; concept of blocking antibodies	1922, 1935
Lowell and Franklin[6]	First double-blind controlled SIT trial with purified extracts	1965
Ishizaka and Ishizaka[7]; Johansson et al[8]	Discovery of IgE	1967
Hunt et al[9]	Venom SIT vs whole-body extracts for Hymenoptera SIT	1978
Passalacqua et al[10]	Double-blind controlled SLIT trial for dust mite	1998
Durham et al[11,12]	Sustained efficacy of both SCIT and SLIT using grass pollen	1999, 2010

Abbreviations: IgE, immunoglobulin E; SCIT, subcutaneous immunotherapy; SLIT, sublingual immunotherapy.

harmless."[3] Galen (AD 130–200), the celebrated Greek physician, observed that oral ingestion of snake venom avoids systemic toxicity; this insight may have inspired snake charmers of the era to swim in snake-infested waters in an attempt to ingest minute amounts of venom to afford protection against the occupational hazards of their profession.[1] By the 11th century, Chinese healers attempted the first efforts at active immunization against disease by instilling dried materials recovered from the pustules of patients with smallpox into the recipients' nostrils, known as variolation.[1]

Although variolation remained in practice for centuries, it was Edward Jenner, a rural English physician in the 18th century, who provided one of the keystone moments and ushered in the modern era of immunology. His acclaimed contribution is the first experimental demonstration of vaccination, in which he inoculated the fluid from cowpox lesions to protect against smallpox. This carefully documented experiment confirmed anecdotal reports from the time that milkmaids with cowpox were much less vulnerable to contracting smallpox and gave the procedure its name, vaccination, from the Latin word vaccinus (pertaining to a cow). Perhaps more relevant to practicing allergists/immunologists, however, he also provided the first description of cutaneous hypersensitivity on revaccination.[3] Although formal epicutaneous and intradermal allergen testing were still more than 100 years away, Jenner's astute observation that the degree of inflammation on reexposure to the cowpox inoculum reflected the relative immunity to smallpox showed remarkable insight. Although highly honored after his celebrated discovery, he remained in rural practice as a country doctor for the rest of his life.

A contemporary of Jenner from Great Britain, John Bostock, provided the first description of what is now termed seasonal allergic rhinoconjunctivitis. Dr Bostock's designation for the affliction in his original 1819 article was the lyrical and descriptive catarrhus aestivus, roughly translated as summer flow. He describes his own symptoms in this work in which he experienced ocular irritation, paroxysms of sneezing, and tightness of the chest (ie, "a feeling of want of room to receive the air necessary for respiration"), which began every summer in June.[3,13]

Although Bostock provided an important but limited descriptive contribution to allergic diseases, it is Dr Charles Blackley who substantially extended these observations to the cause and possible treatment of allergic rhinitis in his 1873 volume, *Experimental Researches on the Cause and Nature of Catarrhus Aestivus*. Dr Blackley, experimenting on himself, concluded that pollen was the responsible agent for his hay fever, the lay term that he preferred. He performed a series of experiments in which he instilled increasing amounts of pollen (initially rye grass but expanded to multiple other pollens) into his nostril and observed that "a profuse coryza came on in less than a minute after the application. In thirty minutes the nostril was completely occluded, so that it was quite impossible to pass any air through it."[2] Furthermore, he correlated the severity of his symptoms with the quantity of airborne pollen, having fabricated numerous devices of his own invention for the collection and quantification of atmospheric pollens. Out of desperation for a satisfactory treatment to alleviate his own suffering, he attempted medical management with a wide variety of agents, including quinine, arsenic, and belladonna, none with satisfactory results; however, he did acknowledge that one possibility for palliation would be a suitable change of locality. Finally, Dr Blackley made what can be regarded as the first investigational attempt at SIT by repeatedly applying pollen to his abraded skin in an effort to decrease local reactivity; however, no change was observed.[2]

After Blackley's seminal observations and innovations in the area of allergic rhinitis, there followed an important period of discovery into the concepts of antitoxin and the therapeutic use of antisera in passive immunization. Dr Henry Sewall, in 1887 at the University of Michigan, demonstrated in an animal model that protection against lethal envenomation from snakebites can be conferred by repeated inoculation of sublethal venom doses, giving rise to the concept of antitoxin.[1,14] By 1890, Shibasabura Kitasato and Emil von Behring, working collaboratively in the Robert Koch's laboratory in Berlin, developed tetanus and diphtheria antisera for therapeutic use.[3] However, it was not until 1897 that Paul Erlich had refined and standardized the production of diphtheria antitoxin that it found widespread commercial use.[1] Dr Erlich, of course, made a remarkable array of contributions not only in antitoxin research but also with the staining and identification of both mast cells and eosinophils, which would later be recognized to be fundamental to the pathogenesis of allergic diseases. At the dawn of the 20th century, several further attempts in passive immunization and experiments in anaphylaxis heralded the development of SIT. Drawing from the experience of Kitasato and von Behring, William Dunbar in 1902 described his attempts at passive SIT using a horse- and rabbit-derived antipollen antitoxin for hay fever in humans. This technique was performed by instilling a powder or an ointment preparation of the antitoxin into the eyes, nose, and mouth for rhinitis symptoms and via inhalation for asthma.[3,15] In the same year, Charles Richet and Paul Portier provided the first experimental description of anaphylaxis while immunizing dogs with sea anemone toxin, a discovery for which Richet was awarded the Nobel Prize in Medicine.[3,16] Alexandere Besredka of the Pasteur Institute in 1907 furthered the knowledge of anaphylaxis by demonstrating that progressively increasing the doses of antigen resulted in protection from an anaphylactic challenge in a guinea pig model.[1]

With the foundational work now complete in establishing pollen as the cause of hay fever, success in passive protection via antisera, and the evolving understanding of the immune response to vaccination, the stage was set for Noon and Freeman's seminal investigation into active SIT. In 1911, both Noon and Freeman were working in Sir Almroth Wright's laboratory at St Mary's Hospital, London. Noon subscribed to the conceptual bases of Dunbar's earlier work, namely, that a toxin component of the pollen was responsible for generating the symptom constellation of hay fever and that a pollen antitoxin would be protective from these effects. However, unlike Dunbar's attempts to passively transfer the antitoxin, Noon and Freeman developed a protocol of subcutaneous injections of pollen extracts with increasing doses according to a defined schedule for patients with hay fever. By so doing, they pioneered the first successful SIT trial. Beyond that, they recognized several fundamental tenets of SIT that continue to hold true in current clinical practice: the optimal dose interval is initially 1 to 2 weeks and that allergen overdose may induce anaphylaxis.[1] Although Noon died of tuberculosis prematurely in 1913 at 36 years, Freeman completed a trial of 84 patients with their SIT regimen, which was reported in the *Lancet* in 1914. Although not rigorously controlled, the trial nevertheless showed that allergen-SIT was effective in allergic patients and that it seemed to confer an acquired immunity lasting for at least 1 year after cessation of treatment.[4] After the success of Noon and Freeman, acceptance and incorporation of SIT expanded rapidly in clinical practice. Dr Chandler Walker established one of the first dedicated clinics for allergic patients at the Peter Bent Brigham Hospital in Boston, which was followed shortly by Dr Robert Cooke's clinic at New York Hospital in 1918.[1] Dr Cooke made numerous contributions to the nascent field of SIT, including the development of intradermal skin testing (extending Oscar Schoss's original scratch test, first established in 1912), the discovery with Mary Loveless of blocking antibodies in response to allergen-SIT, the introduction of the protein nitrogen unit for extract standardization, and the identification of house dust as a ubiquitous allergen.[3,5] Furthermore, he was a dedicated teacher and leader who provided crucial leadership as allergy/immunology began to be recognized as a distinct medical subspecialty and was vital to establishing the first training programs in this emerging field.[3]

By the 1920s, allergen-SIT was established as a viable and effective treatment of allergic conditions, including allergic rhinitis and asthma. Dr Arthur Coca was an influential force in the field during this decade, developing a reagent to extract allergens for use in skin testing. He founded the *Journal of Immunology* and is credited with coining the term atopy (derived from the Greek term "strangeness") into the allergic lexicon.[3,17] In addition, Otto Prausnitz and Heinz Küstner deserve mention during this time for their demonstration of passive transfer of hypersensitivity (in this case, fish hypersensitivity via intradermal injection of Küstner's serum into Prausnitz and challenge 24 hours later with intradermal injection of fish antigen). The eponymous P-K reaction refers to the reaction that occurs on allergen challenge after passive transfer of what is now known to be allergen-specific IgE (termed "atopic reagin" at the time by Coca) into a nonallergic subject.[3]

As SIT practice evolved, the technique was adapted for treatment of conditions beyond hay fever. In 1956, Dr Mary Loveless, mentioned earlier in connection with Cooke in the discovery of blocking antibodies, performed uncontrolled studies using SIT for Hymenoptera hypersensitivity. She found that whole-body insect extracts versus the use of pure isolated venom were ineffective to treat this disease.[3,18] She also devoted substantial effort to emulsified depot preparations of allergen for SIT, but it was later discovered that the emulsion preparation induced plasma cell dyscrasias in animal models and its use was not pursued further.[1] Bernard Levine and Charles Parker, working independently in the 1960s, defined the antigenic determinants responsible for penicillin hypersensitivity, which ultimately led to successful desensitization protocols for allergic patients requiring this crucial antibiotic.[3,19,20]

Perhaps equal in significance to the Noon and Freeman's first clinical trial of SIT is the discovery of the fundamental molecule of allergy, IgE. Two research teams working via dissimilar experimental avenues arrived at the same conclusion that a new class of immunoglobulin molecules must be the cause implicated in hypersensitivity. The husband and wife team of Kimishige and Teruko Ishizaka isolated a novel immunoglobulin fraction from a patient with extreme ragweed hypersensitivity and demonstrated its ability to fixed radiolabeled allergen.[7,21] They designated this molecule gamma E globulin, for its ability to create erythema in the skin in a P-K reaction. Separately, Hans Bennich and SGO Johansson isolated a unique immunoglobulin from a patient with myeloma, terming it IgND, so named for the patient's initials.[8] Translating this finding to atopic individuals, IgND was elevated in patients suffering from allergic rhinitis or allergic asthma. In 1968, the World Health Organization (WHO) convened an international conference in Lausanne for comparative analysis of the collective data from these two research groups and determined that both groups had discovered the same molecule. The conference concluded with the designation of a new immunoglobulin class, IgE.[21] This milestone represents a watershed moment in the immunology of allergic diseases, because IgE is the fundamental triggering factor for mediators released by mast cells and basophils. Its impact resonates still with the development of omalizumab, a targeted anti-IgE monoclonal antibody that has proved invaluable in severe allergic asthma.

By the late 1960s, allergen-SIT was in common practice, although its efficacy had not yet been rigorously demonstrated in controlled trials. The first double-blind controlled trial was reported in 1965 by Lowell and Franklin,[6] establishing efficacy of SIT using ragweed extract in adult patients with allergic rhinitis. Fontana and colleagues[22] followed in 1966 with the first controlled study of SIT in the pediatric population, which did not show a difference between the treatment and control groups (although this study looked only at the presence or absence of symptoms, as opposed to the degree of severity). However, in 1969, Sadan and colleagues[23] published a controlled trial in children, unequivocally demonstrating a marked decrease in the symptom severity scores and an increase in blocking antibody levels in pediatric patients given SIT to ragweed extract for seasonal allergic rhinitis. Norman and colleagues[24] extended these observations, showing that SIT with antigen E (now known as Amb a 1, the major ragweed antigen) was equal in efficacy to that with whole ragweed extracts in ragweed-sensitive patients and was better tolerated, generating fewer systemic and local reactions.

By the 1970s, SIT for stinging insects was investigated by many groups. A landmark study was published in 1979 by the Hopkins group, led by Larry Lichtenstein, showing the clinical superiority of venom SIT versus whole-body extracts in insect hypersensitivity.[9] In 1974, Dr Richard Lockey was among the first to recognize in an international medical journal that hypersensitivity to imported fire ants and other stinging ants can cause a systemic reaction identical to that seen with other Hymenoptera.[25] Dr Lockey and his colleagues extended their findings to the identification of fire ant venom allergens prepared from whole-body extracts using sera from sensitized patients via immunoblotting.[26] Finally, the largest longitudinal study to date of venom SIT using US Federal Drug Administration standardized extracts was completed from 1979 to 1990, with the enrollment of more than 1400 patients into a venom immunotherapy (VIT) program. The results of this broad study demonstrated the overall safety of VIT, with a net incidence of 12% treatment-related systemic reactions, none of which were fatal.[27]

Although the 1970s and 1980s saw considerable work in demonstrating the efficacy and safety of SIT, the development of standardized extracts over the last 20 years has greatly enhanced the ability of allergists to deliver SIT of an accurate and consistent bioactivity. In the United States, there are now 19 standardized extracts, whose production is governed by current good manufacturing practice and whose potency is assured via standardized assays. The responsibility for the oversight of these procedures rests with the Center for Biologics Evaluation and Testing, a division of the US

Food and Drug Administration. In essence, there are two vital components to the standardization of a given allergen in the United States: an initial reference assessment of allergenicity known as the ID_{50} EAL method, which uses highly allergic individuals to a given allergen to comprise a reference standard, and a lot release limit assay, which is an in vitro assay (often a competition enzyme-linked immunosorbent assay) designed to ensure bioequivalence between different lots of standardized allergen. The situation in Europe is markedly different, where the onus is on the manufacturer to provide assurance of lot-to-lot consistency, without the use of an external reference standard.[28] There is, however, an ongoing effort in the European Union (the CREATE project) to develop international reference allergen standards.[29]

In 1998, WHO released a position paper that validated the accumulating body of work into the safety, efficacy, and standardization of allergen-SIT. Despite SIT being in practice for more than 80 years, this approbation nevertheless represented a landmark moment in the field, as members of all the major allergy and immunology organizations convened in Geneva to discuss the current state of the knowledge in the field and formulate the position paper. The committee concluded that allergen immunotherapy is safe (but noted the risk of anaphylaxis) and is indicated for allergic rhinitis/conjunctivitis, Hymenoptera hypersensitivity, and allergic asthma. They stressed the importance of appropriate patient selection, in particular those who had failed pharmacotherapy because of either intolerance or inadequate symptom control, and cautioned that SIT should only be prescribed by a knowledgeable allergist and administered in a clinical setting equipped to deal with the rare (but real) risk of systemic reaction.[30]

One lingering question that remained by the late 1990s revolved around the persistence of the clinical efficacy of SIT after treatment cessation, that is, whether a lasting modification of the immunologic response to a given antigen could be induced. The general recommendation had been for a treatment period of 3 to 5 years (including those of the WHO position paper, mentioned earlier), but data for the continued suppression of symptoms were lacking until Durham and colleagues[11] published a double-blind controlled trial in the New England Journal of Medicine in 1999 to address this question. Their work demonstrated a persistent reduction in symptom score and T-cell skin infiltration for up to 3 years after discontinuation of SIT; these changes were indistinguishable from the control group who remained on SIT during the same time frame. More recently, Jacobsen and colleagues[31] have demonstrated that a 3-year course of immunotherapy shows persistent improvement in rhinoconjunctivitis up to 7 years after the cessation of therapy and may also prevent the development of asthma in the pediatric population.

Thus far, this history has focused on subcutaneous immunotherapy (SCIT), but it should be noted that sublingual immunotherapy (SLIT) has become a recognized and accepted part of allergy practice in many parts of the world. Although limited in scope, Scadding and Brostoff[32] reported the first double-blind controlled trial with SLIT in 1986, wherein they reported improvement in symptoms and nasal flow rate after treating a small cohort of dust mite allergic patients. Passalacqua and colleagues[10] confirmed and extended these findings, noting not only decreased symptom scores in patients treated with dust mite SLIT but also diminished conjunctival inflammatory cell infiltrate and intercellular adhesion molecule 1 expression. Since 1986, there have been more than 60 controlled clinical trials with SLIT, most of which have used monomeric therapy to either dust mite or grass pollen. A 2009 World Allergy Organization position paper confirmed the efficacy and safety of SLIT for grass allergens in both adults and children.[33] Finally, the Durham group demonstrated lasting clinical efficacy of SLIT, observing sustained symptom control in grass-allergic subjects for 1 year after cessation of a 3-year treatment period.[12]

Although allergen-SIT, as is currently administered, has proved enormously beneficial to a broad spectrum of allergic patients, there is clearly a lack of uniformity in response to therapy and there remains the small but real risk of systemic reactions (including life-threatening anaphylaxis) during subcutaneous injection. This risk was documented in the almost simultaneous reports by Lockey and colleagues[34] and the British Committee on Safety of Medicines[35] about a number of deaths associated with SCIT. Given the objective of the safest and most effective therapy, there are multiple new investigational approaches that are being explored to deliver SIT. One approach to improving safety has been to add anti-IgE treatment (omalizumab) during initiation of SCIT. Initial trials of this approach indicate improved safety, with significantly few systemic reactions in the omalizumab group.[36] Another strategy is immune modification via targeting of toll-like receptors (TLRs). A TLR4 agonist (Pollinex) has been licensed in the United Kingdom and shown to reduce symptom scores, skin reactivity, and allergen-specific IgE levels in both adults and children with sensitivities to grasses, trees, or ragweed. However, initial trials in the United States have been suspended because of an ongoing investigation of an adverse event with this product.[36] TLR9 is also a potential therapeutic target via administration of cytidine-phosphate-guanosine (CpG) immunostimulatory sequences either in conjugation with allergen or alone. Initial trials with CpG-conjugated Amb a 1 were promising, but there were problems with the study design that led to inconclusive data.[37,38] Trials using CpG sequences packaged as virus-like particles are ongoing.[36] Both recombinant and peptide allergens have been actively investigated, with the goal to increase the safety of administration while preserving the immunomodulatory properties of the allergen preparation. Alternative administration routes beyond SCIT and SLIT represent another possibility for allergen delivery. The most novel among these is intralymphatic injection of allergens, which in a study of 165 grass-allergic subjects showed comparable symptom reduction with 3 intranodal doses (given over two months) versus standard SIT administered over three years.[39]

Although it is impossible to mention every individual who contributed to the development of allergen-SIT, many of the highlights in the progress toward and since the advent of SIT have been reviewed and moreover, we hope, have engendered a sense of respect and admiration for the physicians and scientists who labored diligently to provide a novel and effective technique to alleviate the suffering of those with allergic conditions. Many mysteries still abound in the understanding and treatment of immunologic disease. While we acknowledge the contributions of those whose experiments lead to an efficacious and enduring therapy for over one hundred years, new innovative modalities will incorporate genomic and molecular advances as progress continues toward the ultimate goal of safe, specific, and even curative treatments for allergic disease.

ACKNOWLEDGMENTS

The authors gratefully acknowledge Dr Sheldon Cohen who has written extensively on the history of our specialty and whose very detailed historical perspective of immunotherapy provided outstanding source and reference material for this review.[1]

REFERENCES

1. Cohen SG, Evans R III. Allergen immunotherapy in historical perspective. In: Lockey RF, Ledford DK, editors. Allergens and allergen immunotherapy. 4th edition. New York: Informa Health Care; 2008. p. 1–29.

2. Blackley C. Hay fever; its causes, treatment, and effective prevention. London: Balliere; 1880.

3. Cohen SG, Samter M. Excerpts from classics in allergy. Carlsbad (CA): Symposia Foundation; 1992.

4. Freeman J. Vaccination against hay fever; report of results during the last three years. Lancet 1914;1:1178.

5. Cooke RA. Studies in specific hypersensitiveness. New etiologic factors in bronchial asthma. J Immunol 1922;7:147.

6. Lowell FC, Franklin W. A double-blind study of the effectiveness and specificity of injection therapy in ragweed hay fever. N Engl J Med 1965;273:675–9.

7. Ishizaka K, Ishizaka T. Identification of gamma-E antibodies as a carrier of reaginic antibody. J Immunol 1967;99:1187.

8. Johansson SG, Bennich H, Wide L. A new class of immunoglobulin in human serum. Immunology 1968;14(2):265–72.

9. Hunt KJ, Valentine MD, Sobotka AK, et al. A controlled trial of immunotherapy in insect hypersensitivity. N Engl J Med 1978;299(4):157–61.

10. Passalacqua G, Albano M, Fregonese L, et al. Randomised controlled trial of local allergoid immunotherapy on allergic inflammation in mite-induced rhinoconjunctivitis. Lancet 1998;351(9103):629–32.

11. Durham SR, Walker SM, Varga EM, et al. Long-term clinical efficacy of grass-pollen immunotherapy. N Engl J Med 1999;341(7):468–75.

12. Durham SR, Emminger W, Kapp A, et al. Long-term clinical efficacy in grass pollen-induced rhinoconjunctivitis after treatment with SQ-standardized grass allergy immunotherapy tablet. J Allergy Clin Immunol 2010;125(1):131–8.

13. Bostock J. Case of a periodical affection of the eyes and chest. Med Chir Trans 1819;10:161.

14. Sewall H. Experiments on the preventive inoculation of rattlesnake venom. J Physiol 1887;8:205.

15. Dunbar WP. The present state of our knowledge of hay-fever. J Hyg 1902;13:105.

16. Portier P, Richet C. De l'action anaphylactique de certains venins. CR Soc Biol 1902;54:170.

17. Coca AF, Cooke RA. On the classification of the phenomena of hypersensitiveness. J Immunol 1923;8:163.

18. Loveless M, Fackler W. Wasp venom allergy and immunity. Ann Allergy 1956;14:347.

19. Levine B, Redmond A. Minor haptenic determinant-specific reagins of penicillin hypersensitivity in man. Int Arch Allergy Appl Immunol 1969;35:445.

20. Parker C, Shapiro J, Kern M, et al. Hypersensitivity to penicillenic acid derivatives in human beings with penicillin allergy. J Exp Med 1962;115:821.

21. Harper S. Footnotes on allergy. Uppsala (Sweden): Pharmacia; 1980.

22. Fontana VJ, Holt LE Jr, Mainland D. Effectiveness of hyposensitization therapy in ragweed hay-fever in children. JAMA 1966;195(12):985–92.

23. Sadan N, Rhyne MB, Mellits ED, et al. Immunotherapy of pollinosis in children: investigation of the immunologic basis of clinical improvement. N Engl J Med 1969;280(12):623–7.

24. Norman PS, Winkenwerder WL, Lichtenstein LM. Immunotherapy of hay fever with ragweed antigen E: comparisons with whole pollen extract and placebos. J Allergy 1968;42(2):93–108.

25. Lockey RF. Systemic reactions to stinging ants. J Allergy Clin Immunol 1974;54(3):132–46.

26. Nordvall SL, Johansson SG, Ledford DK, et al. Allergens of the imported fire ant. J Allergy Clin Immunol 1988;82(4):567–76.

27. Lockey RF, Turkeltaub PC, Olive ES, et al. The Hymenoptera venom study. III: Safety of venom immunotherapy. J Allergy Clin Immunol 1990;86(5):775–80.
28. Slater JE, Esch RE, Lockey RF. Preparation and standardization of allergen extracts. In: Adkinson NF, Bochner BS, Busse WW, et al, editors. Middleton's allergy: principles and practice. 7th edition. Philadelphia: Elsevier; 2009. p. 557–68.
29. Chapman MD, Ferreira F, Villalba M, et al, CREATE consortium. The European Union CREATE project: a model for international standardization of allergy diagnostics and vaccines. J Allergy Clin Immunol 2008;122(5):882–9.
30. Bousquet J, Lockey R, Malling HJ. Allergen immunotherapy: therapeutic vaccines for allergic diseases. A WHO position paper.
31. Jacobsen L, Niggemann B, Dreborg S, et al. Specific immunotherapy has long-term preventive effect of seasonal and perennial asthma: 10-year follow-up on the PAT study. Allergy 2007;62(8):943–8.
32. Scadding GK, Brostoff J. Low dose sublingual therapy in patients with allergic rhinitis due to house dust mite. Clin Allergy 1986;16(5):483–91.
33. Canonica GW, Bousquet J, Casale T, et al. Sub-lingual immunotherapy: World Allergy Organization Position Paper 2009. Allergy 2009;64(Suppl 91):1–59.
34. Lockey RF, Benedict LM, Turkeltaub PC, et al. Fatalities from immunotherapy (IT) and skin testing (ST). J Allergy Clin Immunol 1987;79(4):660–77.
35. CSM update: desensitising vaccines. Br Med J (Clin Res Ed) 1986;293:948.
36. Casale TB, Stokes JR. Future forms of immunotherapy. J Allergy Clin Immunol 2011;127(1):8–15.
37. Creticos PS, Schroeder JT, Hamilton RG, et al. Immunotherapy with a ragweed-toll-like receptor 9 agonist vaccine for allergic rhinitis. N Engl J Med 2006; 355(14):1445–55.
38. Dynavax reports interim TOLAMBA ragweed allergy results from DARTT trial [press release January 8, 2007]. Berkeley (CA): Dynavax Technologies; 2007.
39. Senti G, Prinz Vavricka BM, Erdmann I, et al. Intralymphatic allergen administration renders specific immunotherapy faster and safer: a randomized controlled trial. Proc Natl Acad Sci U S A 2008;105(46):17908–12.

Immunotherapy: The Meta-Analyses. What have we Learned?

Moisés A. Calderón, MD, PhD[a],*, Robert J. Boyle, MD, PhD[b], Martin Penagos, MD, MSc[c], Aziz Sheikh, MD, FRCP, FRCGP[d]

KEYWORDS

- Specific allergen immunotherapy • Meta-analysis • Rhinitis
- Asthma

Since the first publication of clinical experimental work on the efficacy of specific allergen immunotherapy (SIT) in humans 100 years ago,[1] the interest of the medical community in this particular kind of treatment for allergic diseases has increased.

SIT is being delivered and investigated for a variety of allergic conditions, including rhinitis, conjunctivitis, asthma, Hymenoptera venom allergy, eczema, food allergy, latex allergy, and drug allergy. SIT is targeted at a large and variable range of allergens. The use of SIT as therapy for allergic respiratory diseases has been recognized in different international guidelines[2–5] and by the World Health Organization.[2,6]

Different routes for SIT have been evaluated, such as the subcutaneous, sublingual, oral, nasal, bronchial, and intralymphatic,[7] the first 2 of these routes being the most commonly used today in clinical practice. Subcutaneous immunotherapy (SCIT) is still the most commonly used route for the treatment of allergic rhinitis and allergic asthma in adults and children. Sublingual immunotherapy (SLIT) was introduced as an alternative to SCIT in the late 1970s. Allergen extracts for SLIT can be administered as drops

Financial disclosures: Moises Calderon has received consulting fees, honoraria for lectures, and/or research funding from ActoGeniX, ALK-Abelló, Allergy Therapeutics, Schering-Plough, and Stallergenes. Robert Boyle and Martin Penagos have no relevant financial disclosures to declare. Aziz Sheikh has received support to attend educational meetings and honoraria from ALK- Abelló.

[a] Department of Allergy and Respiratory Medicine, Imperial College, National Heart and Lung Institute, Royal Brompton and Harefield Trust, Dovehouse Street, London SW3 6LY, UK
[b] Department of Paediatrics, Imperial College, St Mary's Hospital, Praed Street, London W2 1PG, UK
[c] Department of Paediatric Allergy, St Thomas' Hospital, Westminster Bridge Road, London SE1 7EH, UK
[d] Allergy and Respiratory Research Group, Centre for Population Health Sciences, The University of Edinburgh Medical School, Doorway 3, Teviot Place, Edinburgh EH8 9AG, UK
* Corresponding author.
E-mail address: m.calderon@imperial.ac.uk

or fast-dissolving tablets. At present, its prescription by allergists is becoming more frequent in several countries worldwide, mainly within Europe.[8]

The increased interest of the medical community in the use of SIT is reflected by the large number of published randomized double-blind, placebo-controlled trials (RCTs) using standardized products and validated outcome measures that have been published in recent years. These publications have enabled the undertaking of systematic reviews investigating the effectiveness of SIT.[9,10] Some of the data in these systematic reviews have been found to be suitable for meta-analysis. Several different clinical and research/laboratory outcomes have been evaluated in each review. The selection of specific outcomes was established according to the interests of the reviewers, the most commonly used being symptom scores and rescue medication scores.

The clinical area that has received the greatest attention in relation to systematic reviews and meta-analyses is that of chronic allergic respiratory disease, in particular allergic rhinoconjunctivitis and allergic asthma; therefore, these areas represent the focus of this review. While concentrating on SIT for allergic airway disease, the authors nonetheless, where relevant, seek to draw lessons from systematic reviews and meta-analyses in other clinical areas. In other allergic diseases a small number of systematic reviews have been undertaken: there is a Cochrane review and one other systematic review of SIT for eczema in progress[11,12] but none published; there are 2 published meta-analyses of SIT for venom allergy[13,14] and one Cochrane review in progress[15]; there is one published Cochrane review of desensitization for drug allergy[16]; and there is one published meta-analysis of immunotherapy for food allergy recently.[17] These other allergic conditions are not discussed directly in this article, which aims to describe the lessons learned from meta-analyses of allergic rhinitis and asthma.

SYSTEMATIC REVIEWS AND META-ANALYSES

The terms systematic review and meta-analysis are often used interchangeably, but they do not mean exactly the same thing. A systematic review attempts to bring together all empirical evidence that fits specific inclusion criteria to answer a research question. It uses explicit, reproducible methods that are selected with a view to minimizing bias, thus generating valid findings.[18] Not all systematic reviews include meta-analysis, but this step may be included as part of a systematic review if data can meaningfully be combined and are furthermore available in an appropriate form. A meta-analysis comprises the use of statistical methods to estimate an average, or common effect, over several studies.[18,19] By combining information from all relevant clinical trials, meta-analyses can increase the precision of the summary estimates that is typically obtained through small studies, thus allowing a more objective appraisal of the evidence than a traditional narrative synthesis of findings. Meta-analysis also facilitates investigations of the consistency of evidence and the exploration of differences across studies, and enables exploration of controversies arising from apparently conflicting studies.[18] A meta-analysis also allows exploration of, and in some cases explanation of, heterogeneity between studies.

The effect size of the intervention is extracted/calculated for each study and for each outcome. The effect size is a statistical measure for the magnitude of the difference between two interventions adjusted by some estimate of variability. Outcomes are commonly reported using categorical (most commonly dichotomous) and continuous data.[18,20] For dichotomous outcomes, the main options are relative risks (RR), odds ratios (OR), or risk differences (RD). For continuous outcomes, the options are the mean difference (MD) or standardized mean difference (SMD) between the interventions tested.[19] This latter measure is important because different scales are commonly used by different investigators, and if this is so the results derived from these different scales need to be standardized to be able to combine the different studies in a meta-analysis by a common unit. The disadvantage of SMDs is that they are difficult to interpret: one commonly used interpretation of the SMD is to consider the effect size as trivial if the SMD is between 0.0 and 0.2, small for 0.2 to 0.5, moderate for 0.5 to 0.8 and large for greater than 0.8.[18,20,21]

Meta-analyses are usually displayed in graphical form by using "forest plots," which present the findings for all studies plus the combined results. The combined effect appears as a diamond at the bottom of the forest plot. The center of the diamond is equal to the average effect and the extremes of the diamond are equal to the 95% confidence interval (CI) of the average effect. The diamond or average effect is obtained from combining the summary measures collected for all included studies.[19] **Fig. 1** summarizes the main features of a meta-analysis presented in the form of a forest plot.

There are two models for combining studies: the fixed-effect model and the random-effects model. The fixed-effect model considers the variability between the studies as exclusively due to random variation. In other words, the assumption is that if the individual studies were infinitely large they would all produce the same result. By contrast, the random-effects model assumes a different underlying effect for each study and takes this into consideration as an additional source of variation. Under this assumption, if the studies were infinitely large they would still give different results of the effect of the intervention. The effects of the studies are assumed to be randomly distributed, and the central point of this distribution is the focus of the combined (pooled) effect estimate.[19]

HETEROGENEITY

Any kind of variability among studies in a systematic review may be termed "heterogeneity." There are different sources of heterogeneity: (1) clinical heterogeneity (variability in the participants, interventions and outcomes), (2) methodological heterogeneity (variability in study design and risk of bias), and (3) statistical heterogeneity (a consequence of clinical or methodological diversity, or both, among the studies) (**Box 1**). Statistical heterogeneity manifests itself in the observed intervention effects being more different from each other than one would expect if due to random error alone.[18]

If the results of the studies differ greatly then it may not be appropriate to combine the results using meta-analysis. There are available tests to assess heterogeneity across studies. The chi-squared (χ^2 or Chi^2) test assesses whether observed differences in results are compatible with chance alone. A low P value provides evidence of heterogeneity of intervention effects (variation in effect estimates beyond chance). Because of the low power of this test, a P value of .10, rather than the conventional level of .05, is sometimes used to determine statistical significance.[18]

A useful statistic for quantifying inconsistency is the I^2 test. This test describes the percentage of the variability in effect estimates that is due to heterogeneity rather than sampling error (chance). I^2 lies between 0% and 100%; a value of 0% indicates no heterogeneity, and larger values show increasing heterogeneity. Thresholds for the interpretation of I^2 can be misleading, because the importance of inconsistency depends on several factors. A rough guide to interpretation is as follows: 0% to 40%: might not be important, 30% to 60%: may represent moderate heterogeneity, 50% to 90%: may represent substantial heterogeneity, and 75% to 100% considerable heterogeneity.[18] If the I^2 test shows homogeneous results (<40%) then the differences between studies are assumed to be a consequence of sampling variation, and

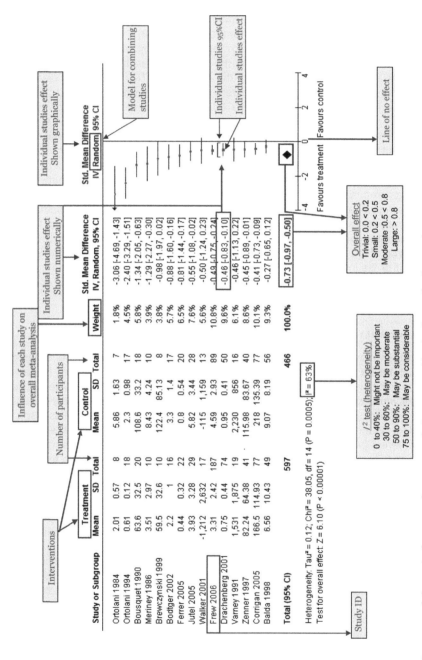

Fig. 1. Summary of the main features of a meta-analysis presented in the form of a forest plot.

| **Box 1** |
| **Types of heterogeneity** |

1. Clinical heterogeneity

   Variability in the participants

   Variability in interventions

   Variability in outcomes

2. Methodological heterogeneity

   Variability in trial design

   Variability in study quality

   Variability in allergen extracts

   Variability in dose schedules

3. Statistical heterogeneity

   Due to clinical and/or methodological diversity

the use of a fixed-effect model is appropriate. If, however, the test shows that significant heterogeneity exists between study results, a random-effects model is advocated.[18,22]

Heterogeneity should not simply be ignored after a statistical test is applied; rather, it should be scrutinized, with an attempt to explain it.[18,22] For example, sensitivity analyses may identify specific causes of statistical heterogeneity in a meta-analysis.

META-ANALYSES OF SIT

At present, 12 meta-analyses evaluating the effect of SIT on allergic rhinitis[23–31] and allergic asthma[29,30,32–37] have been published.

Allergic Rhinitis

The results of meta-analyses of SCIT or SLIT for treating allergic rhinitis are summarized in **Table 1**, and are described in detail here.

SCIT

The first "meta-analysis" on SCIT was published in German and included 43 RCTs published between 1980 and 1997 investigating the effect of SCIT on clinical and immunologic treatment used in patients with allergic rhinoconjunctivitis.[23] SCIT was shown to be an effective treatment in allergic rhinoconjunctivitis, decreasing symptoms, the need for medication, and reactivity in specific nasal and conjunctival provocation tests, as well as inflammatory markers. This study was more a "general literature review" rather than a formal systematic review, as no search design methodology was presented and no statistical meta-analyses were conducted. However, the investigators did thoroughly review possible mechanisms involved in SIT and concluded that the efficacy of SIT is dependent on the allergen to which the individual patient is sensitive, the quality and total amount of the allergen applied, and the SIT schedule.

A second "analysis" of SIT for treating allergic rhinitis was conducted on 16 prospective, single-blind or double-blind, placebo-controlled studies published between 1966 and 1996. This review included 759 patients (546 adults, 53 children, 160 all ages).[24] The investigators explained that because experimental designs varied considerably from one study to another, it was not possible to reduce the entire

Table 1
Meta-analyses of RCTs of SIT for treating allergic rhinitis

Study,[Ref.] Year	Patients	Allergens	Symptom Scores SMD (95% CI)	Medication Scores SMD (95% CI)	Comment
Calderon et al,[25] 2007	2871 adults	SCIT Seasonal	−0.73 (−0.97, −0.50) $I^2 = 63\%$	−0.57 (−0.82, −0.33) $I^2 = 64\%$	No children included No fatalities reported Moderate heterogeneity
Radulovic et al,[27] 2010	4589 adults & children	SLIT Seasonal and perennial	−0.49 (−0.64, −0.34) $I^2 = 81\%$	−0.32 (−0.43, −0.21) $I^2 = 50\%$	Considerable heterogeneity despite inclusion of large trials
Penagos et al,[28] 2006	484 children	SLIT Seasonal and perennial	−0.56 (−1.01, −0.10) $I^2 = 81\%$	−0.76 (−1.46, −0.06) $I^2 = 86\%$	Considerable heterogeneity
Olaguibel and Alvarez Puebla,[29] 2005	232 children	SLIT Seasonal and perennial	−0.44 (−1.22, 0.35) I^2 = not reported	Not reported	Small numbers Heterogeneity not reported
Compalati et al,[30] 2009	382 adults and children	SLIT House dust mite	−0.95 (−1.77, −0.14) $I^2 = 92\%$	−1.88 (−3.65, −0.12) $I^2 = 95\%$	Considerable heterogeneity despite focus on a single allergen
Di Bona et al,[31] 2010	2971 adults and children with rhinitis	SLIT Grass pollen	−0.32 (−0.44, −0.21) $I^2 = 56\%$	−0.33 (−0.50, −0.16) $I^2 = 78\%$	Moderate heterogeneity

database to a single format for statistical analysis. Therefore, OR and 95% CI were calculated using a random-effects model for a variety of clinical outcomes. All but one study concluded that SIT was effective in terms of reducing symptoms of allergic rhinitis (OR 1.81, 95% CI 1.48–2.23) compared with placebo.

At present, there is only one Cochrane meta-analysis evaluating the effect of allergen injection immunotherapy on seasonal allergic rhinitis.[25] This review examined 51 RCTs published between 1984 and 2006 and included a total of 2871 patients (1645 active, 1226 placebo), each receiving on average 18 injections. A wide range of allergens were administered in these studies: ragweed (n = 12 trials), mixed grass (n = 16 trials), timothy (n = 5 trials), *Parietaria* (n = 6 trials), birch (n = 4 trials), orchard (n = 2 trials), cedar (n = 3 trials), bermuda (n = 1 trial), *Juniperus ashei* (n = 1 trial), and *Cocos nucifera* (n = 1 trial). Six studies specified that patients did not experience coexistent asthma; in 27 studies patients had mild to moderate seasonal allergic asthma; 18 studies did not specify the asthmatic status of their participants. The types of vaccines used were extracts (n = 38 studies), allergoids (n = 12 studies), and non-specified (n = 1 study). The duration of maintenance treatment and the period of follow-up varied considerably between studies, largely reflecting preseasonal, coseasonal, and postseasonal administration. Duration of immunotherapy varied from 3 days (minimum duration) to 3 years (maximum duration). Six studies did not mention the duration of treatment. It was not possible from most of the studies to determine accurately the dose of allergen given in terms of micrograms of major allergen. Doses given were quantified in many different units including BU, PNU, BU, SQ-U, μg Ag, SE-U, AUeq, SU/mL, TU, wt/vol, and HEP. Symptom score data from 15 trials were suitable for meta-analysis and showed an overall reduction in the immunotherapy group (SMD −0.73, 95% CI −0.97 to −0.50; I^2 = 63%). Medication score data from 13 trials showed an overall reduction in the immunotherapy group (SMD −0.57, 95% CI −0.82 to −0.33; I^2 = 64%).

SLIT

The effectiveness of SLIT has been studied in 5 meta-analyses.[26–31] The first Cochrane analysis looked at 22 studies published between 1990 and 2002.[26] This systematic review and meta-analyses was updated in 2010[27] to include 49 RCTs (involving a total of 4589 participants: 2333 active and 2256 placebo), 34 studies were performed in adults and 15 in children. Allergens used were grass pollen (n = 23 trials); *Parietaria* (n = 5 trials), ragweed (n = 2 trials); trees (n = 9 trials): olive (n = 2 trials), cypress (n = 3 trials), birch pollen (n = 2 trials), mixed trees (n = 2 trials); house dust mite (n = 8 trials); and cat (n = 1 trial). Symptom score data showed an overall reduction in the immunotherapy group (SMD −0.49, 95% CI −0.64 to −0.34, $P<.00001$); there was significant heterogeneity between the studies (Chi^2 = 256.76, $P<.00001$, I^2 = 81%). Medication score data from 38 trials showed an overall reduction in the immunotherapy group (SMD −0.32, 95% CI −0.43 to −0.21, $P<.00001$). Significant heterogeneity was indicated (Chi^2 = 73.32, P = .0003, I^2 = 50%). The predetermined subgroup analyses performed in this review show that SLIT is highly effective in both seasonal and perennial allergic rhinitis and that treatment is effective, whatever the duration, although the effect size is greatest with the treatment lasting more than 12 months for both symptoms (SMD −0.70, 95% CI −1.19 to −0.21) and medication scores (SMD −0.44, 95% CI −0.84 to −0.04). Similarly to the previous version of this Cochrane review, the investigators were unable to identify a significant reduction in either symptoms or medication scores in children.

A separate systematic review focused only on the pediatric use of SLIT in studies published between 1990 and 2004.[28] Ten studies provided enough data for meta-analyses and included 484 children (245 SLIT and 239 placebo). Allergens included were mites (n = 4 trials), grass mix (n = 3 trials), olive (n = 1 trial), *Parietaria* (n = 1 trial), and *Phleum poa* (n = 1 trial). There was a significant reduction in both symptoms (SMD −0.56, 95% CI −1.01 to −0.10, I^2 = 81%) and medication use (SMD −0.76, 95% CI −1.46 to −0.06, I^2 = 85%) after SLIT compared with placebo. The subgroup analyses performed for treatment duration and type of allergen showed that SLIT for longer than 18 months and with pollen extracts was effective compared with SLIT courses shorter than 18 months and with mites. Duration of treatment varied between 3 and 36 months.

Six pediatric trials were included in a systematic review and meta-analysis to assess the effect of SLIT compared with placebo (117 children in SLIT and 115 placebo).[29] Allergens included were house dust mite (n = 3 trials), grass mixed (n = 1 trial), olive (n = 1 trial), and *Parietaria* (n = 1 trial). Using a random-effect model there was a reduction in nasal symptoms scores (SMD −0.44, 95% CI −1.22 to 0.35; I^2 = not reported).

The effectiveness of SLIT with house dust mite extracts for allergic rhinitis was independently meta-analyzed in 9 trials published up to March 1, 2008 with a total of 403 participants (194 active, 209 placebo).[30] A significant reduction in symptoms of allergic rhinitis (SMD −0.95, 95% CI −1.77 to −0.14, I^2 = 92%) and rescue medication (SMD −1.88, 95% CI −3.65 to −0.12, I^2 = 95%) was found in the SLIT group compared with the placebo group.

More recently, the effect of SLIT with grass allergens in adults and children with seasonal allergic rhinitis was separately evaluated in 19 trials; this review included 2971 patients (1518 receiving SLIT and 1453 placebo).[31] In this analysis there was a significant reduction in both symptoms (SMD −0.32, 95% CI −0.44 to −0.21, I^2 = 56%) and medication use (SMD −0.33, 95% CI −0.50 to −0.16, I^2 = 78%) compared with placebo. The investigators concluded that the treatment seems to be more efficacious in adults than in children, and prolonging the duration of preseasonal treatment for more than 12 weeks improves the treatment efficacy.

Allergic Asthma

The results of meta-analyses of SCIT or SLIT for treating allergic asthma are summarized in **Table 2**, and are described in detail here.

SCIT

The clinical efficacy of SCIT in asthma was firstly summarized by a meta-analysis of 20 trials for asthma published between 1954 and 1990.[32] Subsequently this systematic review was updated as a Cochrane meta-analysis to include 75 trials published between 1954 and 2001.[33] The last update looked at 81 trials.[34] Allergens used were house dust mite (n = 42 trials), pollen (n = 27 trials), animal dander (n = 10 trials), *Cladosporium* mold (n = 2 trials), latex (2 trials), and multiple allergens (n = 6). Overall, there was a significant reduction in asthma symptoms and medication and improvement in bronchial hyperreactivity following immunotherapy. There was a significant improvement in asthma symptom scores (SMD −0.59, 95% CI −0.83 to −0.35) and it would have been necessary to treat 3 (95% CI 3–5) patients with immunotherapy to avoid one deterioration in asthma symptoms. Overall, it would have been necessary to treat 4 (95% CI 3–6) patients with immunotherapy to avoid one requiring increased medication. Allergen immunotherapy significantly reduced allergen specific bronchial hyperreactivity, with some reduction in nonspecific bronchial hyperreactivity as well. There was, however, no consistent effect on lung function. The investigators stated that the benefits of allergen immunotherapy could be overestimated because of unpublished negative studies, and suggested that additional studies would be necessary to overturn these results. It was concluded that

Table 2
Meta-analyses of RCTs of SIT for treating allergic asthma

Study	Patients	Allergens	Symptom Scores SMD (95% CI)	Medication Scores SMD (95% CI)	Comment
Abramson et al,[34] 2010	3459 children and adults	SCIT Seasonal or perennial	−0.59 (−0.83, −0.35) $I^2 = 90\%$	−0.53 (−0.80, −0.27) $I^2 = 67\%$	Open trials included No detailed evaluation of safety Considerable heterogeneity
Calamita et al,[36] 2006	1706 adults and children	SLIT Seasonal and perennial	−0.38 (−0.79, 0.03) $I^2 = 64\%$	−0.91 (−1.94, 0.12) $I^2 = 92\%$	Considerable heterogeneity Weak methodology Open trials included
Penagos et al,[37] 2008	441 children	SLIT Seasonal and perennial	−1.14 (−2.10, −0.18) $I^2 = 94\%$	−1.63 (−2.83, −0.44) $I^2 = 95\%$	Considerable heterogeneity
Olaguibel and Alvarez Puebla,[29] 2005	193 children	SLIT Seasonal and perennial	−1.42 (−2.51, −0.34) $I^2 =$ not reported	Not reported	Small numbers Heterogeneity not reported
Compalati et al,[30] 2009	476 adults and children	SLIT House dust mite	−0.95 (−1.74 −0.15) $I^2 = 93\%$	−1.48 (−2.70, −0.26) $I^2 = 96\%$	Considerable heterogeneity despite focus on a single allergen

allergen immunotherapy is a treatment option in highly selected patients with extrinsic ("allergic") asthma.

Ross and colleagues[35] extracted data from 24 prospective trials published between 1966 and 1998 in allergic asthmatics. Using a random-effects model, the SCIT patients group showed an improvement compared with the placebo group for symptoms of asthma (OR 2.76, 95% CI 2.22–3.42), for pulmonary function (OR 2.87, 95% CI 1.82–4.52), protection against bronchial challenge (OR 1.81, 95% CI 1.32–2.49), and reduced need for medications (OR 2.00, 95% CI 1.46–2.72).

SLIT

The efficacy of SLIT in mild to moderate asthmatics was evaluated in a meta-analyses of 25 studies published between 1991 and 2005 (total 1706 patients).[36] The effect of SLIT on asthma symptoms (SMD -0.38, 95% CI -0.79 to 0.03; $I^2 = 64\%$) and asthma medication use (SMD -0.91, 95%CI -1.94 to 0.12, $I^2 = 92\%$) were not statistically significant. This review has some methodological issues, which make interpretation difficult. First, there were no restrictions in relation to inclusion criteria for trial selection; the review thus included both open and blinded trials. Second, the outcomes analyzed were not clearly defined. Finally, statistical analysis included qualitative assessments instead of a quantitative approach for some outcomes.

Another meta-analysis focused on allergic asthma in children (3–18 years of age)[37] and included 9 studies published between 1990 and May 2006 with total of 441 patients. The effect of SLIT was significant for both improvement of asthma symptoms (SMD -1.14, 95% CI -2.10 to -0.18, $I^2 = 94\%$) and reduction in asthma medication use (SMD -1.63, 95% CI -2.83 to -0.44, $I^2 = 95\%$) compared with placebo. The investigators concluded that SLIT with standardized vaccines reduces both symptom scores and rescue medication use in children with allergic asthma compared with placebo.[24] Nonetheless, in this meta-analysis the heterogeneity was very significant (>94%), with a wide 95% CI for SMD in both outcomes. This variation indicates the diverse methodology used throughout studies. More studies are required to make a robust conclusion.

Five pediatric RCTs were included in another systematic review and meta-analyses to assess the effect of SLIT compared with placebo.[29] Allergens included were house dust mite (4 trials) and olive (1 trial). Using a random-effects model, there was a significant reduction in bronchial symptoms scores (SMD -1.42, 95% CI -2.51 to -0.34; $I^2 = $ not recorded).

Compalati and colleagues[30] undertook a review of the effect of house dust mite SLIT for treating allergic asthma. These investigators found a significant reduction for symptom scores (SMD -0.95, CI 95% -1.74 to -0.15, $I^2 = 93\%$) and rescue medication use (SMD -1.48, 95% CI -2.70 to -0.26, $I^2 = 96\%$) in the SLIT group compared with the placebo group.

COMPARING SCIT WITH SLIT USING META-ANALYSES

There are very few trials comparing SCIT with SLIT for the same allergen within the same study; a direct comparison is not possible because of the absence of well-designed primary studies. It is also problematic, however, to use the results obtained in one systematic review and meta-analysis for comparison with the results obtained in separate meta-analysis, for example of SCIT versus SLIT for treating allergic rhinoconjunctivitis. The effect size of one particular outcome is related to that particular meta-analysis, which is based on the data extracted from a specific systematic review. The high clinical and methodological heterogeneity (more than 50%) found in the various meta-analyses makes comparisons even more difficult. However, efforts have been made to quantify any differences in clinical efficacy between SLIT and SCIT. For example, a set of parallel meta-analyses of SCIT (n = 6 trials), SLIT (drops; n = 12 trials) and SLIT (tablets; n = 6 trials) in a total of 3629 patients with grass pollen rhinitis found the level of efficacy was greater for SLIT tablets (SMD −0.41, 95% CI −0.51 to −0.31) and SCIT (SMD −0.46, 95% CI −0.62 to −0.31) than for SLIT drops (SMD −0.14, 95% CI −0.25 to −0.02). Tests for heterogeneity were nonsignificant for SLIT tablets and SCIT (P = .23 and P = .99, respectively), but significant for the SLIT drop analysis (P = .002). Results were similar with a random-effects model.[38]

SAFETY EVALUATIONS IN META-ANALYSES

Systematic reviews have shown that SCIT is safe when prescribed to selected patients in a specialist clinic with adequate facilities and trained health personnel. SCIT can produce both local and systemic adverse reactions; however, in the majority of cases these symptoms are readily reversible if recognized early and with prompt treatment. Adverse effects may occur with all allergen preparations whether using standardized extracts, allergoids, or recombinant allergens.[39] In the only Cochrane systematic review and meta-analyses on SCIT for seasonal allergic rhinitis,[25] 22% of SCIT versus 8% of placebo had mild (European Academy of Allergy and Clinical Immunology [EAACI] Grade II) and 7% of SCIT versus 1% had moderate to severe (EAACI Grade III) allergic reactions at some time during their course of SCIT. Anaphylaxis (EAACI Grade IV) was reported only in 3 cases in the SCIT group (0.72%) versus 1 case in the placebo group (0.33%). Adrenaline was used in 3.4% of participants (19/557 patients; 0.13% of 14,085 injections) in the SCIT group versus 0.25% (1/404 patients; 0.01% of 8278 injections) in the placebo group. This review suggests that adverse reactions serious enough to require treatment with adrenaline (epinephrine) occur approximately once in every 770 immunotherapy injections. There were no fatalities.[25]

The safety profile of SLIT seems to be superior to that for SCIT; however, it is difficult to compare safety data between different meta-analyses, because different trials and meta-analyses use different grading systems for severity. Although there is recent consensus on an immunotherapy adverse event grading system, this was not used for the studies included in the meta-analyses published to date.[39,40]

WHAT HAVE WE LEARNED FROM THE META-ANALYSES?

It is important to step back and reflect on what this body of work has contributed to advancing our understanding of the management of people with allergic airway disease. Some key over-arching lessons include the following observations.

- *Systematic reviews and meta-analyses are powerful tools for synthesizing clinical trial data in a format that is easily accessible to trained clinicians.* One hundred years after the discovery of SIT, there is now a substantial body of trial evidence available to draw on in this field, and investigators have on the whole been very generous in sharing their data for meta-analysis.
- *Meta-analyses have shown that SCIT and SLIT are effective in the treatment of allergic rhinitis and allergic asthma.* Meta-analyses of SIT based on properly well performed systematic reviews represent the highest level of evidence. Meta-analyses of SCIT and SLIT for allergic rhinitis[23–31] and allergic asthma[29,30,32–37] show that these forms of treatment are clinically efficacious when compared with placebo. Because of the high level of heterogeneity present in the meta-analyses of SLIT and SCIT particularly for allergic asthma, caution is needed in

drawing conclusions. Some of this heterogeneity can be attributed to variation in study design and methodological limitations in the clinical trials themselves. The inclusion of weak study designs (eg, open trials) in systematic reviews and meta-analyses would bias in favor of demonstrating a beneficial effect associated with treatment.

- *SIT is a relatively safe form of treatment for allergic rhinitis*. In the modern age and with appropriate safeguards in place, SIT is a relatively safe form of treatment, particularly if given through nonparenteral routes. However, clinical trials and meta-analyses are not a good way to assess the risk of rare adverse events such as fatal anaphylaxis, due to insufficient statistical power and less than optimal safety monitoring, which usually occur within a clinical trial setting. Moreover, reporting of safety outcomes has been limited in many clinical trials and some meta-analyses of SIT, particularly meta-analysis of SCIT for treating allergic asthma.

- *Future SIT meta-analyses should focus on specific allergens, populations, and outcomes*. SIT is being delivered and investigated for a variety of allergic conditions such as asthma, allergic rhinitis, eczema, and food allergy through a variety of routes (mainly subcutaneous and sublingual). It is important that some boundaries are drawn and a focus is found when researchers conduct a systematic review and meta-analyses, due to the unavoidable clinical and methodological heterogeneity in reviews that include a wide range of differing studies. This approach will allow us to reach conclusions that are more specific and with less heterogeneity.

- *The quality of systematic reviews and meta-analyses is critical for making reliable and valid conclusions about the therapeutic intervention*. The need for high-quality RCTs is well recognized, but the literature on quality assessment for systematic reviews and meta-analyses is at an earlier stage of development. Poor published quality reviews and meta-analyses can be misleading, and criteria have been developed for the assessment of systematic review quality.[41,42] Common weaknesses include lack of a priori systematic review design, a comprehensive literature review, a quality assessment of included studies (for example using GRADE criteria[43]), and inappropriate statistical methods for meta-analysis. Considering that meta-analysis is a statistical procedure that incorporates the results of pooled independent studies, the reader must be critical and objective in the interpretation of its results, and data should be carefully scrutinized for adequate study design.[39,44]

- *Selection and grading of the primary end points in SIT trials is necessary*. There are clear discrepancies in the selection and grading of the primary end points for assessing the response to SIT in allergic rhinitis and allergic asthma. Recommendations have been made to unify these criteria[45]; however, many of the studies included in the systematic reviews and therefore in the meta-analyses were conducted prior to these recommendations. There is a need for further trials and meta-analyses that report more global outcome measures than symptom and medication scores, such as quality of life and health economic assessments. There is also a lack of studies looking at long-term outcomes (eg, immune tolerance), health economic evaluations, and head-to-head studies with other active treatments (eg, intranasal steroids).

- *Adequate study size and power calculations are needed for future SIT trials, to limit heterogeneity between trials included in meta-analyses*. Inclusion of multiple small trials in a single meta-analysis may increase the risk of overestimating or underestimating the true treatment effect.[45] Many studies of small numbers of participants are included in the current systematic reviews and in meta-analyses. Power calculation should be determined before initiation of any particular therapeutic intervention.

- *There may be a need for a publicly accessible immunotherapy trials data repository, to facilitate updates/follow-on systematic reviews and meta-analyses.* It is very important that the results of both positive and negative trials are reported, as this may reduce the risk of publication bias.[39,46] Studies with so-called negative results are more often not submitted for publication or for report to regulatory authorities, and take longer to be published.[46] The lack of this information may be reflected in the data included for meta-analyses that might lead to an overestimation of beneficial effects of SIT. Trials need to be reported in accordance with CONSORT guidelines.[47]

REFERENCES

1. Noon L. Prophylactic inoculation against hay fever. Lancet 1911;i:1572.
2. Bousquet J, Lockey R, Malling HJ. Allergen immunotherapy: therapeutic vaccines for allergic diseases. A WHO position paper. J Allergy Clin Immunol 1998;102(4 Pt 1):558–62.
3. International Consensus Report on diagnosis and management of asthma. International Asthma Management Project. Allergy 1992;47:S1–61.
4. Bousquet J, Van Cauwenberge P, Khaltaev N. Allergic rhinitis and its impact on asthma. J Allergy Clin Immunol 2001;108:S147–334.
5. Cox L, Li JT, Nelson H, et al. Allergen immunotherapy: a practice parameter second update. J Allergy Clin Immunol 2007;120:S25–85.
6. Bateman ED, Hurd SS, Barnes PJ, et al. Global strategy for asthma management and prevention: GINA executive summary. Eur Respir J 2008;31(1):143–78.
7. Passalacqua G, Compalati E, Canonica GW. Advances in allergen-specific immunotherapy. Curr Drug Targets 2009;10(12):1255–62.
8. Canonica GW, Bousquet J, Casale T, et al. Sub-lingual immunotherapy: world allergy organization position paper 2009. Allergy 2009;64(Suppl 91):1–59.
9. Calderon MA. Meta-analyses of specific immunotherapy trials. Drugs Today (Barc) 2008;44:S31–4.
10. Compalati E, Penagos M, Tarantini F, et al. Specific immunotherapy for respiratory allergy: state of the art according to current meta-analyses. Ann Allergy Asthma Immunol 2009;102:22–8.
11. Calderon MA, Boyle R, Nankervis H, et al. Specific allergen immunotherapy for the treatment of atopic eczema (Protocol). Cochrane Database Syst Rev 2010; 10:CD008774.
12. Compalati E, Massimo L, Anthi R, et al. Meta-analysis of immunotherapy for atopic dermatitis. Allergy 2010;65:S92.
13. Watanabe AS, Fonseca LA, Galvão CE, et al. Specific immunotherapy using Hymenoptera venom: systematic review. Sao Paulo Med J 2010;128(1): 30–7.
14. Ross RN, Nelson HS, Finegold I. Effectiveness of specific immunotherapy in the treatment of hymenoptera venom hypersensitivity: a meta-analysis. Clin Ther 2000;22(3):351–8.
15. Elremeli M, Bulsara MK, Daniels M, et al. Venom immunotherapy for preventing allergic reactions to insect stings (Protocol). Cochrane Database Syst Rev 2010;11:CD008838.

16. Lin D, Li WK, Rieder MJ. Cotrimoxazole for prophylaxis or treatment of opportunistic infections of HIV/AIDS in patients with previous history of hypersensitivity to cotrimoxazole. Cochrane Database Syst Rev 2007;2:CD005646.

17. Fisher HR, Toit G, Lack G. Specific oral tolerance induction in food allergic children: is oral desensitisation more effective than allergen avoidance? a meta-analysis of published RCTs. Arch Dis Child 2011;96(3):259–64.

18. Higgins JPT, Green S, editors. Cochrane handbook for systematic reviews of interventions, version 5.1.0 [updated March 2011]. The Cochrane Collaboration; 2011. Available at: www.cochrane-handbook.org. Accessed February 26, 2011.

19. Perera R, Heneghan C. Interpreting meta-analyses in systematic reviews. Ann Intern Med 2009;150:JC2–2, JC2–3.

20. Leucht S, Kissling W, Davis JM. How to read and understand and use systematic reviews and meta-analyses. Acta Psychiatr Scand 2009;119:443–50.

21. Cohen J. Statistical power analysis for the behavioral sciences. 2nd edition. Hillsdale (NJ): Lawrence Erlbaum Associates; 1988.

22. Egger M, Smith GD, Phillips AN. Meta-analysis: principles and procedures. BMJ 1997;315:1533–7.

23. Klimek L, Malling HJ. [Specific immunotherapy (hyposensitization) in allergic rhinoconjunctivitis. Meta-analysis of effectiveness and side effects]. HNO 1999; 47(7):602–10 [in German].

24. Ross RN, Nelson HS, Finegold I. Effectiveness of specific immunotherapy in the treatment of allergic rhinitis: an analysis of randomized, prospective, single- or double-blind, placebo-controlled studies. Clin Ther 2000;22(3): 342–50.

25. Calderon MA, Alves B, Jacobson M, et al. Allergen injection immunotherapy for seasonal allergic rhinitis. Cochrane Database Syst Rev 2007;1:CD001936.

26. Wilson DR, Lima MT, Durham ST. Sublingual immunotherapy for allergic rhinitis: systematic review and meta-analysis. Allergy 2005;60:4–12.

27. Radulovic S, Calderon MA, Wilson D, et al. Sublingual immunotherapy for allergic rhinitis. Cochrane Database Syst Rev 2010;12:CD002893.

28. Penagos M, Compalati E, Tarantini F, et al. Efficacy of sublingual immunotherapy in the treatment of allergic rhinitis in pediatric patients 3 to 18 years of age: a meta-analysis of randomized, placebo-controlled, double-blind trials. Ann Allergy Asthma Immunol 2006;97:141–8.

29. Olaguíbel JM, Alvarez Puebla MJ. Efficacy of sublingual allergen vaccination for respiratory allergy in children. Conclusions from one meta-analysis. J Investig Allergol Clin Immunol 2005;15:9–16.

30. Compalati E, Passalacqua G, Bonini M, et al. The efficacy of sublingual immunotherapy for house dust mites respiratory allergy: results of a GA2LEN meta-analysis. Allergy 2009;64:1570–9.

31. Di Bona D, Plaia A, Scafidi V, et al. Efficacy of sublingual immunotherapy with grass allergens for seasonal allergic rhinitis: a systematic review and meta-analysis. J Allergy Clin Immunol 2010;126(3):558–66.

32. Abramson MJ, Puy RM, Weiner JM. Is allergen immunotherapy effective in asthma? A meta-analysis of randomized controlled trials. Am J Respir Crit Care Med 1995;151(4):969–74.

33. Abramson MJ, Puy RM, Weiner JM. Allergen immunotherapy for asthma. Cochrane Database Syst Rev 2003;4:CD001186.

34. Abramson MJ, Puy RM, Weiner JM. Injection allergen immunotherapy for asthma. Cochrane Database Syst Rev 2010;8:CD001186.

35. Ross RN, Nelson HS, Finegold I. Effectiveness of specific immunotherapy in the treatment of asthma: a meta-analysis of prospective, randomized, double-blind, placebo-controlled studies. Clin Ther 2000;22(3):329–41.

36. Calamita Z, Saconato H, Pela AB, et al. Efficacy of sublingual immunotherapy in asthma: systematic review of randomized-clinical trials using the Cochrane Collaboration method. Allergy 2006;61:1162–72.

37. Penagos M, Passalaqua G, Compalati E, et al. Metaanalysis of the efficacy of sublingual immunotherapy in the treatment of allergic asthma in pediatric patients, 3 to 18 years of age. Chest 2008;133:599–609.

38. Calderon M, Strodl Andersen J, Lawton S. Meta-analysis supports the efficacy of grass allergy immunotherapy tablets is comparable to subcutaneous immuno-therapy. Available at: http://eaaci.net/images/files/Abstract_Books/2010/Abstract_Book_ERAM-SERIN2010.pdf. Accessed February 26, 2011.

39. Calderón MA, Casale TB, Togias A, et al. Allergen-specific immunotherapy for respiratory allergies: from meta-analysis to registration and beyond. J Allergy Clin Immunol 2011;127(1):30–8.

40. Cox L, Larenas-Linnemann D, Lockey R, et al. Speaking the same language: the world allergy organization subcutaneous immunotherapy systemic reaction grading system. J Allergy Clin Immunol 2010;125(3):569–74.

41. Shea BJ, Hamel C, Wells GA, et al. AMSTAR is a reliable and valid measurement tool to assess the methodological quality of systematic reviews. J Clin Epidemiol 2009;62(10):1013–20.

42. Kung J, Chiappelli F, Cajulis OO, et al. From systematic reviews to clinical recom-mendations for evidence-based health care: validation of Revised Assessment of Multiple Systematic Reviews (R-AMSTAR) for grading of clinical relevance. Open Dent J 2010;16(4):84–91.

43. Brożek JL, Akl EA, Compalati E, et al, GRADE Working Group. Grading quality of evidence and strength of recommendations in clinical practice guidelines Part 3 of 3. The GRADE approach to developing recommendations. Allergy 2011. DOI: 10.1111/j.1398-9995.2010.02530.x. [Epub ahead of print].

44. Moher D, Liberati A, Tetzlaff J, et al, PRISMA Group. Preferred reporting items for systematic reviews and meta-analyses: the PRISMA Statement. Ann Intern Med 2009;151:264–9.

45. Casale TB, Canonica GW, Bousquet J, et al. Recommendations for appropriate sublingual immunotherapy clinical trials. J Allergy Clin Immunol 2009;124:665–70.

46. Nieto A, Mazon A, Pamies R, et al. Sublingual immunotherapy for allergic respi-ratory diseases: an evaluation of meta-analyses. J Allergy Clin Immunol 2009;124:157–61.

47. Bousquet PJ, Calderón MA, Demoly P, et al. The Consolidated Standards of Re-porting Trials (CONSORT) Statement applied to allergen-specific immunotherapy with inhalant allergens: a Global Allergy and Asthma European Network (GA(2) LEN) article. J Allergy Clin Immunol 2011;127(1):49–56.

Mechanisms of Subcutaneous Allergen Immunotherapy

Ozge U. Soyer, MD[a], Mubeccel Akdis, MD, PhD[b],
Cezmi A. Akdis, MD[b],*

KEYWORDS

- Allergy • Allergen immunotherapy • T regulatory cells
- Interleukin 10 • Transforming growth factor β
- Immune tolerance

Allergic inflammation takes place because of the development of an adaptive immune response induced by noninfectious environmental substances (allergens) in sensitized subjects, leading to several diseases including asthma, allergic rhinoconjunctivitis, anaphylaxis, urticaria, and atopic dermatitis.[1] Sensitization to an allergen depends on the capacity of the allergen to prime the helper T (T_H) subtype 2 cell response, during which interleukin (IL)-4 and IL-13 drive IgE antibody production by initiating IgE class switch in B cells. Binding of IgE to its high-affinity receptor (FcεRI) on mast cells and basophils results in secretion of biologically active compounds, mainly histamine, lipid-derived mediators, newly synthesized cytokines, chemokines, and growth factors associated with the immediate phase of allergic reaction.[2–6] In addition, binding of IgE to FcεRI on dendritic cells and monocytes and to the low-affinity receptor of IgE (FcεRII) on B cells increases the uptake of allergen by antigen-presenting cells (APCs). These APCs present the allergen's T-cell epitope peptides and activate allergen-specific CD4[+] T cells, which orchestrate the late-phase allergic immune response.[7]

Changes in the balance between allergen-specific T regulatory (Treg) cells and T_H2 and/or T_H1 cells are critical in the development and treatment of allergic diseases.[8,9] In addition, recently identified T-cell subsets, such as T_H17, T_H22, and T_H9, have been found to play a role in allergic diseases, and data regarding their relationship with

The authors' laboratories are supported by the Swiss National Foundation grants and Christine Kühne-Center for Allergy Research and Education (CK-CARE).

[a] Department of Pediatric Allergy, Ankara Education and Research Hospital, Ministry of Health, Ulucanlar Street, No 11, Ankara, Turkey 06080
[b] Department of Dermatology, Swiss Institute of Allergy and Asthma Research (SIAF), University of Zurich, Obere Strasse 22, CH7270 Davos, Switzerland
* Corresponding author.
E-mail address: akdisac@siaf.uzh.ch

Immunol Allergy Clin N Am 31 (2011) 175–190
doi:10.1016/j.iac.2011.02.006
0889-8561/11/$ – see front matter © 2011 Elsevier Inc. All rights reserved.

immunology.theclinics.com

allergic inflammation continue to accumulate.[10–13] Antihistamines, leukotriene receptor antagonists, and glucocorticoids used for the management of allergic diseases provide a temporary relief of symptoms and signs because of the transient suppression of inflammation in allergic diseases.[14] However, a long-term cure can be achieved by allergen-specific immunotherapy (SIT) with a disease-modifying effect, which might also lead to a decrease in the requirement of antiinflammatory and symptomatic medications.[15] The basic principle of allergen-SIT depends on a desensitization strategy by the repeated administration of increased doses of the causative allergen to induce a state of tolerance through the constitution of allergen-specific Treg cells (**Fig. 1**).[8,16–18]

TREG CELLS IN IMMUNE RESPONSE

In healthy individuals, immune response to allergens has included unresponsiveness of T cells or active peripheral tolerance induction by the subsets of Treg cells.[19–21] Peripheral blood mononuclear cells (PBMCs) of healthy subjects secrete higher levels of IL-10 and transforming growth factor β (TGF-β) after allergen stimulation, leading to active suppression of specific T cell responses.[22] In addition, in nonatopic individuals, active suppression against allergens is mediated by Tr1 cells or $CD4^+CD25^+$ Treg cells.[23,24]

Forkhead box protein 3 (FOXP3) transcription factor is critical for the function of $CD4^+CD25^+$ Treg cells and the maintenance of peripheral immunologic tolerance.[25–27] X-linked immune dysregulation, polyendocrinopathy, and enteropathy (IPEX) syndrome was described as because of mutations in FOXP3, resulting in nonfunctional $CD4^+CD25^+$ Treg cells.[26] The hallmark features of IPEX syndrome are enteropathy characterized by severe and refractory diarrhea; autoimmune endocrinopathies, which usually include early-onset insulin-dependent diabetes mellitus, thyroiditis, or both; hemolytic anemia; thrombocytopenia as autoimmune manifestations and chronic dermatitis; and elevated IgE levels as allergic manifestations.[28] Similar genotypes do not always accompany similar phenotypes in terms of disease presentation and severity, and FOXP3 expression does not correlate with disease severity.[29]

The role of immune suppressive function of $CD4^+CD25^+FOXP3^+$ Treg cells in allergic diseases has been described during the last decade.[30] In acute atopic dermatitis lesions, impaired skin infiltration of $CD4^+CD25^+FOXP3^+$ Treg cells is observed.[31] There are also higher frequencies of circulating $CD4^+CD25^+FOXP3^+$ Treg cells, which correlate with atopic dermatitis severity and peripheral blood eosinophil counts.[32,33] During bronchoalveolar lavage, $CD4^+FOXP3^+$ Treg cells are increased in patients with moderate to severe asthma compared with those with mild asthma and controls.[34] After systemic glucocorticoid treatment, there is an increase in the frequency of $CD25^+$ memory $CD4^+$ T cells and FOXP3 messenger RNA expression by $CD4^+$ T cells.[35] During pollen season, there is a decrease in the allergen-specific suppressive capacity of $CD4^+CD25^+$ Treg cells in cell cultures obtained from patients with hay fever.[36] In murine models, transfer of $CD4^+CD25^+FOXP3^+$ Treg cells suppresses the house dust mite–induced allergic airway inflammation in an IL-10–independent way.[37] The recruitment of $FOXP3^+$ Treg cells in local draining lymph nodes of the lung is associated with spontaneous resolution of chronic asthma. In a mouse model of antigen-induced lung inflammation, $CD4^+CD25^+$ Treg cells promote migration of mast cell progenitors to the lungs.[38]

Two subtypes of $CD25^{high}$ T cells were defined because of the differential expression of the chemokine receptor CCR6. In contrast to regulatory activities, the activated $CD25^{high}$ T cells that lack the expression of CCR6 enhance T_H2 responses.[39] There is an increase in $CD4^+CD25^{high}$ T cells in the peripheral blood of allergic children after pollen exposure.[40] However, in patients with severe refractory asthma, the baseline $CD4^+CD25^{+high}$ Treg cells in the peripheral blood are low compared with healthy subjects. During exacerbations, both in blood and in situ, there is further decrease in the number and function of $CD4^+CD25^{+high}$ Treg cells with a decrease in IL-10 gene expression.[41] The number of allergen-specific $CD4^+CD25^{high}FOXP3^+$ Treg cells does not show any difference between atopic and nonatopic subjects.[42] $CD4^+CD25^{high}CD127^{low}$ Treg cells have been included in the recovery of allergic inflammation. It was shown that in allergic asthma, $CD4^+$ invariant natural killer T cells selectively killed $CD4^+CD25^{high}CD127^{low}$ Treg cells in cocultures, and this cytotoxicity was positively correlated with asthma severity.[43] In allergic diseases, the function of Treg cells depends on the concentration and type of the eliciting agent, with different thresholds for individual allergens and patients with different genetic and immunologic backgrounds.[44] In addition, the stage of the disease, such as acute or chronic; remission or exacerbation; and affected tissue versus peripheral blood analysis show substantial differences. Furthermore, analysis methods and the type of antibody used have caused discrepancies in the previous findings.

Repeated exposure of nonallergic beekeepers to bee venom antigens during the beekeeping season provides a suitable model to understand the mechanisms of T-cell tolerance induction in healthy immune response. On bee venom exposure, an immediate switch of allergen-specific T cells from T_H1 and T_H2 cells to IL-10–secreting Tr1 cells occurs. This leads to diminished T-cell–related cutaneous late-phase responses in parallel to decreased allergen-specific T-cell proliferation and T_H1 and T_H2 cytokine secretion. At the end of the beekeeping season, peripheral T-cell response returns to baseline level within 2 to 3 months.[23] Another role of $CD4^+CD25^+$ Treg cells in a healthy immune response to allergens has been demonstrated in cow's milk allergy. Children with cow's milk allergy who became tolerant had increased number of circulating $CD4^+CD25^+$ T cells and decreased in vitro proliferative responses to bovine β-lactoglobulin in PBMCs compared with children who still had clinically active allergy.[45]

In patients with persistent allergic rhinitis, allergen-specific IL-10–secreting type 1 Treg cells are decreased in the peripheral blood, but the number and function of $CD4^+CD25^+$ Treg cells are not impaired.[46] When $CD4^+$ inducible Treg cells are transferred to cockroach-sensitized and -challenged mice, the cells differentiated to IL-10–producing $CD4^+$ type 1 cells in the lung and reversed airway hyperresponsiveness and airway inflammation via TGF-β, IL-10, interferon γ (IFN-γ), and cell surface receptor programmed death-1.[47]

ROLE OF IL-10 AND TGF-β IN ALLERGEN TOLERANCE

IL-10 and TGF-β, the suppressive cytokines of T-cell proliferation and cytokine production, are necessary in peripheral tolerance to allergens, autoantigens, transplantation antigens, and tumor antigens.[30,48–50] Transfer of ovalbumin (OVA) peptide–specific $CD4^+CD25^+$ T cells to OVA-sensitized mice resulted in an IL-10–dependent decrease in airway hyperreactivity, recruitment of eosinophils, and T_H2 cytokines to airways after allergen challenge. After transfer of $CD4^+CD25^+$ T cells, increased lung expression of IL-10 was detected and regulation was reversed by anti–IL-10R antibody.[51] IL-10 directly affects APC functions by downregulating the expression of major histocompatibility complex class II and costimulatory molecules on the surface of macrophages and monocytes.[30] IL-10 inhibits the expression of a large number of proinflammatory cytokines and chemokines and many chemokine receptors.[52] In addition to these indirect effects, IL-10 directly affects T-cell activation through suppression of CD28, CD2, and

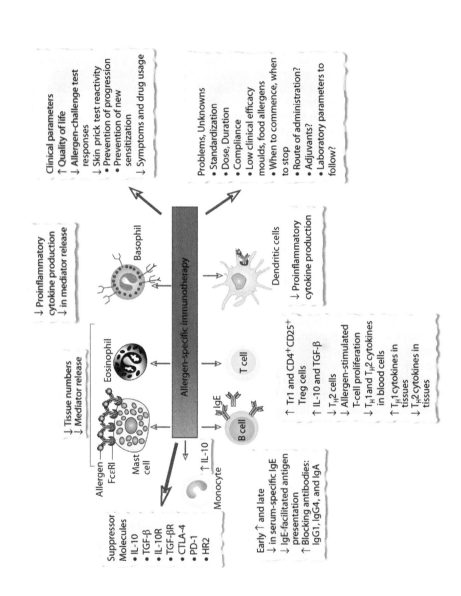

inducible T-cell costimulator signaling via Src homology 2 domain–containing protein tyrosine phosphatase-1.[53] IL-10 suppresses the production of allergen-specific and total IgE and increases the level of IgG4, resulting in a decrease in allergic inflammation.[49] The cells that produce IL-10 also include dendritic cells[54] and B cells.[55] There is a 2-sided interaction between Treg cells and IL-10. The differentiation of Tr1 cells by tolerogenic dendritic cells necessitates the IL-10–dependent immunoglobulin-like transcript 4/human leukocyte antigen-G pathway.[56]

TGF-β superfamily has many immunoregulatory functions that are important for angiogenesis, cancer,[57] and wound healing.[58] TGF-β induces FOXP3 expression, leading to the conversion of naive $CD4^+CD25^-$ T cells into $CD4^+CD25^+$ T cells.[59] TGF-β signaling is, also, required for in vivo expansion and immunosuppressive capacity of $CD4^+CD25^+$ T cells.[60] TGF-β not only contributes to the differentiation of suppressive Treg cells but also is involved in the differentiation of inflammatory T_H17 cells through SMAD2 receptor.[61] TGF-β induces the expression of some other molecules involving runt-related transcription factors 1 and 3, which are associated with the development and suppressive functions of $FOXP3^+$ inducible Treg cells.[62] The role of TGF-β in the pathogenesis of asthma, particularly in airway remodeling and fibrosis, has been emphasized.[63] TGF-β1 induces epithelial-mesenchymal transition in primary airway epithelial cells. However, the number of cells undergoing epithelial-mesenchymal transition is higher in airway epithelial cultures from patients with asthma.[64] Administration of anti–TGF-β antibody or neutralizing TGF-β through SMAD3 significantly reduces peribronchial fibrosis, airway smooth muscle proliferation, and mucus production, but the intensity of accompanying airway inflammation does not change.[65,66] The extracellular TGF-β released from airway epithelial cells stimulates autocrine synthesis of collagen-I,[67] whereas TGF-β decreases the production of enzymes such as collagenase.[68] Furthermore, in cytotoxic T lymphocytes and natural killer cells, TGF-β is an antagonist of IFN-γ production and cytolytic activity. In addition, TGF-β has a negative regulator effect on B-cell proliferation and differentiation[69] and on most immunoglobulins, except mucosal IgA, which is increased.[70] Coexpression of TGF-β1 and IL-10 permitted Treg cells to completely suppress airway hyperreactivity in a mouse model of asthma.[71]

ALLERGEN-SIT AND TREG CELLS

Allergen-SIT results in the generation of allergen-specific Treg cells and suppressive cytokines.[72–74] There is no well-defined distinction between the subsets of Treg cells in humans in whom $CD4^+CD25^+$ Treg cells and IL-10- and TGF-β–secreting Tr1 cells represent overlapping populations in the circulation.[75]

Changes in the frequencies of antigen-specific T cells with a loss of IL-4–producing T cells and acquisition of IL-10–producing $CD4^+CD25^+$ T cells are associated with allergen-SIT.[76,77] There is increase in local $FOXP3^+CD25^+$ T cells in the nasal mucosa,

◀ ───

Fig. 1. Clinical and immunologic effects of allergen-SIT. Allergen-SIT induces the development of Treg cells and suppressive cytokines IL-10 and transforming growth factor β; decreases tissue numbers and mediator release of mast cells and eosinophils; increases IgG4 and decreases IgE; and decreases proinflammatory cytokine production of dendritic cells. Clinically, allergen-SIT decreases symptoms and medication use and prevents the development of new allergic sensitizations. There are still some problems and still unknowns about allergen-SIT; standardization of allergens, optimal dose and duration of allergen-SIT, most efficient and convenient route of administration, laboratory parameters (predictors) to decide to start, optimum time to stop and follow the efficacy. CTLA-4, cytotoxic T-lymphocyte antigen 4; HR2, heptad repeat 2; PD-1, programmed death-1.

which correlates with the clinical efficacy after pollen immunotherapy.[78] When PBMCs were stimulated with Der p 2 after 1 year of immunotherapy with house dust mite, IL-10–secreting CD4+CD25+ Treg cells increased more than the control group together with downregulation of nuclear factor κB expression.[79] In OVA-sensitized mice with asthma, the depletion of CD4+CD25+ T cells hampers tolerance induction.[80] Immunotherapy might lead to differential induction of Treg cells. At the end of the SIT induction phase, increased number of IL-10–secreting Tr1 cells has been shown followed by a reduced ratio of allergen-specific T$_H$2/IFN-γ+ T$_H$1 cells by 1 year.[81] The differential T-cell activation and regulatory patterns induced by SIT depend on the severity of the underlying allergic sensitization. The increment in natural and acquired Treg cells develops earlier and reaches higher levels in less severe subjects.[82] CD8+CD25+FOXP3+ Treg cells expressing IL-10 also increased in response to house dust mite SIT in patients with asthma (**Fig. 2**).[83] Grass pollen immunotherapy increased the expression of mucosal and peripheral T-cell IL-10[84] and TGF-β.[85] Similarly, peptide-based immunotherapies were also able to induce peripheral T-cell tolerance by decreasing the systemic T$_H$1 and T$_H$2 cell response to allergens via induction of Treg cells.[86–88] Venom peptide (phospholipase A$_2$) immunotherapy increased the production of IL-10 and transcription of the suppressor of cytokine signaling (*Socs*) 3 gene in mild honey bee allergy.[89]

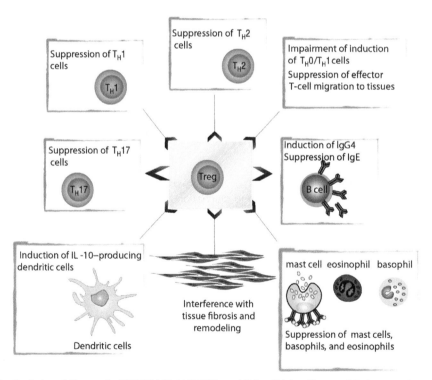

Fig. 2. Roles of Treg cells (FOXP3+CD4+CD25+ and Tr1 cells) in allergen-SIT. Suppression of T$_H$1, T$_H$2, and T$_H$17 cells; induction of IL-10–producing dendritic cells; suppression of mast cells, basophils, and eosinophils; interference with tissue fibrosis and remodeling; suppression of allergen-specific IgE; and induction of IgG4 and/or IgA.

ALLERGEN-SIT AND SPECIFIC ANTIBODY RESPONSE

In some of the nonatopic healthy individuals, there is no detectable antibody response or is low. However, in high dose of allergen exposure, relatively high amounts of specific IgG4 and specific IgG1 and IgA have been observed in response to allergen with no or low specific IgE response.[90] Although low amounts of antigen exposure might lead to immunologic ignorance resulting in no antibody response in mice,[91] very low dose (eg, a single bee sting) is sufficient to induce IgE and/or IgG production against phospholipase A_2 in humans.[92]

Activation of the complement cascade is an important feature of IgG subclass of immunoglobulins except IgG4. IgG4 fails to fix complement and binds only FcγRII and FcγRIII weakly, but it does not induce immune complex formation.[93] It is a dynamic molecule with a continuous exchange of heavy and light chains, referred as Fab-arm exchange. This exchange enables the expression of 2 different antigen-binding sites on a single IgG4 molecule. The increase in systemic IgG4 levels indicates that antiinflammatory, tolerance-inducing mechanisms have been activated and are associated with a decrease in allergic symptoms.[94,95] Nonallergic beekeepers have approximately 1000 times high ratio of specific IgG4 to specific IgE compared with allergic individuals.[96] There is a positive correlation between bee venom–specific IgG4 and the number of annual stings and years spent in beekeeping. Nearly half of the beekeepers who were stung less than 25 times a year had a history of systemic allergic reactions to bee venom, compared with no allergy in those with more than 200 stings per year.[92] However, there are controversial data in other forms of sensitizations. In a longitudinal study, after high exposure to cats, 2 groups of individuals were observed: 1 group developing high IgG responses to cat allergen without sensitization and wheeze and the other group with sensitization, IgG, and respiratory symptoms.[97] The degree of exposure to the allergen might affect the sensitization. In an adult population, the prevalence of sensitization to cat was significantly decreased in the lowest and highest cat-exposed groups.[98]

During allergen-SIT, IL-10 production occurs early with low doses of allergen at 2 to 4 weeks, but the increase in serum allergen-specific IgG4, IgA, and IgE occurs later at 6 to 12 weeks, which takes place at higher allergen doses leading to inhibition of early skin responses.[99] IgG4 suppresses IgE-mediated degranulation of mast cells and basophils, antigen presentation by direct allergen competition, and inhibitory FcγRIIb IgG receptors and mediates inhibition of basophil activation by FcγRIIa and IgG FcγRIIb receptors. It also reduces the number of allergen-specific memory B cells that have undergone class switching to IgE.[100–104] There is a transient increase in serum-specific IgE, followed by gradual decrease over months or years of treatment.[105,106] The seasonal increase in IgE decreases after the buildup phase of allergoid immunotherapy.[107] The increase in antigen-specific IgG4 is more than the increase in IgE; therefore, the ratio of specific IgE to IgG4 significantly decreases from 6 months to 3 years.[106] In predicting the clinical response, higher pretreatment ratio of allergen-specific IgE to total IgE is associated with an effective clinical response at the end of the SIT period.[108] Allergen-SIT also induces a serum-blocking activity, presumed to be because of allergen-specific IgG that blocks the formation of allergen-IgE complexes and binding to CD23[+] B cells, which results in the inhibition of IgE-facilitated allergen presentation to T cells.[84]

Other antibody classes might also contribute to clinical efficacy of SIT. The increase in TGF-β observed during house dust mite SIT is associated with a significant increase in specific IgA to Der p 1.[22] The IgA response to allergen-SIT is selective for IgA2. It correlates with increased nasal mucosal TGF-β expression and enhanced monocyte IL-10 expression.[85]

Both allergen-specific IL-10–secreting Tr1 cells and $CD4^+CD25^+$ Treg cells from healthy individuals induce IgG4 and suppress IgE production in the PBMCs and purified B-cell cultures of humans. This effect is particularly because of IL-10 production by these cells.[109] In contrast, IgA production is independent of T-cell help, and the role of Tr1 or Treg cells is limited, whereas it was highly induced by direct B-cell activation via toll-like receptor (TLR)7 and TLR9.

These data suggest that Treg cells may contribute to the suppression of allergic diseases by suppression of IgE and induction of IgG4, whereas IgA production is enhanced by B-cell activation via TLR7 and TLR9.

ALLERGEN-SIT AND MAST CELLS, EOSINOPHILS, AND BASOPHILS AS EFFECTOR CELLS

Allergen-SIT efficiently modulates the thresholds for mast cell and basophil activation and decreases IgE-mediated histamine release. Long-term venom immunotherapy resulted in a continuous decrease in serum mast cell tryptase concentration over time, which might involve a decrease in the function or number of mast cells.[110] Treg cells directly inhibit the $Fc\gamma RI$-dependent mast cell degranulation through cell-cell contact involving OX40-OX40L interactions between Treg cells and mast cells, respectively. Activated mast cells show increased cyclic adenosine monophosphate concentrations and reduced Ca^{++} influx in the presence of Treg cells. The in vivo depletion or inactivation of Treg cells causes enhancement of the anaphylactic response.[111] Loss of interaction between mast cells and Treg cells may contribute to more severe allergic reactions.

Allergen-SIT has been associated with a decrease in the influx of activated eosinophils and activated $CD4^+$ T cells into target tissues after allergen stimulation. Decreased number and activation of circulating basophils have also been observed after allergen-SIT.[112–114] Inhibition of seasonal increases in both nasal mast cells and eosinophils, which correlates with symptomatic improvement because of the reduced local expression of IL-5 and IL-9.[115,116] IL-10 downregulates eosinophil function and activity and suppresses IL-5 production by human resting T_H0 and T_H2 cells.[117] During SIT, reduced plasma levels of eosinophil cationic protein and chemotactic factors for eosinophils and neutrophils correlated with decreased bronchial hyperreactivity.[118] Allergen-SIT also prevented seasonal rises in the number of cells expressing eotaxin and regulated on activation, normal T-expressed, and presumably secreted (RANTES).[119]

Effects of allergen-SIT on dendritic cells have also been identified. In allergic patients, human blood dendritic cells have impaired IFN-α production by CpG stimulation through TLR9. During maintenance phase, allergen-SIT leads to increase in concentrations of IFN-α in response to CpG in PBMC, suggesting the contribution of allergen-SIT in dendritic cell TLR9-mediated innate immune function.[120] The T-cell immunoglobulin and mucin domain (TIM)4 molecule, expressed by dendritic cells, is the natural ligand of TIM1. Dendritic cell–derived TIM4 can bind TIM1 on $CD4^+$ T cells and drive them to develop into T_H2 cells. Allergen-SIT suppresses TIM4 expression in dendritic cells of patients with allergic rhinitis, resulting in suppression of T_H2 responses. In addition, interaction of antigen-specific IgG and $Fc\gamma RII$ downregulates TIM4 production by dendritic cells.[120]

Long-term allergen-SIT is associated with the reduction of not only the immediate response to allergen provocation but also the late-phase reaction in the nasal and bronchial mucosa or in the skin. The mechanism of late-phase reaction involves the recruitment, activation and persistence of eosinophils, and activated T cells at the sites of allergen exposure. Successful allergen-SIT is concerned with decreased responses to nonspecific stimulation so that bronchial, nasal, and conjunctival hyper-reactivities to nonspecific stimuli, which seems to reflect the underlying mucosal inflammation, decrease after allergen-SIT and correlate with clinical improvement.[121]

SUMMARY

Different types of Treg cells, the naturally occurring, thymic-selected $CD4^+CD25^+FOXP3^+$ Treg cells[122] and the inducible type 1 Treg cells,[23,123] control diverse steps of inflammation in various diseases[124,125] and allergen-specific immune response via suppression of APCs[126]; inhibition of the development of T_H2, T_H1, and T_H17 responses[123,127,128]; suppression of allergen-specific IgE and induction IgG_4 and IgA^{109}; suppression of mast cells, basophils, and eosinophils[111]; interference with tissue fibrosis and remodelling[129]; and impairment of induction of T_H0/T_H1 cells (see **Fig. 2**).[130]

Peripheral tolerance to allergens induced by allergen-SIT involves control of allergen-specific immune response in multiple steps, which are being investigated for the achievement of safer approaches and more efficient ways of allergen-SIT. In addition, targeting of T cells through allergen-specific therapy leads to modification of the balance between T_H1, T_H2, and Treg cells. Better understanding of all these mechanisms will provide a basis for the development of novel therapeutic and also prophylactic modalities in the future.

REFERENCES

1. Galli SJ, Tsai M, Piliponsky AM. The development of allergic inflammation. Nature 2008;454(7203):445–54.
2. Larche M, Akdis CA, Valenta R. Immunological mechanisms of allergen-specific immunotherapy. Nat Rev Immunol 2006;6(10):761–71.
3. Akdis M, Akdis CA. Mechanisms of allergen-specific immunotherapy. J Allergy Clin Immunol 2007;119(4):780–91.
4. Jutel M, Akdis M, Akdis CA. Histamine, histamine receptors and their role in immune pathology. Clin Exp Allergy 2009;39(12):1786–800.
5. Akdis CA, Jutel M, Akdis M. Regulatory effects of histamine and histamine receptor expression in human allergic immune responses. Chem Immunol Allergy 2008;94:67–82.
6. Akdis M, Burgler S, Crameri R, et al. Interleukins from 1 to 37 and interferon-gamma. J Allergy Clin Immunol 2011;127:701–21, e70.
7. Robinson DS, Larche M, Durham SR. Tregs and allergic disease. J Clin Invest 2004;114(10):1389–97.
8. Akdis CA. Allergy and hypersensitivity: mechanisms of allergic disease. Curr Opin Immunol 2006;18(6):718–26.
9. Akdis M, Verhagen J, Taylor A, et al. Immune responses in healthy and allergic individuals are characterized by a fine balance between allergen-specific T regulatory 1 and T helper 2 cells. J Exp Med 2004;199(11):1567–75.
10. Louten J, Boniface K, de Waal Malefyt R. Development and function of TH17 cells in health and disease. J Allergy Clin Immunol 2009;123(5):1004–11.
11. Akdis M. The cellular orchestra in skin allergy; are differences to lung and nose relevant? Curr Opin Allergy Clin Immunol 2010;10(5):443–51.
12. Burgler S, Ouaked N, Bassin C, et al. Differentiation and functional analysis of human T(H)17 cells. J Allergy Clin Immunol 2009;123(3):588–95, e581–7.

13. Akdis CA. T cells in health and disease. J Allergy Clin Immunol 2009;123(5): 1022–3.

14. Bousquet J, Bachert C, Canonica GW, et al. Unmet needs in severe chronic upper airway disease (SCUAD). J Allergy Clin Immunol 2009;124(3):428–33.

15. Zielen S, Kardos P, Madonini E. Steroid-sparing effects with allergen-specific immunotherapy in children with asthma: a randomized controlled trial. J Allergy Clin Immunol 2010;126(5):942–9.

16. Palomares O, Yaman G, Azkur AK, et al. Role of Treg in immune regulation of allergic diseases. Eur J Immunol 2010;40(5):1232–40.

17. Akdis M, Akdis CA. Therapeutic manipulation of immune tolerance in allergic disease. Nat Rev Drug Discov 2009;8(8):645–60.

18. Akdis CA, Akdis M. Mechanisms of allergen-specific immunotherapy. J Allergy Clin Immunol 2011;127:18–27.

19. Akdis M. Immune tolerance in allergy. Curr Opin Immunol 2009;21(6):700–7.

20. Ozdemir C, Akdis M, Akdis CA. T regulatory cells and their counterparts: masters of immune regulation. Clin Exp Allergy 2009;39(5):626–39.

21. Akdis CA. New insights into mechanisms of immunoregulation in 2007. J Allergy Clin Immunol 2008;122(4):700–9.

22. Jutel M, Akdis M, Budak F, et al. IL-10 and TGF-beta cooperate in the regulatory T cell response to mucosal allergens in normal immunity and specific immuno-therapy. Eur J Immunol 2003;33(5):1205–14.

23. Meiler F, Zumkehr J, Klunker S, et al. In vivo switch to IL-10-secreting T regula-tory cells in high dose allergen exposure. J Exp Med 2008;205(12):2887–98.

24. Ling EM, Smith T, Nguyen XD, et al. Relation of CD4+CD25+ regulatory T-cell suppression of allergen-driven T-cell activation to atopic status and expression of allergic disease. Lancet 2004;363(9409):608–15.

25. Hori S, Nomura T, Sakaguchi S. Control of regulatory T cell development by the transcription factor Foxp3. Science 2003;299(5609):1057–61.

26. Bennett CL, Christie J, Ramsdell F, et al. The immune dysregulation, polyendoc-rinopathy, enteropathy, X-linked syndrome (IPEX) is caused by mutations of FOXP3. Nat Genet 2001;27(1):20–1.

27. Siegmund K, Ruckert B, Ouaked N, et al. Unique phenotype of human tonsillar and in vitro-induced FOXP3+CD8+ T cells. J Immunol 2009;182(4):2124–30.

28. Wildin RS, Smyk-Pearson S, Filipovich AH. Clinical and molecular features of the immunodysregulation, polyendocrinopathy, enteropathy, X linked (IPEX) syndrome. J Med Genet 2002;39(8):537–45.

29. Gambineri E, Perroni L, Passerini L, et al. Clinical and molecular profile of a new series of patients with immune dysregulation, polyendocrinopathy, enteropathy, X-linked syndrome: inconsistent correlation between Forkhead box protein 3 expression and disease severity. J Allergy Clin Immunol 2008;122(6):1105–12 e1.

30. Akdis CA, Akdis M. Mechanisms and treatment of allergic disease in the big picture of regulatory T cells. J Allergy Clin Immunol 2009;123(4):735–46 [quiz: 747–8].

31. Verhagen J, Akdis M, Traidl-Hoffmann C, et al. Absence of T-regulatory cell expression and function in atopic dermatitis skin. J Allergy Clin Immunol 2006;117(1):176–83.

32. Ito Y, Adachi Y, Makino T, et al. Expansion of FOXP3-positive CD4+CD25+ T cells associated with disease activity in atopic dermatitis. Ann Allergy Asthma Immunol 2009;103(2):160–5.

33. Zimmermann M, Koreck A, Meyer N, et al. TWEAK and TNF-alpha cooperate in the induction of keratinocyte apoptosis. J Allergy Clin Immunol 2011;127:200–7, e1–10.

34. Smyth LJ, Eustace A, Kolsum U, et al. Increased airway T regulatory cells in asthmatic subjects. Chest 2010;138(4):905–12.

35. Karagiannidis C, Akdis M, Holopainen P, et al. Glucocorticoids upregulate FOXP3 expression and regulatory T cells in asthma. J Allergy Clin Immunol 2004;114(6):1425–33.

36. Anderson AE, Mackerness KJ, Aizen M, et al. Seasonal changes in suppressive capacity of CD4+ CD25+ T cells from patients with hayfever are allergen-specific and may result in part from expansion of effector T cells among the CD25+ population. Clin Exp Allergy 2009;39(11):1693–9.

37. Leech MD, Benson RA, De Vries A, et al. Resolution of Der p1-induced allergic airway inflammation is dependent on CD4+CD25+Foxp3+ regulatory cells. J Immunol 2007;179(10):7050–8.

38. Jones TG, Finkelman FD, Austen KF, et al. T regulatory cells control antigen-induced recruitment of mast cell progenitors to the lungs of C57BL/6 mice. J Immunol 2010;185(3):1804–11.

39. Reefer AJ, Satinover SM, Solga MD, et al. Analysis of CD25hiCD4+ "regulatory" T-cell subtypes in atopic dermatitis reveals a novel T(H)2-like population. J Allergy Clin Immunol 2008;121(2):415–22, e3.

40. Jartti T, Burmeister KA, Seroogy CM, et al. Association between CD4(+) CD25(high) T cells and atopy in children. J Allergy Clin Immunol 2007; 120(1):177–83.

41. Mamessier E, Nieves A, Lorec AM, et al. T-cell activation during exacerbations: a longitudinal study in refractory asthma. Allergy 2008;63(9):1202–10.

42. Maggi L, Santarlasci V, Liotta F, et al. Demonstration of circulating allergen-specific CD4+CD25highFoxp3+ T-regulatory cells in both nonatopic and atopic individuals. J Allergy Clin Immunol 2007;120(2):429–36.

43. Nguyen KD, Vanichsarn C, Nadeau KC. Increased cytotoxicity of CD4+ invariant NKT cells against CD4+CD25hiCD127lo/- regulatory T cells in allergic asthma. Eur J Immunol 2008;38(7):2034–45.

44. Bellinghausen I, Konig B, Bottcher I, et al. Regulatory activity of human CD4 CD25 T cells depends on allergen concentration, type of allergen and atopy status of the donor. Immunology 2005;116(1):103–11.

45. Karlsson MR, Rugtveit J, Brandtzaeg P. Allergen-responsive CD4+CD25+ regulatory T cells in children who have outgrown cow's milk allergy. J Exp Med 2004;199(12):1679–88.

46. Han D, Wang C, Lou W, et al. Allergen-specific IL-10-secreting type I T regulatory cells, but not CD4(+)CD25(+)Foxp3(+) T cells, are decreased in peripheral blood of patients with persistent allergic rhinitis. Clin Immunol 2010;136(2): 292–301.

47. McGee HS, Agrawal DK. Naturally occurring and inducible T-regulatory cells modulating immune response in allergic asthma. Am J Respir Crit Care Med 2009;180(3):211–25.

48. O'Garra A, Barrat FJ, Castro AG, et al. Strategies for use of IL-10 or its antagonists in human disease. Immunol Rev 2008;223:114–31.

49. Akdis CA, Blesken T, Akdis M, et al. Role of interleukin 10 in specific immunotherapy. J Clin Invest 1998;102(1):98–106.

50. Ozdemir C, Akdis M, Akdis CA. Nature of regulatory T cells in the context of allergic disease. Allergy Asthma Clin Immunol 2008;4(3):106–10.

51. Kearley J, Barker JE, Robinson DS, et al. Resolution of airway inflammation and hyperreactivity after in vivo transfer of CD4+CD25+ regulatory T cells is interleukin 10 dependent. J Exp Med 2005;202(11):1539–47.

52. De Waal Malefyt R, Abrams J, Bennett B, et al. Interleukin 10 (IL-10) inhibits cytokine synthesis by human monocytes: an autoregulatory role of IL-10 produced by monocytes. J Exp Med 1991;174:1209–20.

53. Taylor A, Akdis M, Joss A, et al. IL-10 inhibits CD28 and ICOS costimulations of T cells via src homology 2 domain-containing protein tyrosine phosphatase 1. J Allergy Clin Immunol 2007;120(1):76–83.

54. Le T, Tversky J, Chichester KL, et al. Interferons modulate Fc epsilon RI-dependent production of autoregulatory IL-10 by circulating human monocytoid dendritic cells. J Allergy Clin Immunol 2009;123(1):217–23.

55. Amu S, Saunders SP, Kronenberg M, et al. Regulatory B cells prevent and reverse allergic airway inflammation via FoxP3-positive T regulatory cells in a murine model. J Allergy Clin Immunol 2010;125(5):1114–24, e1118.

56. Gregori S, Tomasoni D, Pacciani V, et al. Differentiation of type 1 T regulatory cells (Tr1) by tolerogenic DC-10 requires the IL-10-dependent ILT4/HLA-G pathway. Blood 2010;116(6):935–44.

57. Cunha SI, Pardali E, Thorikay M, et al. Genetic and pharmacological targeting of activin receptor-like kinase 1 impairs tumor growth and angiogenesis. J Exp Med 2010;207(1):85–100.

58. Shephard P, Martin G, Smola-Hess S, et al. Myofibroblast differentiation is induced in keratinocyte-fibroblast co-cultures and is antagonistically regulated by endogenous transforming growth factor-beta and interleukin-1. Am J Pathol 2004;164(6):2055–66.

59. Chen W, Jin W, Hardegen N, et al. Conversion of peripheral CD4+CD25-naive T cells to CD4+CD25+ regulatory T cells by TGF-beta induction of transcription factor Foxp3. J Exp Med 2003;198(12):1875–86.

60. Huber S, Schramm C, Lehr HA, et al. Cutting edge: TGF-beta signaling is required for the in vivo expansion and immunosuppressive capacity of regulatory CD4+CD25+ T cells. J Immunol 2004;173(11):6526–31.

61. Malhotra N, Robertson E, Kang J. SMAD2 is essential for TGF beta-mediated Th17 cell generation. J Biol Chem 2010;285(38):29044–8.

62. Klunker S, Chong MM, Mantel PY, et al. Transcription factors RUNX1 and RUNX3 in the induction and suppressive function of Foxp3+ inducible regulatory T cells. J Exp Med 2009;206(12):2701–15.

63. Broide DH. Immunologic and inflammatory mechanisms that drive asthma progression to remodeling. J Allergy Clin Immunol 2008;121(3):560–70 [quiz: 571–2].

64. Hackett TL, Warner SM, Stefanowicz D, et al. Induction of epithelial-mesenchymal transition in primary airway epithelial cells from patients with asthma by transforming growth factor-beta1. Am J Respir Crit Care Med 2009;180(2):122–33.

65. Le AV, Cho JY, Miller M, et al. Inhibition of allergen-induced airway remodeling in Smad 3-deficient mice. J Immunol 2007;178(11):7310–6.

66. McMillan SJ, Xanthou G, Lloyd CM. Manipulation of allergen-induced airway re-modeling by treatment with anti-TGF-beta antibody: effect on the Smad signaling pathway. J Immunol 2005;174(9):5774–80.

67. Coutts A, Chen G, Stephens N, et al. Release of biologically active TGF-beta from airway smooth muscle cells induces autocrine synthesis of collagen. Am J Physiol Lung Cell Mol Physiol 2001;280(5):L999–1008.

68. Wynn TA. Common and unique mechanisms regulate fibrosis in various fibroproliferative diseases. J Clin Invest 2007;117(3):524–9.

69. Lebman DA, Edmiston JS. The role of TGF-beta in growth, differentiation, and maturation of B lymphocytes. Microbes Infect 1999;1(15):1297–304.

70. Borsutzky S, Cazac BB, Roes J, et al. TGF-beta receptor signaling is critical for mucosal IgA responses. J Immunol 2004;173(5):3305–9.
71. Presser K, Schwinge D, Wegmann M, et al. Coexpression of TGF-beta1 and IL-10 enables regulatory T cells to completely suppress airway hyperreactivity. J Immunol 2008;181(11):7751–8.
72. Akdis CA, Akdis M, Blesken T, et al. Epitope-specific T cell tolerance to phospholipase A2 in bee venom immunotherapy and recovery by IL-2 and IL-15 in vitro. J Clin Invest 1996;98(7):1676–83.
73. Jutel M, Akdis CA. T-cell regulatory mechanisms in specific immunotherapy. Chem Immunol Allergy 2008;94:158–77.
74. Akdis M. T-cell tolerance to inhaled allergens: mechanisms and therapeutic approaches. Expert Opin Biol Ther 2008;8(6):769–77.
75. Akdis M, Blaser K, Akdis CA. T regulatory cells in allergy: novel concepts in the pathogenesis, prevention, and treatment of allergic diseases. J Allergy Clin Immunol 2005;116(5):961–8 [quiz: 969].
76. Aslam A, Chan H, Warrell DA, et al. Tracking antigen-specific T-cells during clinical tolerance induction in humans. PLoS One 2010;5(6):e11028.
77. Pereira-Santos MC, Baptista AP, Melo A, et al. Expansion of circulating Foxp3+) D25bright CD4+ T cells during specific venom immunotherapy. Clin Exp Allergy 2008;38(2):291–7.
78. Radulovic S, Jacobson MR, Durham SR, et al. Grass pollen immunotherapy induces Foxp3-expressing CD4+ CD25+ cells in the nasal mucosa. J Allergy Clin Immunol 2008;121(6):1467–72, e1461.
79. Tsai YG, Chiou YL, Chien JW, et al. Induction of IL-10+ CD4+ CD25+ regulatory T cells with decreased NF-kappaB expression during immunotherapy. Pediatr Allergy Immunol 2009;21(1 Pt 2):e166–73.
80. Boudousquie C, Pellaton C, Barbier N, et al. CD4+CD25+ T cell depletion impairs tolerance induction in a murine model of asthma. Clin Exp Allergy 2009;39(9):1415–26.
81. Mobs C, Slotosch C, Loffler H, et al. Birch pollen immunotherapy leads to differential induction of regulatory T cells and delayed helper T cell immune deviation. J Immunol 2010;184(4):2194–203.
82. Mamessier E, Birnbaum J, Dupuy P, et al. Ultra-rush venom immunotherapy induces differential T cell activation and regulatory patterns according to the severity of allergy. Clin Exp Allergy 2006;36(6):704–13.
83. Tsai YG, Yang KD, Niu DM, et al. TLR2 agonists enhance CD8+Foxp3+ regulatory T cells and suppress Th2 immune responses during allergen immunotherapy. J Immunol 2010;184(12):7229–37.
84. Nouri-Aria KT, Wachholz PA, Francis JN, et al. Grass pollen immunotherapy induces mucosal and peripheral IL-10 responses and blocking IgG activity. J Immunol 2004;172(5):3252–9.
85. Pilette C, Nouri-Aria KT, Jacobson MR, et al. Grass pollen immunotherapy induces an allergen-specific IgA2 antibody response associated with mucosal TGF-beta expression. J Immunol 2007;178(7):4658–66.
86. Muller U, Akdis CA, Fricker M, et al. Successful immunotherapy with T-cell epitope peptides of bee venom phospholipase A2 induces specific T-cell anergy in patients allergic to bee venom. J Allergy Clin Immunol 1998;101(6 Pt 1):747–54.
87. Haselden BM, Kay AB, Larche M. Immunoglobulin E-independent major histocompatibility complex-restricted T cell peptide epitope-induced late asthmatic reactions. J Exp Med 1999;189(12):1885–94.

88. Oldfield WL, Larche M, Kay AB. Effect of T-cell peptides derived from Fel d 1 on allergic reactions and cytokine production in patients sensitive to cats: a randomised controlled trial. Lancet 2002;360(9326):47–53.

89. Tarzi M, Klunker S, Texier C, et al. Induction of interleukin-10 and suppressor of cytokine signalling-3 gene expression following peptide immunotherapy. Clin Exp Allergy 2006;36(4):465–74.

90. Pereira EA, Silva DA, Cunha-Junior JP, et al. IgE, IgG1, and IgG4 antibody responses to Blomia tropicalis in atopic patients. Allergy 2005;60(3):401–6.

91. Zinkernagel RM, Ehl S, Aichele P, et al. Antigen localisation regulates immune responses in a dose- and time-dependent fashion: a geographical view of immune reactivity. Immunol Rev 1997;156:199–209.

92. Bilo BM, Rueff F, Mosbech H, et al. Diagnosis of Hymenoptera venom allergy. Allergy 2005;60(11):1339–49.

93. Schroeder HW Jr, Cavacini L. Structure and function of immunoglobulins. J Allergy Clin Immunol 2010;125(2 Suppl 2):S41–52.

94. Aalberse RC, Stapel SO, Schuurman J, et al. Immunoglobulin G4: an odd antibody. Clin Exp Allergy 2009;39(4):469–77.

95. Uermosi C, Beerli RR, Bauer M, et al. Mechanisms of allergen-specific desensitization. J Allergy Clin Immunol 2010;126(2):375–83.

96. Carballido JM, Carballido-Perrig N, Kagi MK, et al. T cell epitope specificity in human allergic and nonallergic subjects to bee venom phospholipase A2. J Immunol 1993;150(8 Pt 1):3582–91.

97. Lau S, Illi S, Platts-Mills TA, et al. Longitudinal study on the relationship between cat allergen and endotoxin exposure, sensitization, cat-specific IgG and development of asthma in childhood—report of the German Multicentre Allergy Study (MAS 90). Allergy 2005;60(6):766–73.

98. Custovic A, Hallam CL, Simpson BM, et al. Decreased prevalence of sensitization to cats with high exposure to cat allergen. J Allergy Clin Immunol 2001; 108(4):537–9.

99. Francis JN, James LK, Paraskevopoulos G, et al. Grass pollen immunotherapy: IL-10 induction and suppression of late responses precedes IgG4 inhibitory antibody activity. J Allergy Clin Immunol 2008;121(5):1120–5, e1122.

100. Mothes N, Heinzkill M, Drachenberg KJ, et al. Allergen-specific immunotherapy with a monophosphoryl lipid A-adjuvanted vaccine: reduced seasonally boosted immunoglobulin E production and inhibition of basophil histamine release by therapy-induced blocking antibodies. Clin Exp Allergy 2003;33(9):1198–208.

101. Wachholz PA, Soni NK, Till SJ, et al. Inhibition of allergen-IgE binding to B cells by IgG antibodies after grass pollen immunotherapy. J Allergy Clin Immunol 2003;112(5):915–22.

102. Kepley CL, Taghavi S, Mackay G, et al. Co-aggregation of FcgammaRII with FcepsilonRI on human mast cells inhibits antigen-induced secretion and involves SHIP-Grb2-Dok complexes. J Biol Chem 2004;279(34):35139–49.

103. Cady CT, Powell MS, Harbeck RJ, et al. IgG antibodies produced during subcutaneous allergen immunotherapy mediate inhibition of basophil activation via a mechanism involving both FcgammaRIIA and FcgammaRIIB. Immunol Lett 2010;130(1-2):57–65.

104. Achatz G, Nitschke L, Lamers MC. Effect of transmembrane and cytoplasmic domains of IgE on the IgE response. Science 1997;276(5311):409–11.

105. Van Ree R, Van Leeuwen WA, Dieges PH, et al. Measurement of IgE antibodies against purified grass pollen allergens (Lol p 1, 2, 3 and 5) during immunotherapy. Clin Exp Allergy 1997;27(1):68–74.

106. Gleich GJ, Zimmermann EM, Henderson LL, et al. Effect of immunotherapy on immunoglobulin E and immunoglobulin G antibodies to ragweed antigens: a six-year prospective study. J Allergy Clin Immunol 1982;70(4):261–71.
107. Keskin O, Tuncer A, Adalioglu G, et al. The effects of grass pollen allergoid immunotherapy on clinical and immunological parameters in children with allergic rhinitis. Pediatr Allergy Immunol 2006;17(6):396–407.
108. Di Lorenzo G, Mansueto P, Pacor ML, et al. Evaluation of serum s-IgE/total IgE ratio in predicting clinical response to allergen-specific immunotherapy. J Allergy Clin Immunol 2009;123(5):1103–10, e1101–4.
109. Meiler F, Klunker S, Zimmermann M, et al. Distinct regulation of IgE, IgG4 and IgA by T regulatory cells and toll-like receptors. Allergy 2008;63(11): 1455–63.
110. Dugas-Breit S, Przybilla B, Dugas M, et al. Serum concentration of baseline mast cell tryptase: evidence for a decline during long-term immunotherapy for Hymenoptera venom allergy. Clin Exp Allergy 2010;40(4):643–9.
111. Gri G, Piconese S, Frossi B, et al. CD4+CD25+ regulatory T cells suppress mast cell degranulation and allergic responses through OX40-OX40L interaction. Immunity 2008;29(5):771–81.
112. Durham SR, Ying S, Varney VA, et al. Grass pollen immunotherapy inhibits allergen-induced infiltration of CD4+ T lymphocytes and eosinophils in the nasal mucosa and increases the number of cells expressing messenger RNA for interferon-gamma. J Allergy Clin Immunol 1996;97(6):1356–65.
113. Wilson DR, Irani AM, Walker SM, et al. Grass pollen immunotherapy inhibits seasonal increases in basophils and eosinophils in the nasal epithelium. Clin Exp Allergy 2001;31(11):1705–13.
114. Wurtzen PA, Lund G, Lund K, et al. A double-blind placebo-controlled birch allergy vaccination study II: correlation between inhibition of IgE binding, histamine release and facilitated allergen presentation. Clin Exp Allergy 2008;38(8): 1290–301.
115. Nouri-Aria KT, Pilette C, Jacobson MR, et al. IL-9 and c-Kit+ mast cells in allergic rhinitis during seasonal allergen exposure: effect of immunotherapy. J Allergy Clin Immunol 2005;116(1):73–9.
116. Wilson DR, Nouri-Aria KT, Walker SM, et al. Grass pollen immunotherapy: symptomatic improvement correlates with reductions in eosinophils and IL-5 mRNA expression in the nasal mucosa during the pollen season. J Allergy Clin Immunol 2001;107(6):971–6.
117. Schandene L, Alonso-Vega C, Willems F, et al. B7/CD28-dependent IL-5 production by human resting T cells is inhibited by IL-10. J Immunol 1994; 152(9):4368–74.
118. Rak S, Hakanson L, Venge P. Immunotherapy abrogates the generation of eosinophil and neutrophil chemotactic activity during pollen season. J Allergy Clin Immunol 1990;86(5):706–13.
119. Plewako H, Holmberg K, Oancea I, et al. A follow-up study of immunotherapy-treated birch-allergic patients: effect on the expression of chemokines in the nasal mucosa. Clin Exp Allergy 2008;38(7):1124–31.
120. Zhao CQ, Li TL, He SH, et al. Specific immunotherapy suppresses Th2 responses via modulating TIM1/TIM4 interaction on dendritic cells. Allergy 2010;65(8):986–95.
121. Rak S, Lowhagen O, Venge P. The effect of immunotherapy on bronchial hyper-responsiveness and eosinophil cationic protein in pollen-allergic patients. J Allergy Clin Immunol 1988;82(3 Pt 1):470–80.

122. Wing K, Larsson P, Sandstrom K, et al. CD4+ CD25+ FOXP3+ regulatory T cells from human thymus and cord blood suppress antigen-specific T cell responses. Immunology 2005;115(4):516–25.

123. Cottrez F, Hurst SD, Coffman RL, et al. T regulatory cells 1 inhibit a Th2-specific response in vivo. J Immunol 2000;165(9):4848–53.

124. Chen Y, Kuchroo VK, Inobe J, et al. Regulatory T cell clones induced by oral tolerance: suppression of autoimmune encephalomyelitis. Science 1994;265(5176): 1237–40.

125. Clark RA, Huang SJ, Murphy GF, et al. Human squamous cell carcinomas evade the immune response by down-regulation of vascular E-selectin and recruitment of regulatory T cells. J Exp Med 2008;205(10):2221–34.

126. Lewkowich IP, Herman NS, Schleifer KW, et al. CD4+CD25+ T cells protect against experimentally induced asthma and alter pulmonary dendritic cell phenotype and function. J Exp Med 2005;202(11):1549–61.

127. Bellinghausen I, Konig B, Bottcher I, et al. Inhibition of human allergic T-helper type 2 immune responses by induced regulatory T cells requires the combination of interleukin-10-treated dendritic cells and transforming growth factor-beta for their induction. Clin Exp Allergy 2006;36(12):1546–55.

128. Jaffar Z, Ferrini ME, Girtsman TA, et al. Antigen-specific Treg regulate Th17-mediated lung neutrophilic inflammation, B-cell recruitment and polymeric IgA and IgM levels in the airways. Eur J Immunol 2009;39(12):3307–14.

129. Kitani A, Fuss I, Nakamura K, et al. Transforming growth factor (TGF)-beta1-producing regulatory T cells induce Smad-mediated interleukin 10 secretion that facilitates coordinated immunoregulatory activity and amelioration of TGF-beta1-mediated fibrosis. J Exp Med 2003;198(8):1179–88.

130. Trautmann A, Schmid-Grendelmeier P, Kruger K, et al. T cells and eosinophils cooperate in the induction of bronchial epithelial cell apoptosis in asthma. J Allergy Clin Immunol 2002;109(2):329–37.

Mechanisms of Sublingual Immunotherapy

Guy Scadding, MRCP[a,b,*], Stephen R. Durham, MD[a,b]

KEYWORDS

• Sublingual • Immunotherapy • SLIT • Mechanisms • IgG4

The efficacy of sublingual immunotherapy (SLIT) in the treatment of allergic airways disease, particularly seasonal pollen-induced rhinitis, is now well established.[1,2] Applications of SLIT, at least in clinical trial settings, have been extended to include treatment of food allergy and latex allergy.[3–5] SLIT is convenient for patients and seems safe,[6] providing advantages over classic subcutaneous immunotherapy (SCIT), although head-to-head trials are awaited.

The exact mechanisms by which SLIT exerts its effects have yet to be resolved. These mechanisms are likely to overlap considerably with those of SCIT, yet discrepancies exist, particularly concerning the magnitude of systemic immunologic changes. Moreover, these mechanistic effects do not necessarily correlate with clinical efficacy.

SLIT may exploit the naturally protolerogenic milieu of the oral mucosa (a site exposed to numerous innocuous food proteins on a daily basis) but it is not clear to what extent the oral environment is distinct from the rest of the gastrointestinal tract with regards to immune responses. Much progress has been made in elucidating the early interactions between allergen, antigen-presenting cells, and T cells, but the precise cell types involved are unknown.

Strong evidence exists for effects on allergen-specific IgE and IgG levels (similar to those seen with SCIT) but these changes correlate best with allergen dose, rather than clinical efficacy. As for SCIT, researchers have also looked for evidence of reprogramming of T-cell responses, particularly the induction of regulatory T cells, after SLIT.

No conflicts of interest to disclose.

Stephen Durham has received lecture fees and payments for consultancies from ALK Abello, a manufacturer of allergy vaccines, and research grants from ALK Abello via Imperial College London.

[a] Department of Allergy and Clinical Immunology, Imperial College, Exhibition Road, London SW7 2AZ, UK

[b] Allergy Department, Royal Brompton Hospital, 4th Floor, Fulham Road Building, Sydney Street, London SW3 6NP, UK

* Corresponding author. Allergy Department, Royal Brompton Hospital, 4th Floor, Fulham Road Building, Sydney Street, London SW3 6NP, UK.

E-mail address: g.scadding@ic.ac.uk

However, despite much progress, satisfactory biomarkers of the efficacy of SLIT have still to be established. Recent data[7,8] have confirmed long-lasting, tolerogenic effects of SLIT, the immunologic correlates of which require further study. The use of adjuvants to enhance the efficacy of SLIT, and potentially reduce the high allergen doses required, has also been an area of interest.[9–11]

This article considers the possible mechanisms of SLIT, beginning with the processes involved within the oral mucosa. There follows an evaluation of the major studies concerning downstream immunologic events, both locally and systemically. Areas of uncertainty are highlighted.

CURRENT PROPOSED MECHANISM OF SLIT

Fig. 1 illustrates a hypothetical model of the pathway of allergen and downstream effects of SLIT. In this model, allergen is taken up by submucosal dendritic cells (perhaps oral Langerhans cells), which then migrate to local regional lymphoid tissues, including submandibular and cervical lymph nodes. There, dendritic cells present peptide fragments to allergen-specific T cells in a protolerogenic manner, resulting in inhibition of activation and proli,feration of Th2 cells and stimulation of Th1 and/or regulatory T cells. Subsequently, these T cells influence B cells to produce protective antibody responses, including secretion of allergen-specific IgG4 and IgA, and, later, inhibition of IgE. Regulatory T cells may have further suppressive effects on other inflammatory cells, including eosinophils, mast cells, and basophils, either by cytokine secretion or direct cell-to-cell contact. Given the aggregation of antigen-presenting

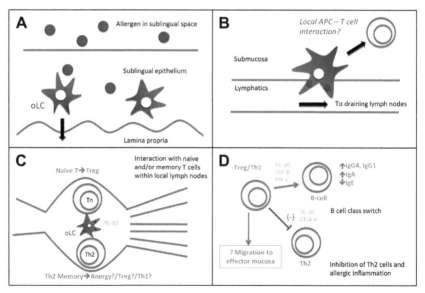

Fig. 1. Postulated mechanisms of sublingual immunotherapy. (*A*) Allergen up-take by dendritic cells, including oral Langerhans' cells, in the sublingual mucosa. (*B*) Dendritic cells transport allergen to regional lymph nodes and/or mucosal T-cell rich areas. (*C*) Within lymph nodes dendritic cells present allergen to T-cells in the context of protolerogenic signals, such as IL-10, leading to the induction of regulatory T cells and Th1 cells, and the inhibition of Th2 cells. (*D*) Regulatory T-cells and Th1-cells suppress Th2-mediated allergic inflammation and induce B cell class switch to IgG4, IgG1 and IgA. (*From* Scadding G, Durham S. Mechanisms of sublingual immunotherapy. J Asthma 2009;46(4):324; with permission.)

cells and lymphocytes in some areas of the oral mucosa itself,[12–14] the possibility of local allergen presentation, bypassing regional lymphoid tissues, is considered.

ALLERGEN UPTAKE AND PRESENTATION IN SLIT

Some years ago, a series of pharmacodynamic studies by Bagnasco and colleagues[15,16] explored the local and systemic distribution of allergen in vivo after application to the human sublingual region. Radiolabeled *Parietaria* allergen was tracked, by both local scintillography and plasma radioactivity, to identify the distribution of allergen after sublingual application, compared with oral (swallowed) allergen. Not only was allergen retained within the sublingual space for several hours, with little direct absorption into the circulation from the mouth (**Fig. 2**), but allergen could also be detected within the mucosa for 20 hours after dosing.

Further similar in vivo human research is lacking; however, several groups have used murine SLIT models and ex vivo human antigen-presenting cells (including those purified from the oral mucosa) to investigate local processes in more detail.[9–11,17–19] Immunostaining of tissue sections from the oral mucosa of mice treated sublingually with labeled ovalbumin has shown the passage of allergen across the epithelium and into the subepithelium over the course of 30 to 60 minutes.[19] At 60 minutes allergen seems to disappear from the submucosa, suggested by the investigators to coincide with uptake by dendritic cells. In a series of experiments, the same group showed allergen uptake, processing, and presentation to T cells in vitro, using dendritic cells purified from the oral mucosa. Furthermore, these dendritic cells appeared to have tolerogenic properties, being capable of inducing T cells secreting interleukin 10 (IL-10) and interferon γ (IFN-γ), and with the ability to suppress T-cell proliferation in vitro.

Previous studies using an ovalbumin-sensitized mouse model of asthma had reported improved efficacy of SLIT using allergen coupled to a mucoadhesive polysaccharide core.[9] Later, using the same SLIT model, the same investigators extracted

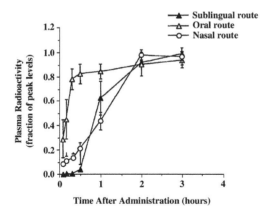

Fig. 2. Average plasma radioactivity curves (mean +/- SEM, normalized to peak levels) observed in three groups of healthy volunteers receiving ^{123}I-Par j 1 (radio-Iodine labelled *Parietaria judaica* major allergen) by sublingual, oral, and nasal routes. Sublingual administration results in negligible direct absorption into the blood stream until after swallowing at 30 minutes. (*From* Bagnasco M, Mariani G, Passalacqua G, et al. Absorption and distribution kinetics of the major *Parietaria judaica* allergen (Par j 1) administered by noninjectable routes in healthy human beings. J Allergy Clin Immunol 1997;100(1):125; with permission.)

allergen-specific T cells with regulatory properties from the cervical lymph nodes of treated mice.[19]

Further murine studies have identified CD11b+CD11c− monocytoid dendritic cells to be the most abundant antigen-presenting cell within the lingual immune system,[13] existing alongside both effector and suppressor CD4+ T cells. The duration of allergen-mucosal contact (longer being more efficacious) and the frequency of administration (more frequent being more efficacious) have been investigated during sublingual treatment in mice.[20,21] A study involving a mouse model of grass pollen-induced allergic rhinitis showed reduced airway inflammation after allergen challenge in sublingually treated animals, associated with impaired T-cell proliferative responses in cervical lymph nodes but not spleens, again suggesting the importance of the local immune response.[22]

Researchers have studied the use of several adjuvants in mouse SLIT models. High molecular weight, charged chitosan particles coupled to ovalbumin-enhanced allergen uptake and presentation in vitro, and had improved efficacy in vivo.[11] Use of certain strains of lactic acid bacteria concurrently with allergen may enhance Th1 and regulatory T-cell responses.[23] Ovalbumin SLIT along with a combination of dexamethasone and vitamin D_3 was also more effective than ovalbumin treatment alone.[10]

Sublingual ovalbumin coupled to cholera toxin subunit B[24,25] has been shown to enhance B-cell-dependent expansion of regulatory T cells and inhibition of effector T cells. The investigators suggest B lymphocytes may play an important role as antigen-presenting cells during tolerance induction by this route, facilitated by the presence of cholera toxin B subunit, which binds to GM1 ganglioside receptors, allowing efficient nonallergen-specific uptake. Similar results were also achieved using intragastric administration of allergen-cholera toxin B complexes.[26]

Studying the local pathway of allergen after sublingual application in human patients is more difficult. However, several studies have used human oral mucosal biopsies (either from fresh cadavers or during intraoral surgery) to investigate local immunologic tissues and the events after allergen application.[12,17,18,27] Oral Langerhans cells (the oral equivalent of the skin Langerhans cell, expressing CD1a and Langerhans cell-specific lectin/CD207) were identified as possible candidate antigen-presenting cells for SLIT, because of their expression of high amounts of major histocompatibility complex (MHC) class I and II, surface IgG receptors, and, most crucially, the high-affinity IgE receptor, FcεRI. Expression of this last receptor was found to be greatest in atopic individuals and to positively correlate with serum total IgE levels.[27] Further evidence suggests possible antiinflammatory effects of this receptor, with cross-linking of FcεRI on monocytes, resulting in the release of IL-10 and production of indoleamine 2,3-dioxygenase.[28,29]

Subsequently, purified oral Langerhans cells have been shown to produce IL-10 in vitro, a process augmented by coligation of toll-like receptor 4 with monophosphoryl lipid A.[17] Moreover, these cells could then induce T cells expressing the prototypic regulatory cell transcription factor Foxp3, and secreting IL-10, transforming growth factor β 1 (TGF-β1) and IFN-γ. These studies led to the hypothesis that allergen was taken up via IgE-FcεRI on the surface of oral Langerhans cells during SLIT in atopic individuals.

However, more recently the same investigators used biopsy material from the vestibular region of the mouth from a larger pool of patients undergoing oral surgery classified according to their atopic and grass pollen allergic status.[18] Using CD1a+ cells as a marker for oral Langerhans cells, these investigators studied allergen uptake and cell migration in an ex vivo model, using fluorescently labeled major grass pollen allergen, Phl p5. They were able to show both dose-dependent and time-dependent saturation kinetics of allergen uptake, as well as IL-10 and TGF-β release from both CD1a+ dendritic cells and cocultured T cells. Such dose-dependent allergen binding fits well with the observed allergen dose-dependency for efficacy in clinical SLIT studies (see later discussion). Moreover, these findings suggest a receptor-mediated allergen uptake process. However, there were no differences between tissues from atopic and nonatopic patients, casting some doubt over the relevance of IgE-FcεRI-mediated uptake. The investigators suggest possible alternative receptor-mediated uptake pathways, such as via IgG-Fcγ receptors or C-type lectins, or by micropinocytosis or macropinocytosis, the last supported by a previous in vitro study of dendritic cell uptake of the grass and birch allergens Phl p1 and Bet v1.[30]

The use of vestibular rather than sublingual mucosal tissue in the study outlined earlier was informed by a previous biopsy study of different regions within the oral cavity, with dendritic cell and mast cell distribution compared within the different regions and with skin tissue.[12] Immunostaining showed a greater concentration of CD1a+ dendritic cells in the oral vestibulum compared with the sublingual region (**Fig. 3**). Immune cells from distinct intraoral mucosal regions and the skin have since been compared in greater detail.[31] CD3+ cells were most abundant in the vestibulo-buccal region. This area, and to a lesser extent the sublingual area, were found to represent potentially protolerogenic environments, as shown by mRNA expression of TGF-β1, IL-10, and Foxp3, plus Th1 gene expression including IFN-γ and Tbet mRNA. These regions also expressed mRNA transcripts of several Th17-type cytokines, not seen in the skin. The relevance of this last finding is unclear.

Investigators have speculated that the oral mucosa has a degree of immune privilege.[32] As well as potentially tolerogenic antigen-presenting cells and T cells, the environment is further protected from inflammatory responses by high levels of secretory IgA, antimicrobial peptides in saliva, and the presence of commensal bacteria. All these factors may be important in facilitating tolerogenic responses to SLIT.

Significant evidence points towards a dominant role for the local mucosa and lymphoid tissues during SLIT. Oral antigen-presenting cells do seem to have natural protolerogenic properties, perhaps further enhanced by various adjuvants. The principal allergen-presenting cell may be the oral Langerhans cell, but other cell types are likely to be involved in addition. The mechanisms of allergen uptake (be they receptor-mediated, allergen-specific, or otherwise) require further confirmation.

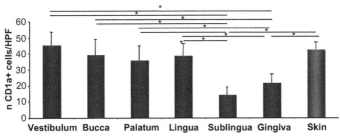

Fig. 3. Higher numbers of oral Langerhans' Cells (oLC) within the vestibulum, bucca, palatum, and lingua compared to sublingual and gingival regions of the oral mucosa. Oral mucosal tissues from different anatomical sites were stained with anti-CD1a antibody for oLC detection. n CD1a+ cells/HPF; mean number of CD1a-positive cells per high powered microscope field. *, $P<.05$. (*From* Allam JP, Stojanovski G, Friedrichs N, et al. Distribution of Langerhans' cells and mast cells within the human oral mucosa: new application sites of allergens in sublingual immunotherapy? Allergy 2008;63(6):725; with permission.)

Evidence does point toward a role for regional lymph glands, although this is largely derived from animal models for obvious reasons. Other areas of uncertainty remain, such as the importance of the tonsils, which have been shown to be rich in regulatory T cells,[14] and may potentially play an important role in SLIT. Moreover, it is perhaps premature to completely rule out a role for other, distal components of the gut immune system. Investigation of allergen uptake and dendritic cell function needs to be extended to the study of human sublingual/vestibular mucosal tissue obtained before and after SLIT in order to determine their relevance to tolerance induction in vivo in man.

DOWNSTREAM IMMUNOLOGIC EFFECTS OF SLIT

In considering the immunologic effects of effective SLIT, it seems prudent to first briefly consider the better-established effects of SCIT.[33,34] SCIT has been shown to have rapid desensitizing effects on mast cells and basophils, providing some protection from anaphylactic responses in days to weeks. Within weeks there is evidence of T-cell tolerance and the induction of regulatory T cells, including cells expressing IL-10 and TGF-β, as well as the prototypic regulatory cell transcription factor Foxp3. B-cell/antibody responses to SCIT appear later, with increases in specific IgG, and in particular IgG4, preceding a decrease in specific IgE that is evident only after 3 to 4 years of treatment [35] (itself usually seen to increase during early stages of treatment). Changes are seen at effector mucosae including reductions in mast cell and eosinophil numbers. In the next section, the evidence for analogous processes in SLIT is considered.

ANTIBODY EFFECTS OF SLIT

Allowing for a break with the proposed chronology of events, as outlined earlier for SCIT, most clinical studies have investigated the effect of SLIT on allergen-specific antibody levels. The observed changes do seem to reflect those of SCIT, albeit at a lower magnitude.

In large, randomized, placebo-controlled trials of grass pollen SLIT significant increases in IgG,[36] IgG4,[14,37] or IgE-blocking antibody[38] have been recorded, becoming significant versus placebo from about 8 weeks of treatment. Moreover, 2 of these studies have shown both dose-dependent increases in IgG/IgG4 and dose-dependent clinical efficacy, although not a direct correlation between antibody titers and clinical response (**Fig. 4**).[36,37]

Levels of specific IgG show a gradual, progressive increase during prolonged treatment with SLIT (**Fig. 5**),[7] whereas specific IgE levels initially increase during treatment, becoming significantly greater than placebo by 2 months, before decreasing to near baseline by about 20 months of treatment (**Fig. 6**).[38,39]

However, similar findings have not been universally reported by investigators. Several studies of house dust mite SLIT in particular, as well as other studies of SLIT with seasonal aeroallergens, have yielded few or no significant changes in specific antibody levels.[40–45] In some cases this finding has been concordant with an absence of significant clinical benefit as per primary outcome measures,[41,44] but in others there is discordance with clinical benefit in the absence of antibody effects.[42,43] A recent study of high-dose house dust mite SLIT[46] produced significant clinical benefit as well as notable T-cell and cytokine responses (discussed later), but produced little in the way of antibody responses, with the only significant finding being an increase specific IgG4 to Der p2 at 2 years of treatment.

These observations raise several questions: foremost, are antibody changes a prerequisite, functional component of successful SLIT or simply a bystander effect,

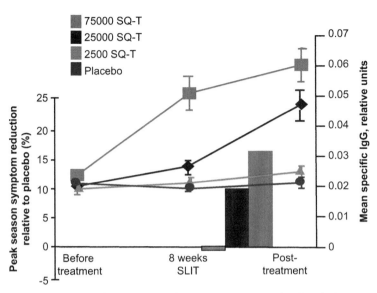

Fig. 4. Serum allergen-specific IgG and peak season symptom reduction during grass pollen SLIT are both dose-dependent. Vertical axis, left; mean peak season symptom reduction relative to placebo in low (2,500 SQ-T/day), medium (25,000 SQ-T/day), and high (75,000 SQ-T/day) dose grass pollen SLIT (histograms). Vertical axis, right; mean allergen-specific IgG in placebo, low, medium and high dose SLIT before, at 8 weeks, and after one year of treatment. (*Data from* Durham SR, Yang WH, Pederson MR, et al. Sublingual immunotherapy with once-daily grass allergen tablets: a randomized controlled trial in seasonal allergic rhinoconjunctivitis. J Allergy Clin Immunol 2006;117(4):806, 807.)

reflecting allergen dose only? Second, are there intrinsic differences between SLIT for house dust mite, a perennial allergen, and for seasonal aeroallergens such as grass pollen? Third, how sensitive are currently used tools such as symptom scores and diaries at measuring the clinical effects of SLIT, particularly in small studies in which allergen exposure between and within individuals is likely to be so variable?

Regarding the first question, there is increasing evidence for a functional role of the induced IgG antibodies. Using an in vitro correlate of B-cell allergen uptake and presentation (facilitated allergen binding [FAB] assay, discussed by Shamji and Durham in detail elsewhere in this issue), it was shown that serum from SLIT-treated patients could inhibit B-cell allergen binding via IgE-FcεRII.[14] The onset of this inhibition paralleled the increase in IgG4, which, in studies of SCIT,[47] has been shown to be the serum factor responsible for this inhibition. However, further work is needed, particularly concerning the possible inhibitory effect of these antibodies on mast cells and basophil activation, such as by assays of allergen-induced basophil activation/histamine release.

Grass pollen SLIT has also recently been shown to significantly increase serum allergen-specific IgA levels.[14,48] Similar changes have been seen after SCIT, and, furthermore, the IgA2 produced was able to induce monocyte IL-10 release in vitro, and positively correlated with nasal TGF-β expression, perhaps reflecting mucosal origin of these antibodies.[49] It is tempting to speculate that the IgA induced during SLIT may also have similar functional properties, although this has yet to be proved. Furthermore, one might hypothesize that changes in IgA may be at least as relevant in SLIT as in SCIT, given the mucosal administration of the former. If so, this finding may in part explain the

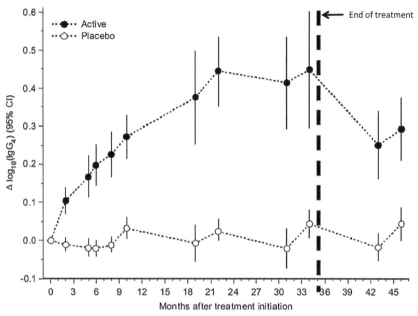

Fig. 5. Change in mean allergen-specific IgG4 level during, and for one season after discontinuation of, 3 years grass pollen SLIT in active and placebo-treated patients. (*From* Durham SR, Emminger W, Kapp A, et al. Long-term clinical efficacy in grass pollen-induced rhinoconjunctivitis after treatment with SQ-standardized grass allergy immunotherapy tablet. J Allergy Clin Immunol 2010;125(1):136; with permission.)

comparable clinical efficacy of the 2 treatment approaches despite the fact that SCIT induces approximately 5 times greater increases in specific IgG than SLIT.[38,47]

T-CELL AND CYTOKINE RESPONSES DURING SLIT

Data concerning the effects of SLIT on T-cell proliferation, cytokine secretion, and on the induction of putative regulatory T cells have been varied and at times conflicting. As with data concerning antibodies, this situation may be the result of different allergens, doses, and treatment regimens, but in addition, may also reflect the increased complexity and variability of the assays used by different researchers.

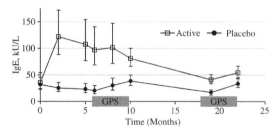

Fig. 6. Allergen-specific IgE levels during 2 years of grass pollen SLIT in active and placebo groups. GPS, grass pollen season. (*From* Dahl R, Kapp A, Colombo G, et al. Sublingual grass allergen tablet immunotherapy provides sustained clinical benefit with progressive immunologic changes over 2 years. J Allergy Clin Immunol 2008;121(2):516; with permission.)

T-cell Proliferation

A detailed account of immune responses during a year-long treatment with birch pollen SLIT was reported several years ago, but remains one of the most informative studies.[50] In vitro peripheral blood mononuclear cell (PBMC) proliferation to major birch pollen allergen Bet v1 was decreased at both 4 and 52 weeks of treatment. Inhibition at 4 weeks was reversible either by neutralizing IL-10 using a monoclonal antibody, or by depleting CD25+ cells. Neither approach had any effect at 52 weeks. These findings were accompanied by an increase in allergen-stimulated gene expression (mRNA level) of IL-10 at 4 weeks, and IFN-γ at 52 weeks.

A recent study of house dust mite immunotherapy reported a progressive inhibition of allergen-induced CD4+ cell proliferation over the course of 2 years.[46] In this case, blocking TGF-β in vitro reversed this inhibition at 6 months, but not significantly at other time points. Several other studies have looked at T-cell proliferative responses, both with[51,52] and without significant positive findings.[41,44]

Cytokine Secretion Profiles

A placebo-controlled trial of tree pollen immunotherapy in a pediatric cohort reported increased allergen-induced PBMC IL-10 mRNA in both high-dose and low-dose SLIT-treated patients at 1 and 2 years, although levels peaked at 1 rather than 2 years of treatment.[53] This finding was accompanied by suppression of IL-5 mRNA in the high-dose group at the same time points, and IL-5 levels were found to correlate with higher symptom scores (**Fig. 7**). The same group later published the finding of raised IL-18 mRNA (a Th1 cytokine) in the actively treated patients.[54]

The effects of 6 months of house dust mite SLIT on PBMC allergen-induced cytokine profiles differed according to the concentration of allergen used in vitro: 10 μg Der p1/mL induced significant IFN-γ release in SLIT-treated but not placebo-treated

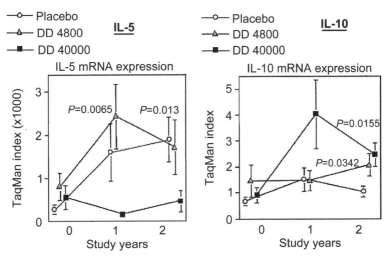

Fig. 7. In vitro allergen-induced IL-5 and IL-10 mRNA expression (real time PCR by TaqMan index) in peripheral blood mononuclear cells from children undergoing a 2 year trial of tree pollen SLIT including placebo, low dose (daily dose 4,800 SQ-U major allergen), and high dose (daily dose 40,000 SQ-U major allergen) treatment. (*Adapted from* Savolainen J, Jacobsen L, Valovirta E. Sublingual immunotherapy in children modulates allergen-induced in vitro expression of cytokine mRNA in PBMC. Allergy 2006; 61(10):1186–97; with permission.)

patients, whereas 0.4 μg Der p1/mL resulted in increased PBMC IL-10 release in the actively treated group.[55] O'Hehir and colleagues[46] reported a decrease in mite allergen-induced PBMC IL-5 secretion at 6 months, with a further decrease by 12 months. Levels at 1 year were less than a quarter of those in placebo-treated patients. Increased allergen-induced IL-10 release in SLIT-treated patients was also seen, but not until after 2 years of treatment.

Bohle and colleagues[50] reported an increase in IL-10 mRNA in allergen-stimulated T cells after only 4 weeks of birch pollen SLIT. However, by 1 year levels had returned to baseline. Conversely, allergen-stimulated IFN-γ gene expression was significantly increased at 1 year, by which point blocking IL-10 or removing CD25+ cells had no effect on allergen-driven T cell proliferation.

Regulatory T cells

Researchers have sought evidence for the generation of regulatory T cells during SLIT. As in SCIT, regulatory T cells may be an important source of antiinflammatory cytokine production, mediators of B-cell class switching, and inhibitors of Th2 cell activation and proliferation. Although in several animal models, particularly those using additional adjuvants, both Foxp3+ and Foxp3− putative regulatory T cells, with demonstrable in vitro effects, have been described,[10,11,19,25] such evidence has proved more elusive in human studies.

O'Hehir and colleagues[46] were able to isolate nondividing, CD25+ CD4+ Foxp3+ cells and show that these cells could inhibit proliferation of CD25− T cells in vitro. However, levels of these cells increased in both SLIT-treated and placebo-treated patients during the trial, without significant difference between the two. However, Bohle and colleagues[50] found no significant changes in T-cell Foxp3 gene expression, but did see trends towards an increase at 4 weeks and a decrease at 52 weeks.

In a recent Finnish study of tree pollen SLIT in children, allergen-induced Foxp3 mRNA levels in PBMC were increased and correlated positively with IL-10 mRNA at 1 and 2 years and with TGF-β mRNA at 1 year.[56] Although symptom scores were improved there was no correlation between Foxp3 gene expression and clinical outcomes.

Making firm conclusions on the effects of SLIT on T-cell responses from even the limited number of studies discussed earlier is not possible. An early IL-10-dependent, regulatory T-cell response, later progressing to a Th1-dominant, IFN-γ-secreting response, is suggested by some studies,[50,55] whereas a more gradual onset regulatory response, with either TGF-β-mediated Th2 suppression (as shown by decreased IL-5) and/or IL-10-mediated inhibition is supported elsewhere.[46,53,56] In addition, there are several other relevant publications in this field. Whereas some have revealed positive findings concerning cytokines such as increased IL-10,[57,58] increased IFN-γ[59] and decreased IL-13,[60] or inhibition of T-cell proliferation,[51,52,57] others have found no significant effects on cytokines and/or T-cell proliferation.[41,44] Discrepancies in laboratory techniques, allergen type and doses, study size, and presence/absence of control groups are all potential confounding factors here. This area warrants further study in larger, controlled trials.

LOCAL MUCOSAL EFFECTS OF SLIT

SCIT has been shown to reduce allergic inflammation at mucosal sites such as the nose and lung, including reductions in mast cell and eosinophil numbers.[61,62] More recently, phenotypic regulatory T cells have been identified in the nasal mucosa of SCIT-treated patients during natural seasonal pollen exposure.[63] These regulatory cells likely have direct antiinflammatory or tolerogenic effects within the target organ. Somewhat less is known regarding local mucosal effects of SLIT.

A placebo-controlled study of house dust mite SLIT used conjunctival allergen provocation tests as an outcome measure.[64] After 1 year of treatment, actively treated patients had fewer neutrophils and eosinophils in conjunctival fluid after allergen challenge compared with placebo-treated patients. The SLIT group also had lower serum eosinophil cationic protein levels at 1 year, as well as lower rhinoconjunctivitis symptom scores. Nasal allergen provocation tests after SLIT for *Parietaria* pollen-induced rhinitis also produced fewer inflammatory cells in nasal secretions of active versus placebo groups.[65] In an open study of birch pollen SLIT, the actively treated group had lower numbers of in-season nasal smear eosinophils as well as higher bronchial metacholine PD20 levels than matched patients treated with pharmacotherapy only.[66] Conversely, a study of house dust mite SLIT failed to detect differences in nasal smear eosinophils between baseline, 6-month, and 12-month recordings.[45]

Only a handful of studies have looked at the effect of SLIT on the oral mucosa during clinical treatment. Two small studies[67,68] investigated biopsy tissue from the sublingual region before and after treatment with grass pollen SLIT, including an individual with persistent local reactions to the allergen.[68] Low numbers of mast cells and eosinophils were found in the tissue, both before and after SLIT. However, the nature and time course of local adverse reactions to SLIT within the mouth is suggestive of mast cell degranulation and allergic inflammation. More recently, 2 larger studies have identified significant numbers of mast cells in sublingual and other regions of the oral mucosal,[12,14] likely in sufficient numbers to be responsible for these commonly seen clinical symptoms. These mild adverse events usually resolve within days to a couple of weeks of initiating treatment; whether this represents early desensitization of effector cells, as reported for SCIT, or simply the exhaustion of local inflammatory cells, is unclear.

Local sublingual Foxp3-expressing cells have been found to be significantly increased in grass pollen SLIT-treated patients compared with placebo.[14] Alongside other findings including antigen-presenting cell abundance, T-cell presence and anti-inflammatory cytokine gene expression,[12–14,31] this finding suggests that local mechanisms, with perhaps local interaction between antigen-presenting cells and T cells, may be relevant. It is uncertain whether regulatory T cells are induced locally within the mucosa or migrate there from regional lymphoid tissue. Similarly, unlike for SCIT, there is no firm evidence for the presence of regulatory T cells at other mucosal sites, such as the nose or lung, after SLIT.

TIME COURSE AND LONG-TERM EFFECTS OF SLIT

The clinical time course of onset of specific immunotherapy can be difficult to measure, especially when aeroallergen exposure can differ from season to season, day to day, and between individuals. A recent study made use of an artificial allergen exposure chamber to expose both grass pollen SLIT and placebo-treated patients to standardized levels of pollen before and then at regular intervals during the course of treatment.[69] Moreover, because the study was entirely conducted outside the pollen season, all other antiallergic medication could reasonably be discontinued to prevent interference.

SLIT-treated patients had significantly lower symptom scores during pollen exposure than placebo-treated patients from 4 weeks onwards; moreover, there was a trend towards a difference at just 1 week (**Fig. 8**).[69] Symptom scores showed progressive improvement to 2 months, with a further slight improvement at 4 months.

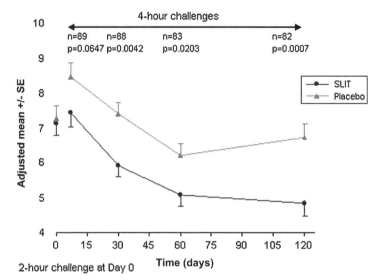

Fig. 8. Time course of effect of grass pollen SLIT versus placebo on symptom scores during exposure to grass pollen allergen within a challenge chamber. Participants were exposed to allergen within the challenge chamber for 2 hours at baseline, and then for 4 hours after one week, 4 weeks, 2 months and 4 months of SLIT or placebo. Average rhinoconjunctivitis total symptom scores (ARTSS, vertical axis) were calculated during the exposure periods. p-values represent difference between SLIT and placebo at each time point. (*From* Horak F, Zieglmayer P, Zieglmayer R, et al. Early onset of action of a 5-grass-pollen 300-IR sublingual immunotherapy tablet evaluated in an allergen challenge chamber. J Allergy Clin Immunol 2009;124(3):474; with permission.)

This latter finding is consistent with previous analyses, suggesting that preseasonal treatment of up to 16 weeks was optimal.[36,70]

There was also a progressive improvement in placebo-treated patients until 2 months, mirroring the large placebo effect seen in seasonal immunotherapy trials, or, alternatively, suggesting a degree of natural desensitization on recurrent exposure.

Regarding mechanisms, specific IgE and IgG levels increased during the 4-month treatment period in the SLIT group only, but no changes were seen in T-cell proliferation or basophil activation studies. Within the actively treated group, those with the greatest relative improvement in symptom scores from baseline to 4 months had greater increases in specific IgG compared with less responsive individuals.

Achieving long-lasting tolerance (clinically shown by symptomatic improvement even after discontinuation of treatment) is a major advantage of allergen immunotherapy compared with pharmacologic treatments. Tolerance is well established for SCIT for several different allergens.[71–73] Two randomized, placebo-controlled studies have confirmed a carry-over effect of grass pollen SLIT for at least 1 year after discontinuation, in both cases after either 3 years or 3 seasons of treatment.[7,8] In the study by Ott and colleagues[8] clinical improvement persisted during a fourth season despite specific IgG4 levels decreasing to baseline values. Specific IgE levels increased sharply in years 1 and 2 before gradually decreasing thereafter, but had not completely returned to baseline levels by year 4.[8] In the study of Durham and colleagues[7] changes in IgG4 were closely paralleled by serum IgE-blocking activity, and were still significantly greater than placebo a year after treatment discontinuation. One important difference between these 2 studies is the use of perennial treatment[7] versus coseasonal treatment only.[8] Although IgG4 levels seem to correlate with treatment and have in vitro blocking activity, an absolute increased level does not seem essential for continued efficacy.

Another study of interest here is a community-based trial of preseasonal and coseasonal grass pollen SLIT carried out in the United Kingdom.[73] After a baseline season, volunteers received either 2 years' placebo, 2 years' SLIT, or 1 year's SLIT followed by a second year of placebo. Both treatment groups showed increases in specific IgE and IgG4 at 1 year; however, a significant symptomatic improvement was seen only in the second year of the group receiving 2 years' SLIT. Specific IgG4 levels in the group receiving only 1 year of SLIT fell in the second year, but did not return completely to baseline levels.

An open study, including follow-up of SLIT-treated patients for up to 15 years, suggested the beneficial effect of house dust mite SLIT on clinical symptoms could persist for up to 7 years after a 3-year treatment.[74] This finding was accompanied by suppression of nasal eosinophils and bronchial hyperreactivity during the same period. In addition, SLIT-treated patients were relatively protected from developing new allergen sensitizations. This finding has been reported previously for SLIT,[75] along with the prevention of asthma development.[76] Such findings in open studies require confirmation in double-blind, placebo-controlled trials.

It remains to be conclusively shown for how long specific IgG changes persist after discontinuation of treatment, and whether this or any other biomarker is useful in reflecting the long-term clinical response. The exact relationship between allergen-specific IgG and IgE levels and clinical efficacy is likely to be more complex than simple quantitative values. For example, relative ratios of specific IgE/IgG may be more important, and, furthermore, the antibody affinity or avidity, rather than the absolute level, is likely to be relevant. Moreover, the persistence of a low titer of specific IgG with high allergen affinity may maintain tolerance even when total specific IgG levels decline. Studies looking at functional antibody assays for several years after treatment discontinuation are needed to assess these matters further.

AREAS OF UNCERTAINTY AND FUTURE STUDY

Although the oral Langerhans cell is an attractive candidate for the role of key antigen-presenting cell in SLIT, it is clear, at least from murine studies, that alternative antigen-presenting cells are also likely involved, including other monocyte-derived dendritic cells, macrophages, and potentially B cells.[19,25] Furthermore, the mechanism of allergen uptake by these cells is as yet uncertain. Further clinical studies using adjuvants are needed, particularly in view of their apparent success in murine models.[9–11,23–25] Grass pollen SLIT along with monophosphoryl lipid A, a toll-like receptor 4 agonist, has been shown to be safe in a proof-of-concept study,[77] but clinical and immunologic effects were modest. A suitable adjuvant would either increase the efficacy of current treatments, or allow maintained efficacy despite lower or less frequent allergen dosing.

The optimum site for allergen application is another area for future study. Trials are required to compare sublingual versus vestibular allergen application given the relative merits of these regions reported in investigational studies.[12,13] Tablet SLIT perhaps has benefits over drops by providing sustained contact in higher concentrations with the mucosa for longer. It remains to be determined if other mucoadhesive formulations can provide further benefit in clinical practice.

Whether the rest of the gastrointestinal tract and mucosal-associated lymphoid tissue plays any part in the mechanism of SLIT is unclear. Although SLIT is considered to exploit an immune mechanism distinct from classic oral tolerance induction there may be considerable overlap. Recent studies of oral tolerance induction to peanut[78,79] and the use of SLIT for hazelnut and the peach lipid transferase protein allergy[3,4] have shown efficacy and may possibly share common mechanisms. It remains to be seen whether either can provide true tolerance (ie, persistence of benefit after treatment discontinuation).

Use of modified recombinant allergens or peptide fragments for SLIT may in future provide safer treatments. Other possibilities to improve efficacy include combining SLIT with anti-IgE or anticytokine drugs, although cost currently makes this approach prohibitive for routine clinical use. The importance of tonsil and adenoidal tissue for sublingual tolerance also warrants further study, as does the role of allergen-specific IgA.

SUMMARY

On a systemic level, current evidence suggests SLIT shares many mechanistic properties in common with SCIT. Evidence points to similar, although less pronounced, effects on specific IgG, IgE, and IgA. Furthermore, IgG antibodies at least seem to be functional. Effects on the T-cell compartment are less certain, but a picture of regulatory and Th1 cell induction and Th2 inhibition is emerging.

Understanding of the local mucosal mechanisms is rapidly progressing, with evidence accumulating for a process involving local antigen-presenting cells as the crucial early mediators of SLIT. Further clarification here may allow for the development of better-targeted vaccines that might simplify, improve, and reduce the costs of treatment. Further such studies will determine whether or not SLIT may replace conventional SCIT as the mainstay of allergen-desensitization treatment.

ACKNOWLEDGMENTS

The authors are grateful to Dr Pablo Rodríguez del Río for the construction of **Fig. 4**.

REFERENCES

1. Wilson DR, Torres Lima M, Durham SR. Sublingual immunotherapy for allergic rhinitis: systematic review and meta-analysis. Allergy 2005;60:4–12.
2. Radulovic S, Calderon MA, Wilson D, et al. Sublingual immunotherapy for allergic rhinitis. Cochrane Database Syst Rev 2010;12:CD002893.
3. Enrique E, Pineda F, Malek T, et al. Sublingual immunotherapy for hazelnut food allergy: a randomized, double-blind, placebo-controlled study with a standardized hazelnut extract. J Allergy Clin Immunol 2005;116(5):1073–9.
4. Fernández-Rivas M, Garrido Fernández S, et al. Randomized double-blind, placebo-controlled trial of sublingual immunotherapy with a Pru p 3 quantified peach extract. Allergy 2009;64(6):876–83.
5. Nettis E, Colanardi MC, Soccio AL, et al. Double-blind, placebo-controlled study of sublingual immunotherapy in patients with latex-induced urticaria: a 12-month study. Br J Dermatol 2007;156(4):674–81.
6. Passalacqua G, Guerra L, Compalati E, et al. The safety of allergen specific sublingual immunotherapy. Curr Drug Saf 2007;2(2):117–23.
7. Durham SR, Emminger W, Kapp A, et al. Long-term clinical efficacy in grass pollen-induced rhinoconjunctivitis after treatment with SQ-standardized grass allergy immunotherapy tablet. J Allergy Clin Immunol 2010;125(1):131–8.

8. Ott H, Sieber J, Brehler R, et al. Efficacy of grass pollen sublingual immuno-therapy for three consecutive seasons and after cessation of treatment: the ECRIT study. Allergy 2009;64(9):1394–401.
9. Razafindratsita A, Saint-Lu N, Mascarell L, et al. Improvement of sublingual immunotherapy efficacy with a mucoadhesive allergen formulation. J Allergy Clin Immunol 2007;120(2):278–85.
10. Van Overtvelt L, Lombardi V, Razafindratsita A, et al. IL-10-inducing adjuvants enhance sublingual immunotherapy efficacy in a murine asthma model. Int Arch Allergy Immunol 2008;145(2):152–62.
11. Saint-Lu N, Tourdot S, Razafindratsita A, et al. Targeting the allergen to oral dendritic cells with mucoadhesive chitosan particles enhances tolerance induc-tion. Allergy 2009;64(7):1003–13.
12. Allam JP, Stojanovski G, Friedrichs N, et al. Distribution of Langerhans cells and mast cells within the human oral mucosa: new application sites of allergens in sublingual immunotherapy? Allergy 2008;63(6):720–7.
13. Mascarell L, Lombardi V, Zimmer A, et al. Mapping of the lingual immune system reveals the presence of both regulatory and effector CD4+ T cells. Clin Exp Allergy 2009;39(12):1910–9.
14. Scadding GW, Shamji MH, Jacobson MR, et al. Sublingual grass pollen immuno-therapy is associated with increases in sublingual Foxp3-expressing cells and elevated allergen-specific immunoglobulin G4, immunoglobulin A and serum inhibitory activity for immunoglobulin E-facilitated allergen binding to B cells. Clin Exp Allergy 2010;40(4):598–606.
15. Bagnasco M, Mariani G, Passalacqua G, et al. Absorption and distribution kinetics of the major *Parietaria judaica* allergen (Par j 1) administered by nonin-jectable routes in healthy human beings. J Allergy Clin Immunol 1997;100(1): 122–9.
16. Bagnasco M, Passalacqua G, Villa G, et al. Pharmacokinetics of an allergen and a monomeric allergoid for oromucosal immunotherapy in allergic volunteers. Clin Exp Allergy 2001;31(1):54–60.
17. Allam JP, Peng WM, Appel T, et al. Toll-like receptor 4 ligation enforces tolero-genic properties of oral mucosal Langerhans cells. J Allergy Clin Immunol 2008;121(2):368–74.
18. Allam JP, Würtzen PA, Reinartz M, et al. Phl p 5 resorption in human oral mucosa leads to dose-dependent and time-dependent allergen binding by oral mucosal Langerhans cells, attenuates their maturation, and enhances their migratory and TGF-beta1 and IL-10-producing properties. J Allergy Clin Immunol 2010;126(3): 638–45.
19. Mascarell L, Lombardi V, Louise A, et al. Oral dendritic cells mediate antigen-specific tolerance by stimulating TH1 and regulatory CD4+ T cells. J Allergy Clin Immunol 2008;122(3):603–9.
20. Kildsgaard J, Brimnes J, Jacobi H, et al. Sublingual immunotherapy in sensitized mice. Ann Allergy Asthma Immunol 2007;98(4):366–72.
21. Rask C, Brimnes J, Lund K. Shorter dosing intervals of sublingual immunotherapy lead to more efficacious treatment in a mouse model of allergic inflammation. Scand J Immunol 2010;71(6):403–12.
22. Brimnes J, Kildsgaard J, Jacobi H, et al. Sublingual immunotherapy reduces allergic symptoms in a mouse model of rhinitis. Clin Exp Allergy 2007;37(4): 488–97.
23. Van Overtvelt L, Moussu H, Horiot S, et al. Lactic acid bacteria as adjuvants for sublingual allergy vaccines. Vaccine 2010;28(17):2986–92.

24. Sun JB, Czerkinsky C, Holmgren J. Sublingual 'oral tolerance' induction with antigen conjugated to cholera toxin B subunit generates regulatory T cells that induce apoptosis and depletion of effector T cells. Scand J Immunol 2007;66(2-3):278–86.

25. Sun JB, Flach CF, Czerkinsky C, et al. B lymphocytes promote expansion of regulatory T cells in oral tolerance: powerful induction by antigen coupled to cholera toxin B subunit. J Immunol 2008;181(12):8278–87.

26. Sun JB, Raghavan S, Sjöling A, et al. Oral tolerance induction with antigen conjugated to cholera toxin B subunit generates both Foxp3+CD25+ and Foxp3-CD25- CD4+ regulatory T cells. J Immunol 2006;177(11):7634–44.

27. Allam JP, Novak N, Fuchs C, et al. Characterization of dendritic cells from human oral mucosa: a new Langerhans' cell type with high constitutive Fc-epsilon RI expression. J Allergy Clin Immunol 2003;112(1):141–8.

28. Novak N, Bieber T, Katoh N. Engagement of Fc epsilon RI on human monocytes induces the production of IL-10 and prevents their differentiation in dendritic cells. J Immunol 2001;167(2):797–804.

29. von Bubnoff D, Matz H, Frahnert C, et al. Fc-epsilonRI induces the tryptophan degradation pathway involved in regulating T cell responses. J Immunol 2002; 169(4):1810–6.

30. Noirey N, Rougier N, André C, et al. Langerhans-like dendritic cells generated from cord blood progenitors internalize pollen allergens by macropinocytosis, and part of the molecules are processed and can activate autologous naive T lymphocytes. J Allergy Clin Immunol 2000;105:1194–201.

31. Allam JP, Duan Y, Winter J, et al. Tolerogenic T cells, Th1/Th17 cytokines and TLR2/TLR4 expressing dendritic cells predominate the microenvironment within distinct oral mucosal sites. Allergy 2011;66(4):532–9.

32. Novak N, Haberstok J, Bieber T, et al. The immune privilege of the oral mucosa. Trends Mol Med 2008;14(5):191–8.

33. Akdis M, Akdis CA. Therapeutic manipulation of immune tolerance in allergic disease. Nat Rev Drug Discov 2009;8(8):645–60.

34. James LK, Durham SR. Update on mechanisms of allergen injection immunotherapy. Clin Exp Allergy 2008;38(7):1074–88.

35. Gleich GJ, Zimmermann EM, Henderson LL, et al. Effect of immunotherapy on immunoglobulin E and immunoglobulin G antibodies to ragweed antigens: a six-year prospective study. J Allergy Clin Immunol 1982;70(4):261–71.

36. Durham SR, Yang WH, Pederson MR, et al. Sublingual immunotherapy with once-daily grass allergen tablets: a randomized controlled trial in seasonal allergic rhinoconjunctivitis. J Allergy Clin Immunol 2006;117(4):802–9.

37. Didier A, Malling HJ, Worm M, et al. Optimal dose, efficacy, and safety of once-daily sublingual immunotherapy with a 5-grass pollen tablet for seasonal allergic rhinitis. J Allergy Clin Immunol 2007;120(6):1338–45.

38. Dahl R, Kapp A, Colombo G, et al. Sublingual grass allergen tablet immunotherapy provides sustained clinical benefit with progressive immunologic changes over 2 years. J Allergy Clin Immunol 2008;121(2):512–8.

39. Lima MT, Wilson D, Pitkin L, et al. Grass pollen sublingual immunotherapy for seasonal rhinoconjunctivitis: a randomized controlled trial. Clin Exp Allergy 2002;32(4):507–14.

40. Aberer W, Hawranek T, Reider N, et al. Immunoglobulin E and G antibody profiles to grass pollen allergens during a short course of sublingual immunotherapy. J Investig Allergol Clin Immunol 2007;17(3):131–6.

41. Rolinck-Werninghaus C, Kopp M, Liebke C, et al. Lack of detectable alterations in immune responses during sublingual immunotherapy in children seasonal

allergic rhinoconjunctivitis to grass pollen. Int Arch Allergy Immunol 2005;136(2): 134–41.

42. Pajno GB, Morabito L, Barberio G, et al. Clinical and immunologic effects of long-term sublingual immunotherapy in asthmatic children sensitized to mites: a double-blind, placebo-controlled study. Allergy 2000;55(9):842–9.

43. Tonnel AB, Scherpereel A, Douay B, et al. Allergic rhinitis due to house dust mites: evaluation of the efficacy of specific sublingual immunotherapy. Allergy 2004;59(5):491–7.

44. Dehlink E, Eiwegger T, Gerstmayr M, et al. Absence of systemic immunologic changes during dose build-up phase and early maintenance period in effective specific sublingual immunotherapy in children. Clin Exp Allergy 2006;36(1):32–9.

45. Bahceciler NN, Arikan C, Taylor A, et al. Impact of sublingual immunotherapy on specific antibody levels in asthmatic children allergic to house dust mites. Int Arch Allergy Immunol 2005;136(3):287–94.

46. O'Hehir RE, Gardner LM, de Leon MP, et al. House dust mite sublingual immuno-therapy: the role for transforming growth factor-beta and functional regulatory T cells. Am J Respir Crit Care Med 2009;180(10):936–47.

47. Nouri-Aria KT, Wachholz PA, Francis JN, et al. Grass pollen immunotherapy induces mucosal and peripheral IL-10 responses and blocking IgG activity. J Immunol 2004;172(5):3252–9.

48. Skoner D, Gentile D, Bush R, et al. Sublingual immunotherapy in patients with allergic rhinoconjunctivitis caused by ragweed pollen. J Allergy Clin Immunol 2010;125(3):660–6.

49. Pilette C, Nouri-Aria KT, Jacobson MR, et al. Grass pollen immunotherapy induces an allergen-specific IgA2 antibody response associated with mucosal TGF-β expression. J Immunol 2007;178:4658–66.

50. Bohle B, Kinaciyan T, Gerstmayr M, et al. Sublingual immunotherapy induces IL-10-producing T regulatory cells, allergen-specific T-cell tolerance, and immune deviation. J Allergy Clin Immunol 2007;120(3):707–13.

51. Fanta C, Bohle B, Hirt W, et al. Systemic immunological changes induced by administration of grass pollen allergens via the oral mucosa during sublingual immunotherapy. Int Arch Allergy Immunol 1999;120(3):218–24.

52. Fenoglio D, Puppo F, Cirillo I, et al. Sublingual specific immunotherapy reduces PBMC proliferations. Eur Ann Allergy Clin Immunol 2005;37(4):147–51.

53. Savolainen J, Jacobsen L, Valovirta E. Sublingual immunotherapy in children modulates allergen-induced in vitro expression of cytokine mRNA in PBMC. Allergy 2006;61(10):1184–90.

54. Savolainen J, Nieminen K, Laaksonen K, et al. Allergen-induced in vitro expression of IL-18, SLAM and GATA-3 mRNA in PBMC during sublingual immuno-therapy. Allergy 2007;62(8):949–53.

55. Cosmi L, Santarlasci V, Angeli R, et al. Sublingual immunotherapy with Dermato-phagoides monomeric allergoid down-regulates allergen-specific immunoglob-ulin E and increases both interferon-gamma- and interleukin-10-production. Clin Exp Allergy 2006;36(3):261–72.

56. Nieminen K, Valovirta E, Savolainen J. Clinical outcome and IL-17, IL-23, IL-27 and FOXP3 expression in peripheral blood mononuclear cells of pollen-allergic children during sublingual immunotherapy. Pediatr Allergy Immunol 2010;21(1 Pt 2):e174–84.

57. Ciprandi G, Fenoglio D, Cirillo I, et al. Induction of interleukin 10 by sublingual immunotherapy for house dust mites: a preliminary report. Ann Allergy Asthma Immunol 2005;95(1):38–44.

58. Ciprandi G, Cirillo I, Fenoglio D, et al. Sublingual immunotherapy induces spiro-metric improvement associated with IL-10 production: preliminary reports. Int Immunopharmacol 2006;6(8):1370–3.

59. Arikan C, Bahceciler NN, Deniz G, et al. Bacillus Calmette-Guérin-induced interleukin-12 did not additionally improve clinical and immunologic parameters in asthmatic children treated with sublingual immunotherapy. Clin Exp Allergy 2004;34(3):398–405.

60. Ippoliti F, De Santis W, Volterrani A, et al. Immunomodulation during sublingual therapy in allergic children. Pediatr Allergy Immunol 2003;14(3):216–21.

61. Wilson DR, Irani AM, Walker SM, et al. Grass pollen immunotherapy inhibits seasonal increases in basophils and eosinophils in the nasal epithelium. Clin Exp Allergy 2001;31:1705–13.

62. Durham SR, Ying S, Varney VA, et al. Grass pollen immunotherapy inhibits allergen-induced infiltration of CD4+ T lymphocytes and eosinophils in the nasal mucosa and increases the number of cells expressing messenger RNA for inter-feron-gamma. J Allergy Clin Immunol 1996;97(6):1356–65.

63. Radulovic S, Jacobson MR, Durham SR, et al. Grass pollen immunotherapy induces Foxp3-expressing CD4+ CD25+ cells in the nasal mucosa. J Allergy Clin Immunol 2008;121(6):1467–72.

64. Passalacqua G, Albano M, Fregonese L, et al. Randomised controlled trial of local allergoid immunotherapy on allergic inflammation in mite-induced rhinocon-junctivitis. Lancet 1998;351(9103):629–32.

65. Passalacqua G, Albano M, Riccio A, et al. Clinical and immunologic effects of a rush sublingual immunotherapy to *Parietaria* species: a double-blind, placebo-controlled trial. J Allergy Clin Immunol 1999;104(5):964–8.

66. Marogna M, Spadolini I, Massolo A, et al. Clinical, functional, and immunologic effects of sublingual immunotherapy in birch pollinosis: a 3-year randomized controlled study. J Allergy Clin Immunol 2005;115(6):1184–8.

67. Marcucci F, Incorvaia C, Sensi L, et al. Lack of inflammatory cells in the oral mucosa of subjects undergoing sublingual immunotherapy. Int J Immunopathol Pharmacol 2008;21(3):609–13.

68. Marcucci F, Sensi L, Incorvaia C, et al. Oral reactions to sublingual immuno-therapy: a bioptic study. Allergy 2007;62(12):1475–7.

69. Horak F, Zieglmayer P, Zieglmayer R, et al. Early onset of action of a 5-grass-pollen 300-IR sublingual immunotherapy tablet evaluated in an allergen chal-lenge chamber. J Allergy Clin Immunol 2009;124(3):471–7.

70. Dahl R, Kapp A, Colombo G, et al. Efficacy and safety of sublingual immuno-therapy with grass allergen tablets for seasonal allergic rhinoconjunctivitis. J Allergy Clin Immunol 2006;118(2):434–40.

71. Durham SR, Walker SM, Varga EM, et al. Long-term clinical efficacy of grass-pollen immunotherapy. N Engl J Med 1999;341(7):468–75.

72. Golden DB. Long-term outcome after venom immunotherapy. Curr Opin Allergy Clin Immunol 2010;10(4):337–41.

73. Smith H, White P, Annila I, et al. Randomized controlled trial of high-dose sublin-gual immunotherapy to treat seasonal allergic rhinitis. J Allergy Clin Immunol 2004;114(4):831–7.

74. Marogna M, Spadolini I, Massolo A, et al. Long-lasting effects of sublingual immu-notherapy according to its duration: a 15-year prospective study. J Allergy Clin Immunol 2010;126(5):969–75.

75. Acquistapace F, Agostinis F, Castella V, et al. Efficacy of sublingual specific immunotherapy in intermittent and persistent allergic rhinitis in children: an

observational case-control study on 171 patients. The EFESO-children multi-center trial. Pediatr Allergy Immunol 2009;20(7):660–4.

76. Novembre E, Galli E, Landi F, et al. Coseasonal sublingual immunotherapy reduces the development of asthma in children with allergic rhinoconjunctivitis. J Allergy Clin Immunol 2004;114(4):851–7.

77. Pfaar O, Barth C, Jaschke C, et al. Sublingual allergen-specific immunotherapy adjuvanted with monophosphoryl lipid A: a phase I/IIa study. Int Arch Allergy Immunol 2010;154(4):336–44.

78. Jones SM, Pons L, Roberts JL, et al. Clinical efficacy and immune regulation with peanut oral immunotherapy. J Allergy Clin Immunol 2009;124(2):292–300.

79. Clark AT, Islam S, King Y, et al. Successful oral tolerance induction in severe peanut allergy. Allergy 2009;64(8):1218–20.

Subcutaneous Injection Immunotherapy for Optimal Effectiveness

Harold S. Nelson, MD

KEYWORDS

- Immunotherapy • Subcutaneous • Injection • Asthma
- Allergic rhinitis • Atopic dermatitis • Oral allergy syndrome

In 1911, Leonard Noon published in *The Lancet* a description of his treatment of patients suffering from grass pollen–induced hay fever. In keeping with immunologic thinking of the day, he hypothesized that these individuals were uniquely sensitive to a toxin contained in the grass pollen, and that by a series of injections of increasing amounts of grass pollen extract he could induce protective antibodies against this toxin.[1] In an era when there was no effective symptomatic treatment for respiratory allergies, the practice of subcutaneous injection immunotherapy spread rapidly, and was extended to a wide range of allergens and conditions. Thus, in 1930 John Freeman, who had succeeded Noon in the initial treatment at St Mary's Hospital in London,[2] described the method of "Rush Inoculations" with examples, not only of using grass pollen extract but also extracts of horse dander and autogenous house dust, to treat patients with both hay fever and asthma.[3] Subcutaneous immunotherapy has been successfully employed for the entire range of inhalant allergens, including pollens, animal danders, house dust mites, and fungi as well as for allergy to insect stings, especially flying Hymenoptera and various species of ants. Despite this extension of subcutaneous immunotherapy to other allergens and other allergic conditions, the basic approach, that of a series of graded increasing doses followed by a prolonged series of maintenance injections, has changed little over the course of the 100 years that it has been employed.

Funding support: None.

Financial disclosures: Consulting: Genentech, Novartis, Merck, Sepracor, Forest Labs, Pfizer, Planet Biopharmaceuticals, GlaxoSmithKline, AstraZeneca, Abbott Laboratories, DBV Technologies, Vectura. Research Grants: ALK-Abelló.

Department of Medicine, National Jewish Health and University of Colorado School of Medicine, 1400 Jackson Street, Denver, CO 80206, USA

E-mail address: nelsonh@njhealth.org

Immunol Allergy Clin N Am 31 (2011) 211–226

doi:10.1016/j.iac.2011.02.010

0889-8561/11/$ – see front matter © 2011 Elsevier Inc. All rights reserved.

immunology.theclinics.com

DISEASE INDICATIONS FOR SUBCUTANEOUS INJECTION IMMUNOTHERAPY
Allergic Rhinitis and Asthma

Allergic rhinitis and asthma often occur together in response to allergen exposure. When John Bostock first described hay fever, he spoke of "a periodic affection of the eyes and chest."[4] The hay fever patients of Noon and Freeman also often complained of symptoms of asthma, and they reported that there was improvement in both hay fever and asthma with the injections of Timothy pollen extract.[2] The effectiveness of appropriate subcutaneous injection immunotherapy for allergic rhinitis and asthma has been repeatedly confirmed in single studies. Cochrane Collaboration meta-analyses have combined the results from many of these studies. An analysis of 15 randomized controlled trials conducted between 1950 and 2006 in subjects with seasonal allergic rhinitis revealed an overall reduction in symptoms in the immunotherapy group with a standard mean difference (SMD) of −0.73 and in 13 trials an SMD for medication use of −0.57. Both of these reductions were highly significant.[5]

Randomized controlled studies of perennial allergic rhinitis have been conducted less frequently than those for seasonal rhinitis; however, there are studies with house dust mite extracts that suggest clinical efficacy in this condition as well. In a small but carefully conducted study in 36 adults with severe allergic rhinitis due to house dust mite allergy uncontrolled by regular antiallergic drugs, a maintenance dose of *Dermatophagoides pteronyssinus* extract was administered for 12 months.[6] Compared with baseline, respiratory symptoms scores were reduced significantly (58%) in the active group, but not significantly (32%) in the placebo group. Medication scores were not significantly reduced in either the active group (20%) or the placebo group (no change).

The most recent Cochrane Database Systematic Review of injection allergen immunotherapy for asthma included 87 randomized controlled trials published through 2005 in the meta-analysis.[7] The investigators found a significant reduction in asthma symptoms (MSD −0.59) based on findings in 35 studies. There was a reduction of medication requirement (SMD −0.53) based on 21 studies, as well as significantly reduced allergen-specific bronchial hyperreactivity (4.1-fold) with some reduction in nonspecific bronchial hyperreactivity (2.2-fold).

Sensitivity to Insect Stings

Injection immunotherapy with the venoms of the flying Hymenoptera (honeybee, yellowjacket, hornet, and wasp) is of well-established efficacy. This therapy is recommended for all patients who have experienced a systemic reaction to an insect sting and who have specific IgE to venom allergens demonstrated by skin testing or in vitro testing, with the exception of children 16 years and younger whose reactions are limited to cutaneous systemic signs and symptoms.[8,9]

Allergic reactions to ant stings are also common, especially the Imported Fire ant in the southern United States and the Jack Jumper ant in Australia. For these insects whole-body extracts are employed for injection immunotherapy, their efficacy being supported by clinical observations[10] and double-blind studies,[11] respectively.

Systemic reactions to biting insects are occasionally reported, but there are only isolated reports of use of injection immunotherapy for their treatment, and effective commercial extracts are not available.[8]

Atopic Dermatitis

Atopic dermatitis has not traditionally been considered an indication for injection immunotherapy, although it frequently coexists with or precedes allergic rhinitis and asthma and is characterized in many patients by positive skin tests and high IgE levels. The most clearly recognized allergic trigger for atopic dermatitis is food allergy. Roughly a third of infants and young children with atopic dermatitis show relevant sensitivity to one or more foods.[12] The evidence for a role of other allergens either by inhalation or through contact with the skin is more circumstantial.[13] However, in addition to several anecdotal accounts of improvement in atopic dermatitis with injection immunotherapy, at least 3 reports of placebo-controlled studies have been published.[14–16] In the first of these studies, 26 children and adults with atopic dermatitis out of 52 originally randomized completed 2 years of injection therapy with a variety of inhalant allergens including house dust, danders, feathers, molds, and grass.[14] Thirteen of 16 treated with all the allergens to which they reacted improved compared with only 4 of 10 who improved on placebo. One of two monozygotic twins with atopic dermatitis flaring during the grass pollen season was given injections of grass pollen extract while her twin received placebo. After 2 years of blinded treatment, skin symptoms during May improved significantly in the grass-treated patient compared with her placebo-treated twin.[15] Recently, a larger study was reported of 1 year of injection therapy with 3 widely differing doses of house dust mite extract in adults with atopic dermatitis.[16] Treatment was initiated in 89 subjects, 51 of whom completed the study. Doses of house dust mite extract were 1/5000th, 1/50th, and 1/5th the customary monthly injection maintenance dose for respiratory allergy, and were given weekly. The reduction in atopic dermatitis score after 2 months was significantly greater in the highest compared with the lowest dose, and there was less use of topical corticosteroids with the 2 higher doses. The results of these studies suggest that there may be a role for injection immunotherapy in atopic dermatitis. However, further studies are needed to confirm this benefit and also to better define the population likely to respond.

Food Allergy and the Oral Allergy Syndrome

Injection of food extracts as treatment for food allergy was tried repeatedly in the early decades after the introduction of immunotherapy. There were occasional reports of success, such as John Freeman's induction in a young boy of tolerance to cod liver oil by inoculations of fish extract by a rush protocol.[3] However, the overall results were felt to be inconsistent, and parenteral food desensitization was not generally recommended.[17] The possibility was reexamined for peanut allergy as it became evident that this sensitivity was responsible for many of the anaphylactic deaths due to food ingestion, and that there was little tendency for this sensitivity to spontaneously remit.[18] A 1-year randomized, controlled study was conducted, with 6 peanut-allergic subjects receiving rush induction followed by maintenance injections.[19] All treated subjects reached the projected maintenance dose, and experienced increased tolerance to oral peanut challenge and decreased skin test reactivity to peanut; however, a median of 33 injections was required to reach maintenance and there was a median of 9 systemic reactions per subject during the buildup to maintenance. After achieving maintenance, all subjects continued to experience systemic reactions (median 15), and 3 subjects required dose reduction with complete or partial loss of the acquired tolerance to peanut. The conclusion was that injection immunotherapy with unmodified peanut extract was not a clinically viable option.

Patients allergic to several pollens and to latex experience oral symptoms on ingestion of specific fruits and vegetables. Case reports of immunotherapy with pollen mixes and multiple-allergen mixes reported improved tolerance and decreased sensitivity to the implicated fruits and vegetables.[20,21] Several series were reported of the effect of birch pollen immunotherapy on sensitivity to apples.[22–24] These nonrandomized studies reported decreased symptoms in comparison with untreated controls on ingestion of apples and, in one report, hazelnuts. A double-blind, double-dummy placebo-controlled study of both sublingual and subcutaneous immunotherapy with birch pollen extract was conducted in 74 subjects, 69% of whom reported oral allergy symptoms on ingestion of apples.[25] In this study, the oral symptoms on follow-up apple challenge decreased in all groups, but significantly only in those receiving placebo. Thus the final answer on immunotherapy for the oral allergy syndrome remains to be determined.

USE OF SPECIFIC ALLERGENS FOR SUBCUTANEOUS IMMUNOTHERAPY
Pollens

The initial study by Noon and Freeman employed Timothy grass pollen extract. Subsequently many pollen extracts have been proved to be effective when administered in adequate doses by injection. Among the allergens employed in the studies reviewed in the meta-analysis of injection immunotherapy in seasonal allergic rhinitis were ragweed (12 studies), mixed grass (16 studies), Timothy (5 studies), *Parietaria* (6 studies), birch (4 studies), orchard grass (2 studies), cedar (3 studies), and Bermuda and *Juniperus ashei* (1 study each).[7] Pollen extracts were also used in 27 of the studies reviewed in the meta-analysis of injection immunotherapy for asthma, including Bermuda grass, orchard grass, Timothy grass, velvet grass, sweet vernal grass, perennial rye grass, birch, olive and ragweed.[5]

House Dust Mites

In keeping with the importance of house dust mite allergy in asthma, 42 of 88 studies reviewed in the meta-analysis of injection immunotherapy for allergic asthma employed house dust mite extract, in almost all instances *Dermatophagoides pteronyssinus* or *Dermatophagoides farinae*.[7] Extracts of house dust mites have been used in virtually all studies reporting immunotherapy for perennial allergic rhinitis.

Animal Dander

Animal dander extracts, primarily cat or dog, were employed in 10 of the studies reviewed for the meta-analysis of injection immunotherapy for asthma.

Fungi

Three double-blind, placebo-controlled studies have been conducted in Europe with either *Cladosporium* or *Alternaria* extracts.[26–28] All 3 studies were small but used well-defined mold spore seasons and partially purified, standardized extracts. All 3 studies demonstrated significant improvement with active treatment compared with placebo in symptoms, medication use, or both.

It is unclear whether the results of these 3 European studies can be used to support the efficacy of fungal therapy in the United States. Despite the obvious clinical importance of fungal allergy in the United States, there are distinct problems with fungal immunotherapy: (1) the presence of hundreds of thousands of different species of fungi, (2) lack of accurate information on exposure patterns for most fungal species, (3) generally poor quality of commercially available fungal extracts, and (4) lack of commercial extracts for many of the clinically implicated fungal genera.[29,30]

Cockroach

No adequately controlled studies are available to assess the efficacy of cockroach extract. However, 3 commercially available cockroach extracts have been assayed for potency, and found to have potencies of 1735 to 8570 BAU/mL. This level would suggest that therapeutic doses can be achieved, at least with the most potent of the 3 extracts. Only glycerinated extracts of cockroach should be used, because of the high degree of autodigestion in aqueous preparations.

Latex

Four patients with anaphylactic sensitivity to latex underwent injection immunotherapy with a commercial latex extract.[31] All had reduction in skin tests, 3 had latex exposure without symptoms, and the other had reduced symptoms. The same commercial extract was employed in a 6-month study in 24 subjects with urticaria, rhinitis, or asthma due to latex exposure; 16 received active treatment and 8 received placebo.[32] Systemic reactions occurred with 9% of injections. Following treatment there was significant improvement in the latex glove challenge and a strong trend toward improvement in bronchial and nasal symptoms on inhalation challenge in the active treatment group, without improvement in the controls. A different commercial latex extract was employed in a double-blind, placebo-controlled study of 23 latex-allergic subjects, most of whom had asthma.[33] Systemic reactions (SRs) were observed with 30% of injections and in 82% of patients receiving active treatment. Most SRs were mild and no subject withdrew because of SRs. There was no difference in the change from baseline in the diary-reported rhinoconjunctivitis or cutaneous symptoms between the active and placebo groups. On the basis of these reports injection therapy for latex sensitivity cannot be considered an established therapeutic approach, especially in view of the absence of an approved commercial extract in the United States.

EXTRACT DOSING FOR INJECTION THERAPY

A wide range of doses of allergen extracts are employed in subcutaneous injection immunotherapy in the United States.[34] The results of double-blind, placebo-controlled studies of dosing in injection therapy suggest that many of the doses being employed are clinically ineffective.[35,36]

Effective doses of allergen extract for injection immunotherapy can only be determined by placebo-controlled studies. Except for the ragweed studies, most of these studies have been conducted in Europe where there is no common method of extract standardization. Therefore, to be able to combine all of the studies of extract dosing, the only available method is to express the dose as the major allergen content of the extract delivered at maintenance, even though this method presents problems related to differing monoclonal antibodies employed for the determinations. The doses that have been proved to give good clinical responses for those extracts, which have been standardized, are listed in **Table 1**. Also listed are doses that have produced definitely inferior results, sometimes no better than placebo. It must be noted that the range of effective major allergen dosing is fairly narrow; except for house dust mites and *Alternaria*, most values are between 10 and 20 µg.

Information regarding effective dosing by major allergens is useful only if the major allergen content is known for the commercially available allergen extracts. Of the United States standardized or nonstandardized extracts, only those of short ragweed list information on major allergen content. The content is listed in Food and Drug Administration units that are approximately equal to micrograms. Also, the content of major allergen varies quite widely from company to company, even in standardized extracts. Nevertheless, many of the extract-manufacturing companies have analyzed their own and other companies' products for major allergen content, so this information can often be obtained. **Table 2** lists the mean allergen content of multiple samples of United States extracts provided by one extract company.

Table 1
Effective maintenance doses for injection immunotherapy by major allergy content

Allergen Extract	Major Allergen	Range of Effective Doses	Less Effective or Ineffective Doses
Grasses	Phl p 5 or other group 5 allergens	15 µg[37] 18.6 µg[38] 20 µg[39]	2 µg[40]
Birch	Bet v 1	3.28 µg[41] 12 µg[42]	Not determined
Short ragweed	Amb a 1	6 µg[43] 11 µg[44] 12.4 µg[45] 24 µg[46]	0.6 µg[45] 2.0 µg[46]
Dermatophygoides	Der p 1Der f 1	7 µg[47] 10 µg[47]	0.7 µg[48]
Cat dander	Fel d 1	11.3 µg[49] 15 µg[50] 17.3 µg[51]	3 µg[52] 3 µg[53]
Dog dander	Can f 1	15 µg[54]	3 µg[54]
Alternaria	Alt a 1	1.6 µg[28]	Not determined

Multiple Allergen Mixes

The vast majority of controlled studies of injection immunotherapy have employed only a single extract.[5,7] On the other hand, the common practice in the United States is to administer a mixture of allergens.[55] The English and non-English medical literature was searched up to 2007 for reports of multiple allergen immunotherapy. Five studies, all administering extracts by injection, were identified that employed

Table 2
Representative mean content of major allergens in some United States standardized and nonstandardized extracts

Allergen Extract	Concentration	Major Allergen	Mean Content of Major Allergen
Short ragweed	1:10 wt/vol	Amb a 1	520 µg/mL
Timothy grass	100,000 BAU/mL	Phl p 5	660 µg/mL
Kentucky blue grass (June)	100,000 BAU/mL	Poa p 5	300 µg/mL
Orchard grass	100,000 BAU/mL	Dac g 5	740 µg/mL
Bermuda grass	10,000 BAU/mL	Cyn d 1	225 µg/mL
Dermatophagoides pteronyssinus	10,000 AU/mL	Der p 1	67 µg/mL
		Der p 2	69 µg/mL
Dermatophagoides farinae	10,000 AU/mL	Der f 1	65 µg/mL
		Der f 2	80 µg/mL
Cat dander	10,000 BAU/mL	Fel d 1	40 µg/mL
A.P. dog (H.S.)	1:100 wt/vol	Can f 1	140 µg/mL
Dog dander	1:10 wt/vol	Can f 1	5.4 µg/mL

Each mean major allergen content represents analyses of multiple extracts from several extract manufacturers. Data were provided by Greg Plunkett, PhD, ALK-Abelló, Round Rock, TX, September 2010.

more than 2 non–cross-reacting extracts in therapy.[56] Three of the 5 demonstrated clinical efficacy, 2 for allergic rhinitis[35,57] and 1 for asthma in children,[58] while 2 did not.[59,60] In the allergic rhinitis studies showing efficacy, ragweed-allergic subjects were matched for severity of symptoms during one pollen season. The ragweed component of their multiple allergen immunotherapy was then either eliminated or reduced by 95%, in both cases resulting in significant reduction in control of symptoms during the ensuing ragweed pollen season. In the asthma study, children were treated with all inhalants giving positive skin tests, but at several different maintenance doses. The 2 highest doses (1:5000 wt/vol and 1:250 wt/vol for each allergen extract) resulted in many fewer children with asthma at the end of the study, with the higher dose showing the best results.

An additional study of preseasonal immunotherapy for grass pollen–induced rhinitis and asthma[61] was not included in the review of multiallergen immunotherapy. In this study, subjects received 2 to 10 allergens in addition to grass extract or placebo in their treatment mix. Only 18 subjects participated; however asthma symptom-medication scores (SMS) were reduced significantly by immunotherapy (74%) with a trend for improvement in SMSs for rhinitis as well (43%).

Extract Dosing in Children

The study of injection immunotherapy for childhood asthma demonstrated that maximum concentrations of 1:5000 wt/vol resulted in greater reduction in asthma than placebo, but it was less effective than the 1:250 wt/vol dose of each of the extracts included in the treatment.[58] Otherwise there are very few studies of pediatric dosing and no consensus as to whether the dose should be different from that employed in adults. In 2 studies, in which immunotherapy was shown to reduce the incidence of new sensitization, the doses employed were less than those proven effective in adults. Thus, a dose containing 7 μg Der p 1 is recommended in adults,[47,48] whereas in the study in 2- to 6-year-olds the maintenance dose contained 2 μg Der p 1[62] and in the study of 5- to 8-year-olds the maintenance dose contained 3.5 μg Der p 1.[63] It is therefore possible that lower doses than are required by adults may be effective in young children.

SPECIAL CONSIDERATIONS IN CHILDREN
Age for Beginning Immunotherapy

Caution has been advised regarding initiating injection immunotherapy in children younger than age 5 years.[64–66] Among the perceived problems are difficulty in communicating with the child regarding SRs (ie, the health care provider recognizing a systemic reaction) and that injections can be traumatic for very young children.[65] Balanced against these concerns are recent reports from Europe regarding the safety and efficacy of injection immunotherapy in young children[67,68] and the reports of the long-lasting, disease-modifying actions of immunotherapy (**Table 3**). In a report from Spain, data were presented on 239 children aged 1 to 5 years treated with injection therapy. In 6689 injections there was only one systemic reaction, which occurred 90 minutes following an injection of house dust mite extract and which rapidly responded to treatment.[67] A report from Italy gave results from 592 children aged 3.5 to 10.5 years with severe asthma. These children were contrasted with 590 non-atopic children from the clinic.[68] After 3 years, the immunotherapy group showed greater improvement in symptoms, medication use, spirometry, and evidence of sensitivity compared with the drug-treated control group. Clinical adverse events were characterized as mild and transient.

Table 3
Prevention by subcutaneous injection immunotherapy for new sensitizations in monosensitized patients

Study,[Ref.] Year	Condition	Age (years)	Number	Follow-Up	New Sensitization	P Value
Des Roches et al,[62] 1997	Asthma (house dust mite)	2–6	22 treated 22 controls	3 y (end of treatment)	Active 55% Controls 100%	<.001
Purello-D'Ambrosio et al,[69] 2001	Asthma or allergic rhinitis Multiple-single allergens	≥14, mean 22.5	7182 treated 1214 controls	Treated 4 y Follow-up 3 y	Active 26.95% Controls 76.77%	<.0001
Pajno et al,[63] 2001	Asthma (house dust mite)	5–8	75 treated 63 controls	Treated 3 y Follow-up 3 y	Active 24.6% Control 66.7%	.0002
Inal et al,[70] 2007	Asthma or rhinitis (house dust mite)	6–16	45 SCIT 40 SLIT 62 Controls	5 y	Active 29.7% (no difference SCIT/SLIT) Control 53.3%	.002

Modification of Disease

Prevention of new sensitizations in monosensitized patients

Several studies have reported that injection immunotherapy in monosensitized children or young adults decreases the number who develop new sensitivities not only during the course of immunotherapy but also for several years after treatment is discontinued (see **Table 3**). A similar protection has not been reported in polysensitized patients.

Prevention of progression from rhinitis to asthma

The main evidence that injection immunotherapy decreases the likelihood of asthma developing in patients who only have rhinitis comes from the Preventive Allergy Treatment (PAT) study, conducted in 6 European pediatric centers.[71] The children, aged 6 to 14 years, were required to have symptomatic allergic rhinitis only to grass and/or birch and have no asthma during an initial observational year. One hundred and sixty-three children were then randomized to injection immunotherapy with Timothy and/or birch pollen extracts (n = 79) or were untreated controls (n = 72) during 3 years of the treatment phase of the study. At the end of 3 years, asthma had developed in 24% of the 79 children receiving injection immunotherapy and in 44% of the 76 control children. Follow-up observations on the children made 7 years after immunotherapy was discontinued showed no waning of the protective effect, with asthma in 25% of 64 treated subjects and in 45% of 53 control subjects.[72]

DURATION OF TREATMENT AND PERSISTENCE OF EFFECT

Duration of Treatment

The onset of efficacy of injection immunotherapy is quite rapid, with good results reported following a single preseasonal course of treatment.[38] Most randomized studies are of just 1 year; however, in 2 studies of 3 years' duration, there was progressive improvement with each year of treatment.[37,73] A 3-year duration of injection immunotherapy is also supported by studies showing persisting benefit for several years following 3 to 4 years of injection immunotherapy.[62,63,72–76]

Persistence of Benefit After Discontinuation of Treatment

Multiple lines of evidence indicate that the beneficial effects of injection immunotherapy persist after completion of a course of treatment of adequate length and sufficient dosing. The suppression of both development of new sensitivities in monosensitized patients and development of asthma in patients with allergic rhinitis has been shown to persist, with little evidence of diminution for 3 to 7 years.[63,69,72]

Studies have also been conducted that show persisting benefit for the symptoms of allergic rhinitis and allergic asthma. Specific immunotherapy to grass was discontinued after 3 to 4 years of treatment in 108 patients who had responded well to treatment.[75] Each year there was an increased number of patients with recurrent rhinitis symptoms, reaching 31% by the third year after discontinuation. In a placebo-controlled study, 32 subjects who had received grass injection immunotherapy for 3 or 4 years were randomized to continue to receive either maintenance injections of Timothy or placebo.[76] After 3 years, there was no difference in symptoms during the grass pollen season between the 2 groups. A small, open study of injection grass immunotherapy was conducted between 1988 and 1991. The participants were followed up prospectively through the grass pollen seasons of 1997 and 2003, 6 and 12 years after the discontinuation of treatment.[77] After 12 years there were still fewer symptoms, fewer new sensitizations, and a strong trend for less seasonal asthma in the treated group.

Injection immunotherapy was discontinued in a group of patients who had received house dust mite extract for from 12 to 96 months and had become symptom free.[74] Over the 3 years following discontinuation, approximately half the patients relapsed. The likelihood of relapse correlated inversely with both the duration of immunotherapy and the degree of immediate skin test suppression they experienced during treatment. On the basis of these studies the usual recommendation is that immunotherapy be continued for 3 to 5 years before discontinuation is considered.

ADHERENCE TO SUBCUTANEOUS INJECTION IMMUNOTHERAPY

Because injection immunotherapy is usually administered in a medical facility, it is easy to determine whether a patient receives the treatment. Several investigators have examined the percentage of patients who have discontinued the treatment of their own volition before completing the planned 3-year course of injections. In 2 university clinics, approximately half of the patients discontinued treatment; the major contributing factor was the inconvenience of the treatment.[78,79] A much lower rate of discontinuation was reported from a large private clinic where only 12% of 1033 patients prescribed injection immunotherapy failed to complete at least 3 years of treatment.[80] Again inconvenience was a major contributor, as were concurrent medical conditions, change of residence, and adverse reactions. Patient-initiated withdrawals during 3 years of immunotherapy administered intranasally, sublingually, or subcutaneously were compared in 2774 children in southern Italy.[81] Patient withdrawals over the 3 years were 73.2% for intranasal, 21.5% for sublingual, and 10.9% for subcutaneous injection immunotherapy. The principal reason for withdrawal from intranasal was local nasal symptoms (57%). Major reasons for withdrawal from sublingual were cost (36%) and ineffectiveness (25%), and cost (40%) and inconvenience (24%) were reasons for withdrawal from subcutaneous.

COMPARATIVE EFFECTIVENESS OF SUBCUTANEOUS AND SUBLINGUAL IMMUNOTHERAPY

The relative effectiveness of sublingual and subcutaneous immunotherapy either in the short-term or long-term is not established. The data available to assess relative effectiveness consists of meta-analyses of reports of treatment of allergic rhinitis by the two methods, comparative results when the same investigator treated similar patients by the two methods, and studies with patients randomized to treatment by the two methods.

Systematic reviews of published articles on treatment of allergic rhinitis by sublingual immunotherapy (SLIT)[82] and injection immunotherapy (SCIT)[5] were conducted for the Cochrane Collaboration. Twenty-two double-blind, placebo-controlled trials involving 979 patients were included in the SLIT meta-analysis. There was an oval reduction in symptoms (SMD −0.42) and medication use (SMD −0.43). Fifty-one studies with 2871 subjects met the criteria for randomized trials of SCIT. The overall improvement in symptoms was SMD −0.73 and for medications SMD −0.57, suggesting a possible greater efficacy of SCIT over SLIT.

The same United Kingdom group conducted studies on the use of SLIT and SCIT for seasonal allergic rhinitis due to grass pollen. In 1989, they recruited 40 patients with severe hay fever unresponsive to symptomatic therapy.[38] Patients were administered a preseasonal course of either Timothy pollen extract or placebo by injection. During the ensuing grass pollen season, the active-treatment group had a reduction in total symptoms of 61% and reduction of medication use of 79% compared with the placebo-treated group. Fifty-six patients with grass pollen–induced allergic rhinitis were recruited in 1998 and randomized to SLIT or placebo.[83] The SLIT was of 9 to 14 months' duration by the beginning of the grass pollen season, with a monthly cumulative dose of Timothy 225 times that administered in the SCIT study. Reduction in symptoms in the active-treatment group during the grass pollen season of 1999 was 28% and medication use was reduced by 45% compared with placebo, although neither result was statistically significant. Global assessment of improvement was significant in the active group, but the magnitude of the difference from placebo was about half that observed in the previous SCIT study for patient-reported outcomes.

A placebo-controlled comparison study of treatment of allergic rhinitis due to birch pollen, uncontrolled by symptomatic therapy, was conducted in Denmark.[41] Seventy-one subjects were observed during one birch pollen season, then randomized to injection therapy or sublingual therapy with a cumulative monthly dose 225 times that in the SCIT group. Both groups had significant reductions in symptoms and medication compared with the placebo group. There were no statistically significant differences between those receiving SCIT and SLIT. However, compared with the placebo group the reduction in symptoms and medication use in the SCIT group was 70% and 33% greater, respectively, than in the SLIT group.

The response of perennial allergic rhinitis in patients sensitized only to house dust mites to immunotherapy with house dust mite extract administered either by injection or sublingually was compared in 193 patients.[73] The cumulative monthly SLIT dose in this study was only 3 times that used for SCIT. Clinical improvement during 3 years of immunotherapy was progressive and similar in the two groups. After discontinuation, the subjects were followed for an additional 3 years. There was no increase of symptoms in the SCIT group, but symptoms increased significantly in the third follow-up year in the SLIT group. SCIT was also significantly better for reduction in nasal airway resistance and prick skin tests to house dust mites.

Thus by all 3 data sets, there is a suggestion of a superior response to SCIT compared with SLIT; however, this conclusion is very tentative and many more studies are needed.

SUMMARY

Immunotherapy by the subcutaneous injection of increasing doses and then maintenance doses of extracts of inhalant allergens has been practiced with only minor changes for 100 years. Controlled clinical trials have established its efficacy in treating allergic rhinitis, asthma, and stinging insect sensitivity, and there are preliminary data to suggest a favorable response in some patients with atopic dermatitis. It is not recommended for treating primary food allergy, but may benefit the oral allergy symptoms associated with pollen sensitivity. The best documented responses are to extracts of pollens, house dust mites, and animal danders, and to venom and whole-body extracts of stinging insects. There is limited support for its use in fungal and latex allergy, and to date there is no documentation of efficacy with cockroach extracts. The response to subcutaneous injection immunotherapy is very dose dependent, with doses one-fifth or one-twentieth of the effective doses often offering little or no benefit. Dosing is best expressed as the major allergen content of the maintenance dose. This practice is limited by the availability of data on the major allergen content of commercially available extracts in the United States. Treatment with mixtures of non–cross-reacting extracts has been proved to be effective in injection immunotherapy, provided the concentration of each extract is adequate. Among the exciting findings with subcutaneous injection immunotherapy is its disease-modifying actions. These actions include blocking the development of new sensitivities in monosensitized patients, blocking the progression to asthma in patients with allergic rhinitis, and persistence of treatment effects up to 7 to 10 years following discontinuation of a 3-year course of treatment. Studies comparing the outcome with subcutaneous injection and sublingual-swallow approaches to immunotherapy are inadequate, but the limited data available suggest that subcutaneous injection may be somewhat more effective than sublingual administration.

REFERENCES

1. Noon L. Prophylactic inoculation against hay fever. Lancet 1911;i:1572–3.
2. Freeman J. Further observations on the treatment of hay fever by hypodermic inoculations of pollen vaccine. Lancet 1911;ii:814–7.
3. Freeman J. Rush Inoculation with specific reference to hay fever treatment. Lancet 1930;i:744–7.
4. Bostock J. Case of a periodical affection of the eyes and chest. Med Chir Trans 1819;10:161.
5. Calderon MA, Alves B, Jacobson M, et al. Allergen injection immunotherapy for seasonal allergic rhinitis. Cochrane Database Syst Rev 2007;1:CD001936.
6. Varney VA, Tabbah K, Mavroleon G, et al. Usefulness of specific immunotherapy in patients with severe perennial allergic rhinitis induced by house dust mite: a double-blind, randomized, placebo-controlled trial. Clin Exp Allergy 2003;33: 1076–82.
7. Abramson MJ, Puy RM, Weiner JM. Injection allergen immunotherapy for asthma. Cochrane Database Syst Rev 2010;8:CD001186.
8. Golden DB. Insect allergy. Chapter 57. In: Adkinson NF Jr, Bochner BS, Busse WW, et al, editors. Middleton's allergy: principles and practice. 7th edition. Philadelphia (PA): Elsevier, Inc; 2009. p. 1005–17.
9. Moffitt JE, Golden DK, Reisman RE, et al. Stinging insect hypersensitivity: a practice parameter update. J Allergy Clin Immunol 2004;114:869–86.
10. Freeman TM, Highlander R, Ortez A, et al. Imported fire ant immunotherapy: effectiveness of whole body extract. J Allergy Clin Immunol 1992;90:210–5.
11. Brown SG, Wiese MD, Blackman KE, et al. Ant venom immunotherapy: a double-blind placebo-controlled crossover trial. Lancet 2003;361:1001–6.
12. Sicherer SH, Sampson HA. Food hypersensitivity and atopic dermatitis: pathophysiology, epidemiology, diagnosis and management. J Allergy Clin Immunol 1999;104:S114–22.
13. Boguniewicz M, Leung DY. Atopic dermatitis. Chapter 62 in 14. In: Adkinson NF Jr, Bochner BS, Busse WW, et al, editors. Middleton's allergy: principles and practice. 7th edition. Philadelphia (PA): Elsevier, Inc; 2009. p. 1083–103.
14. Kaufman HS, Roth HL. Hyposensitization with alum precipitated extracts in atopic dermatitis: a placebo-controlled study. Ann Allergy 1974;32:321–30.
15. Ring J. Successful hyposensitization treatment in atopic eczema: results of a trial in monozygotic twins. Br J Dermatol 1982;107:597–602.
16. Werfel T, Breuer K, Rueff F, et al. Usefulness of specific immunotherapy in patients with atopic dermatitis and allergic sensitization to house dust mites: a multi-centre, randomized, dose-response study. Allergy 2006;61:202–5.
17. Vaughan WT, Black TH. Practice of allergy. 2nd edition. St Louis (MO): CV Mosby Company; 1948.
18. Oppenheimer JJ, Nelson HS, Bock SA, et al. Treatment of peanut allergy with rush immunotherapy. J Allergy Clin Immunol 1992;90:25–62.

19. Nelson HS, Lahr J, Rule R, et al. Treatment of anaphylactic sensitivity to peanuts by immunotherapy with injections of aqueous peanut extract. J Allergy Clin Immunol 1997;99:44–51.
20. Kelso JM, Jones RT, Tellez R, et al. Oral allergy syndrome successfully treated with pollen immunotherapy. Ann Allergy Asthma Immunol 1995;74:391–6.
21. Asero R. Fennel, cucumber and melon allergy successfully treated with pollen-specific injection immunotherapy. Ann Allergy Asthma Immunol 2000; 84:460–2.
22. Asero R. Effects of birch pollen-specific immunotherapy on apple allergy in birch pollen-hypersensitive patients. Clin Exp Allergy 1998;28:1368–73.
23. Modrzynski M, Zawisza E, Rapiejko P, et al. Specific-pollen immunotherapy in the treatment of oral allergy syndrome in patients with tree pollen hypersensitivity. Przegl Lek 2002;59:1007–10.
24. Bucher X, Pichler WJ, Dahinden CA, et al. Effect of tree pollen specific, subcutaneous immunotherapy on the oral allergy syndrome to apple and hazelnut. Allergy 2004;59:1272–6.
25. Hansen KS, Khinchi MS, Skov PS, et al. Food allergy to apple and specific immunotherapy with birch pollen. Mol Nutr Food Res 2004;48:441–8.
26. Dreborg S, Agrell B, Foucard T, et al. A double-blind multicenter immunotherapy trial in children using a purified and standardized *Cladosporium herbarum* preparation. Allergy 1986;41:131–40.
27. Malling H-J, Dreborg S, Weeke B. Diagnosis and immunotherapy of mould allergy V. Clinical efficacy and side effects of immunotherapy with *Cladosporium herbarum*. Allergy 1986;41:507–19.
28. Horst M, Hejjaoui A, Horst V, et al. Double-blind, placebo-controlled rush immunotherapy with a standardized *Alternaria* extract. J Allergy Clin Immunol 1990; 85:460–72.
29. Salvaggio JE, Burge HA, Chapman JA. Emerging concepts of mold allergy: what is the role of immunotherapy? J Allergy Clin Immunol 1993;92:217–22.
30. Patterson MI, Slater JE. Characterization and comparison of commercially available German and American cockroach allergen extracts. Clin Exp Allergy 2002; 32:721–7.
31. Pereira C, Pedro E, Tavares B, et al. Specific immunotherapy for severe latex allergy. Eur Ann Allergy Clin Immunol 2003;36:217–25.
32. Sastre J, Fernandez-Nieto M, Rico P, et al. Specific immunotherapy with a standardized latex extract in allergic workers: a double-blind, placebo-controlled study. J Allergy Clin Immunol 2003;111:985–94.
33. Tabar AI, Anda M, Bonifazi F, et al. Specific immunotherapy with standardized latex extract versus placebo in latex-allergic patients. Int Arch Allergy Immunol 2006;141:369–76.
34. Nelson HS. The use of standardized extracts in allergen immunotherapy. J Allergy Clin Immunol 2000;106:41–5.
35. Franklin W, Lowell FC. Comparison of two dosages of ragweed extract in the treatment of pollenosis. JAMA 1967;201:915–7.
36. Norman PS. A rational approach to desensitization. J Allergy 1969;44:129–45.
37. Dolz I, Martinez-Cocerac C, Bartolone JM, et al. A double-blind, placebo-controlled study of immunotherapy with grass pollen extract Alutard SQ during a 3-year period with initial rush immunotherapy. Allergy 1996;1:489–500.
38. Varney VA, Gaga M, Frew AJ, et al. Usefulness of immunotherapy in patients with severe summer hay fever uncontrolled by antiallergic drugs. BMJ 1991;302: 265–9.

39. Walker SM, Pajno GB, Lima MT, et al. Grass pollen immunotherapy for seasonal rhinitis and asthma: a randomized, controlled trial. J Allergy Clin Immunol 2004; 107:87–93.

40. Frew AJ, Powell RJ, Corrigan CJ, et al. Efficacy and safety of specific immunotherapy with SQ allergen extract in treatment-resistant seasonal allergic rhinoconjunctivitis. J Allergy Clin Immunol 2006;117:319–28.

41. Khinchi MS, Poulsen LK, Carat F, et al. Clinical efficacy of sublingual and subcutaneous birch pollen allergen specific immunotherapy: a randomized, placebo-controlled, double-blind, double-dummy study. Allergy 2004;59:45–53.

42. Rak S, Heinrich C, Schevnius A. Comparison of nasal immunopathology in patients with seasonal rhinoconjunctivitis treated with topical steroids or specific allergen immunotherapy. Allergy 2006;60:643–9.

43. Creticos PS, Adkinson NF Jr, Kagey-Sobotka A, et al. Nasal challenge with ragweed pollen in hay fever patients: Effect of immunotherapy. J Clin Invest 1989;76:2247–53.

44. Van Metre TE Jr, Adkinson NF Jr, Amodio FJ, et al. A comparative study of the effectiveness of the Rinkel method and the current standard method of immunotherapy for ragweed pollen hay fever. J Allergy Clin Immunol 1979;66:500–13.

45. Creticos PS, Marsh DG, Proud D, et al. Responses to ragweed-pollen nasal challenge before and after immunotherapy. J Allergy Clin Immunol 1989;84: 197–205.

46. Furin MJ, Norman PS, Creticos PS, et al. Immunotherapy decreases antigen-induced eosinophil cell migration into the nasal cavity. J Allergy Clin Immunol 1991;88:27–32.

47. Olsen OT, Larsen KR, Jacobsen L, et al. A 1-year, placebo-controlled, double-blind house-dust-mite immunotherapy study in asthmatic adults. Allergy 1997; 52:853–9.

48. Haugaard L, Dahl R, Jacobsen L. A controlled dose-response study of immunotherapy with standardized, partially purified extract of house dust mite: clinical efficacy and side effects. J Allergy Clin Immunol 1993;91:709–22.

49. Alvarez-Cuesta E, Cuesta-Herranz J, Puyana-Ruiz J, et al. Monoclonal antibody standardized cat extract immunotherapy: risk benefit effects from a double-blind placebo study. J Allergy Clin Immunol 1994;93:556–66.

50. Varney VA, Edwards J, Tabbah K, et al. Clinical efficacy of specific immunotherapy to cat dander: a double-blind placebo-controlled trial. Clin Exp Allergy 1997;27:860–7.

51. Hedlin G, Graff-Lonnevig V, Heilborn H, et al. Immunotherapy with cat- and dog-dander extracts: V. Effects of 3 years of treatment. J Allergy Clin Immunol 1991; 87:955–64.

52. Ewbank PA, Murray J, Sanders K, et al. A double-blind, placebo-controlled immunotherapy dose-response study with standardized cat extract. J Allergy Clin Immunol 2003;111:155–61.

53. Nanda A, O'Connor M, Anand M, et al. Dose dependence and time course of the immunologic response to administration of standardized cat allergen extract. J Allergy Clin Immunol 2004;114:1339–44.

54. Lent A, Harbeck R, Strand M, et al. Immunological response to administration of standardized dog allergen extract at differing doses. J Allergy Clin Immunol 2006;118:1249–56.

55. Esch RE. Specific immunotherapy in the U.S.A. General concept and recent initiatives. Arb Paul Ehrlich Inst Bundesamt Sera Impfstoffe Frankf A M 2003; 94:17–22.

56. Nelson HS. Multiallergen immunotherapy for allergic rhinitis and asthma. J Allergy Clin Immunol 2009;123:763–9.
57. Lowell FC, Franklin W. A double-blind study of the effectiveness and specificity of injection therapy in ragweed hay fever. N Engl J Med 1965;273:675–9.
58. Johnstone DE, Dutton A. The value of hyposensitization therapy for bronchial asthma in children: a14-year study. Pediatrics 1968;42:793–802.
59. Bousquet J, Becker WM, Hejjaoui A, et al. Differences in clinical and immunologic reactivity of patients allergic to grass pollens and to multiple-pollen species. II. Efficacy of a double-blind, placebo-controlled, specific immunotherapy with standardized extracts. J Allergy Clin Immunol 1991;88:43–53.
60. Adkinson NF Jr, Eggleston PA, Eney D, et al. A controlled trial of immunotherapy for asthma in allergic children. N Engl J Med 1997;336:24–31.
61. Reid MJ, Moss RB, Hsu Y-P, et al. Seasonal asthma in northern California: allergic causes and efficacy of immunotherapy. J Allergy Clin Immunol 1986; 78:590–600.
62. Des Roches A, Paradis L, Menardo JL, et al. Immunotherapy with a standardized *Dermatophagoides pteronyssinus* extract. VI. Specific immunotherapy prevents the onset of new sensitization in children. J Allergy Clin Immunol 1997;99:450–3.
63. Pajno GB, Barberio G, De Luca F, et al. Prevention of new sensitizations in asthmatic children monosensitized to house dust mite by specific immunotherapy. A six-year follow-up study. Clin Exp Allergy 2001;31:1392–7.
64. Ownby DR, Adinoff AD. The appropriate use of skin testing and allergen immunotherapy in young children. J Allergy Clin Immunol 1994;94:662–5.
65. Cox L, Li JT, Nelson HS, et al, Joint task Force on Practice Parameters; American Academy of Allergy, Asthma and Immunology; American College of Allergy, Asthma and Immunology; Joint Council of Allergy, Asthma and Immunology. Allergen immunotherapy: a practice parameter second update. J Allergy Clin Immunol 2007;120(Suppl 3):S25–85.
66. Canadian parameters immunotherapy. Can Med Assoc J 2005;173(Suppl 6): S46–50.
67. Rodriquez Perez N, Ambriz Moreno MJ. Safety of immunotherapy and skin tests with allergens in children younger than five years. Rev Alerg Mex 2006;53:47–51.
68. Cantani A, Micera M. A prospective study of asthma desensitization in 1182 children, 592 asthmatic children and 590 nonatopic controls. Eur Rev Med Pharmacol Sci 2005;9:325–9.
69. Purello-D'Ambrosio F, Gangemi S, Merendino RA, et al. Prevention of new sensitizations in monosensitized subjects submitted to specific immunotherapy or not. A retrospective study. Clin Exp Allergy 2001;31:1295–302.
70. Inal A, Altintas DU, Yilmaz M, et al. Prevention of new sensitizations by specific immunotherapy in children with rhinitis and/or asthma monosensitized to house dust mite. J Investig Allergol Clin Immunol 2007;17:85–91.
71. Moller C, Dreborg S, Ferdousi HA, et al. Pollen immunotherapy reduces the development of asthma in children with seasonal rhinoconjunctivitis (the PAT-Study). J Allergy Clin Immunol 2002;109:251–6.
72. Jacobsen L, Niggemann B, Dreborg S, et al. Specific immunotherapy has long-term preventive effect on seasonal and perennial asthma. 10-year follow-up on the PAT study. Allergy 2007;62:943–8.
73. Tahamiler R, Saritzali G, Canakcioglu S, et al. Comparison of the long-term efficacy of subcutaneous and sublingual immunotherapies in perennial rhinitis. ORL J Otorhinolaryngol Relat Spec 2008;70:144–50.

74. Des Roches A, Paradis L, Knani J, et al. Immunotherapy with a standardized *Dermatophagoides pteronyssinus* extract. V. Duration of the efficacy of immunotherapy after its cessation. Allergy 1996;51:30–3.
75. Ebner C, Kraft D, Ebner H. Booster immunotherapy (BIT). Allergy 1994;49:38–42.
76. Durham SR, Walker SM, Varga E-M, et al. Long-term clinical efficacy of grass-pollen immunotherapy. N Engl J Med 1999;341:468–75.
77. Eng PA, Borer-Reinhold M, Heijnen IA, et al. Twelve-year follow-up after discontinuation of preseasonal grass pollen immunotherapy in childhood. Allergy 2006;61:198–201.
78. Lower T, Henry J, Mandik L, et al. Compliance with allergen immunotherapy. Ann Allergy 1993;70:480–2.
79. Cohn JR, Pizzi A. Determinants of patient compliance with allergen immunotherapy. J Allergy Clin Immunol 1993;91:734–7.
80. Rhodes BJ. Patient dropouts before completion of optimal dose, multiple allergen immunotherapy. Ann Allergy Asthma Immunol 1999;82:281–6.
81. Pajno B, Vita D, Caminiti L, et al. Children's compliance with allergen immunotherapy according to administration routes. J Allergy Clin Immunol 2005;116:1380–1.
82. Wilson DR, Torres Lima M, Durham SR. Sublingual immunotherapy for allergic rhinitis. Cochrane Database Syst Rev 2003;12:CD002693.
83. Torres Lima M, Wilson D, Pitkin L, et al. Grass pollen sublingual immunotherapy for seasonal rhinoconjunctivitis: a randomized controlled trail. Clin Exp Allergy 2002;32:507–14.

Allergen Compatibilities in Extract Mixtures

Robert E. Esch, PhD*, Thomas J. Grier, PhD

KEYWORDS

• Allergenic extracts • Stability • Compatibility

INTRODUCTION

A working knowledge of allergen extract stabilities and compatibilities can influence clinical decisions related to developing specific allergen panels for skin testing and optimizing named-patient immunotherapy formulations.[1,2] Inclusion of stock or customized extract mixtures is not uncommon in United States allergy clinics. In most cases, these mixtures consist of extracts from phylogenetically related species that exhibit near-complete allergenic cross-reactivity because of the presence of homologous allergens. The most common examples are the house dust mites mixture containing equal parts *Dermatophagoides farinae* and *D pteronyssinus*; and the ragweed mixture containing short ragweed (*Ambrosia artemisiifolia*) and giant ragweed (*A trifida*). These and other mixtures of allergenic extract are often used for skin testing and treatment in place of extracts derived from a single species. Broader mixtures covering multiple non–cross-reactive allergens have also been incorporated into treatment regimens, but their prudent use is essential to improving the diversity and effectiveness of allergen-specific immunotherapy.

Allergenic extracts lose their allergenic activity during storage and handling, sometimes in complex ways, making it difficult to identify all of the mechanisms involved in a particular situation. Early studies on allergen stability involved thermal stability, dilution, and adsorption to glass surfaces.[3–5] Because allergic patients are not sensitized to the same allergens, an extract may appear to retain its potency when evaluated in patients who are reactive to heat-stable allergens, whereas loss of potency may be evident in patients who are reactive to heat-labile allergens.[6] This differential heat sensitivity of different allergens can be extended to other physical conditions that are known to affect allergen structure and function. Thus, studies have been conducted that evaluated the effect of pH or diluent used to prepare extracts, use of

The authors are employees of Greer Laboratories, Inc, a manufacturer and supplier of allergen products.
Research and Development, Greer Laboratories, Inc, 639 Nuway Circle, Lenoir, NC 28645, USA
* Corresponding author.
E-mail address: esch@greerlabs.com

Immunol Allergy Clin N Am 31 (2011) 227–239
doi:10.1016/j.iac.2011.02.009   **immunology.theclinics.com**

preservatives, and dilution, and all have been shown to have an important role in extract stability.[7–11]

The kinetics of denaturation of an allergen in purified form is different when compared with the same allergen present in an allergen extract. The thermal decay of purified Amb a 1 occurred as a first order reaction, whereas the same allergen as a component of an extract decayed through a more complex reaction.[12] Many enzymes, especially proteases, were known to be present in allergenic extracts,[13,14] but their role in extract stability became apparent only after extracts with high protease content were mixed with extracts with allergens that were susceptible to proteolytic degradation.[15]

Stability is an essential requirement for diagnostic and therapeutic allergen preparations that are routinely diluted, used in multiple-dose vials, and stored for extended periods. Manufacturers' concentrates should be stable at refrigeration temperatures for perhaps several years, and should be stable for periods at higher temperatures that may be encountered during shipment and routine use. Expiration dating based on potency tests is a requirement for standardized extracts licensed in the United States. The dating periods verify that the labeled potency accurately reflects the allergenic activity of the vial contents under specified conditions. Unfortunately, validated potency tests are available only for standardized extracts, and for most commercial allergen products, which are not standardized, expiration dating is based on the rule that gives 36 months for 50% glycerinated extracts and 18 months for extracts containing less than 50% glycerin.

Once the products leave the manufacturer and enter the clinic, the products are frequently diluted or combined with other extracts, sometimes from another manufacturer. The stability of these mixtures is extremely difficult to predict because the combinations vary widely, the diluent used may vary from clinic to clinic, and storage conditions can also vary. Thus, the compositional heterogeneity of allergen extracts and the added complexity of multiextract mixtures present a formidable challenge to optimization and validation of stability-indicating in vivo or in vitro assays displaying appropriate sensitivity and specificity levels. To date, owing primarily to the small number of published studies on extract stability and compatibilities, no consensus exists on the best available experimental approaches, methods, and criteria for studies of this type.

POTENCY TESTS FOR ALLERGEN PRODUCTS

Various methods have been proposed for the potency testing of diagnostic and therapeutic allergen preparations. They range from the measurement of overall allergenicity using quantitative skin testing or competition immunoglobulin E (IgE) enzyme-linked immunosorbent assays (ELISAs) to immunoassays for specific allergen measurements.[16–19] Each of these methods has advantages and disadvantages. Measurements of overall allergenicity are important for labeling purposes but may lack the sensitivity to detect the degradation of selected allergens in an extract or mixture of extracts. Skin testing, when conducted intradermally, can have the sensitivity needed to assess the potency of highly diluted extracts but must be performed in several patients to account for their differences in sensitivities to different allergenic components. In multicenter studies, skin testing at each clinic can yield interesting but conflicting data based on these differences in subject reactivities or allergen exposures.

In the United States, standardization of commercial allergen extract potencies through skin testing involves only the initial (primary) reference extract preparation.

Subsequent batches of reference antigen and all production lots from licensed manufacturers undergo in vitro potency testing, with labeled values based on immunochemical equivalence to the current reference extract. Selection of appropriate and consistent allergic serum pools for competition IgE ELISAs becomes crucial to the accuracy of both lot-release and stability testing of products analyzed in this manner. Failure to maintain well-characterized reference reagents or a drift in their performance characteristics can have a significant impact on the product's clinical efficacy or safety.

Methods for measuring overall allergen activity have limitations in evaluating more complex, multiextract mixtures. Physical interactions between extract constituents in mixtures can lead to unpredictable or inconsistent interpretation of results. For this reason, immunochemical assays offering exquisite allergenic specificity and moderate to high analytical sensitivity have emerged as the preferred methods for most extract compatibility investigations. Allergen-specific monoclonal and polyclonal antibodies can be produced in large quantities, and various immunoassay formats can be configured without the need for a sophisticated laboratory. The analytical performance of these assays can vary depending on the selection and qualification criteria for component reagents, incubation conditions, and data output and reduction procedures.

Small differences among procedures used in different laboratories can result in significant variability in assay results, particularly for sensitive methods requiring relatively high (>1000-fold) sample dilutions to produce parallel dilution-response curves within the desired dynamic range. Monoclonal antibody–based immunoassays can be highly sensitive and reproducible but, paradoxically, can also be too specific to yield clinically relevant information.

Therefore, care must be taken when selecting the suitable method for stability testing, and more than one method is almost always required to generate useful information. Regardless of the methods selected, they must be validated for their intended use and the test results must be carefully interpreted before applying them in clinical settings.

ALLERGEN EXTRACT COMPATIBILITY STUDIES

Since 1990, data and methodologies from eight studies[15,20–26] on allergen extract compatibility have been reported. The specific extract combinations and analytical methods examined in these studies are described in chronologic order in **Tables 1** and **2**, respectively. Unpublished results summarized in meeting abstracts or comments in publications displaying no experimental details and data were excluded from this discussion.

Seven of the eight published studies[15,20,21,23–26] on allergen compatibility were conducted in the United States using source materials, extract concentrates, and diluents produced by multiple manufacturers licensed by the US Food and Drug Administration (FDA). Initial investigations were focused on the IgE-binding potencies of perennial ryegrass extracts based on observations that grass pollen allergens were susceptible to potency reductions during exposures to elevated temperature or after mixing with certain fungal extracts.

Other grass extracts (timothy, meadow fescue) known to be highly cross-reactive with ryegrass were included in subsequent studies[21,24,25] to confirm allergen susceptibilities within a model homologous group for specific grass products used in many allergy clinics across the United States. The wide range of other extracts evaluated for compatibility in the United States studies also reflects the broad spectrum of

Table 1
Extract combinations included in eight published studies on extract compatibility

References	Year	Target Extract	Companion Extracts
Esch[15]	1991	Perennial ryegrass	Cocklebur, sagebrush, marsh elder, ragweed, oak, lamb's quarter, elm, or pigweed
			Cat epithelia, dog epithelia or goat epithelia
			Moth, caddisfly, dust mite *Dermatophagoides farinae*, dust mite *D pteronyssinus*, or American cockroach
			Alternaria alternata, Aspergillus fumigatus, Penicillium notatum, Fusarium moniliforme, Mucor racemosus, Aureobasidium pullulans, Paecilomyces varioti, or *Microsporum canis*
Kordash et al[20]	1993	Perennial ryegrass	Hickory, *D farinae*, cockroach mix or *Helminthosporium interseminatum*
Nelson et al[21]	1996	Timothy grass	*Alternaria alternata, Cladosporium herbarum, Penicillium notatum,* American cockroach, dust mite mix, or mold mix
		Bermuda grass	*Alternaria alternata, C herbarum, Penicillium notatum,* American cockroach, dust mite mix, or mold mix
		Short ragweed	*Alternaria alternata, C herbarum, Penicillium notatum,* American cockroach, dust mite mix, or mold mix
		White oak	*Alternaria alternata, C herbarum, Penicillium notatum,* American cockroach, dust mite mix, or mold mix
		Box elder	*Alternaria alternata, C herbarum, Penicillium notatum,* American cockroach, dust mite mix, or mold mix
		Russian thistle	*Alternaria alternata, C herbarum, Penicillium notatum,* American cockroach, dust mite mix, or mold mix
		Cat	*Alternaria alternata, C herbarum, Penicillium notatum,* American cockroach, dust mite mix, or mold mix
		D farinae	*Alternaria alternata, C herbarum, Penicillium notatum,* American cockroach, dust mite mix, or mold mix
Hoff et al[22]	2002	Timothy grass	*Fusarium culmorum*
		Birch	*F culmorum*
Meier et al[23]	2006	Mountain cedar	Fire ant
Grier et al[24]	2007	Meadow fescue grass	Dust mite *D farinae* or dust mite *D pteronyssinus*
			Alternaria alternata, Aspergillus fumigatus, Aspergillus niger, Penicillium chrysogenum, Penicillium notatum, Bipolaris sorokiniana, C herbarum, C sphaerospermum, Epicoccum nigrum, F moniliforme, F solani, Mucor plumbeus, or *Aureobasidium pullulans*

(continued on next page)

Table 1 *(continued)*			
References	**Year**	**Target Extract**	**Companion Extracts**
		Short ragweed	*Alternaria alternata, Aspergillus fumigatus, Penicillium notatum*, American cockroach, German cockroach
		Cat	*Alternaria alternata, Aspergillus fumigatus, Penicillium notatum*, American cockroach, German cockroach
		D farinae	*Alternaria alternata, Aspergillus fumigatus, Penicillium notatum*, American cockroach, German cockroach
Rans et al[25]	2009	Timothy grass	Fire ant
		Short ragweed	Fire ant
		Cat	Fire ant
		D pteronyssinus	Fire ant
Grier et al[26]	2009	Dog epithelia	*Alternaria alternata, Aspergillus fumigatus, Penicillium notatum*, American cockroach, German cockroach, fire ant
		Dog hair/dander	*Alternaria alternata, Aspergillus fumigatus, Penicillium notatum*, American cockroach, German cockroach, fire ant

allergens recognized by many atopic patients and the resulting use of diverse multiextract mixtures for immunotherapy. The single European study[22] used freeze-dried target pollen extracts (timothy grass, birch) mixed with a protease-rich *Fusarium* extract prepared by the investigators from commercial source materials cultured from a defined strain.

Of the seven United States reports,[15,20,21,23–26] four were authored or coauthored by scientists from one extract manufacturer (Greer, including the authors of this article),[15,24–26] and one study was conducted by investigators from a different extract supplier (Hollister-Stier, formerly Miles Allergy Products).[20] Familiarity and years of experience with the in vitro potency tests listed in **Table 2**, combined with access to or synthesis of specialized allergen and antibody reagents used for these methods, have facilitated the execution of extract compatibility studies in these laboratories. Recent investigations have included mixtures prepared with extracts from multiple United States manufacturers at variable glycerin and human serum albumin (HSA) concentrations. Incorporation of systematic sample designs and diverse test methodologies will continue to drive progress toward improved analytical and clinical assessments of more complex extract mixtures.

The pioneering studies of Esch[15] and Kordash[20] examined the properties of perennial ryegrass extracts mixed with a wide variety of allergenic products known or suspected to possess hydrolytic enzymes capable of altering protein structures and associated allergen activities. Both studies reported proteolytic enzyme activities of the companion extracts using chromogenic substrate (Azocoll) or casein gel digestion methods. Esch compared extracts prepared with multiple pollen, epithelia, insect, and fungal source materials and found protease concentrations ranging from less than 5 μg trypsin equivalent units per milliliter (eight pollens, three epithelia, one insect, three fungi) to more than 4000 units per milliliter (the fungus *Microsporum canis*). Extracts from one insect (American cockroach) and three other fungi (*Fusarium moniliforme, Aspergillus fumigatus*, and *Penicillium notatum*) possessed moderate protease levels between 150 and 250 trypsin equivalent units per milliliter.

Table 2
In vivo and in vitro analytical methods included in eight published studies on extract compatibility

References	Year	Target Extract	Analysis Method
Esch[15]	1991	Perennial ryegrass	IgE ELISA inhibition
			IgE SDS-PAGE immunoblotting
		Companion extracts	Protease assays
Kordash et al[20]	1993	Perennial ryegrass	$ID_{50}EAL$ quantitative intradermal skin testing
			IgE RAST inhibition
			SDS-PAGE
			HPLC
		Companion extracts	Protease casein gel clearing assays
Nelson et al[21]	1996	Timothy grass	IgE ELISA inhibition
		Bermuda grass	IgE ELISA inhibition
		Short ragweed	IgE ELISA inhibition
		White oak	IgE ELISA inhibition
		Box elder	IgE ELISA inhibition
		Russian thistle	IgE ELISA inhibition
		Cat	IgE ELISA inhibition
		D farinae	IgE ELISA inhibition
Hoff et al[22]	2002	Timothy grass	IgE, Phl p 1 mIgG, and Phl p 5 mIgG SDS-PAGE immunoblotting
			Rat basophil leukemia cell-mediator release assay
			SDS-PAGE
		Birch	IgE, Bet v 1 mIgG, and Bet v 2 mIgG SDS-PAGE immunoblotting
			Rat basophil leukemia cell-mediator release assay
			SDS-PAGE
		Fusarium culmorum	Gelatinase zymography and PepTag protease assay
Meier et al[23]	2006	Mountain cedar	SDS-PAGE
Grier et al[24]	2007	Meadow fescue grass	IgE ELISA inhibition
			IgE SDS-PAGE immunoblotting
		Short ragweed	Amb a 1 radial immunodiffusion
		Cat	Fel d 1 radial immunodiffusion
		D farinae	IgE ELISA inhibition
			IgE SDS-PAGE immunoblotting
Rans et al[25]	2009	Timothy grass	IgE ELISA inhibition
			IgE SDS-PAGE immunoblotting
			SDS-PAGE
		Short ragweed	Amb a 1 radial immunodiffusion
			SDS-PAGE
		Cat	Fel d 1 radial immunodiffusion
			SDS-PAGE
		D pteronyssinus	IgE ELISA inhibition
			SDS-PAGE
Grier et al[26]	2009	Dog epithelia	IgE ELISA inhibition
			IgE SDS-PAGE immunoblotting
			Dog albumin rIgG ELISA
		Dog hair/dander	IgE ELISA inhibition
			IgE SDS-PAGE immunoblotting
			Can f 1 mIgG/rIgG ELISA

Abbreviations: HPLC, high-performance liquid chromatography; $ID_{50}EAL$, Intradermal Dilution for 50 mm sum of Erythema diameters determines bioequivalent ALlergy units; mIgG, mouse immunoglobulin G; RAST, radioallergosorbent test; rIgG, rabbit immunoglobulin G; SDS-PAGE, sodium dodecyl sulfate polyacrylamide gel electrophoresis.

A direct correlation was observed between total protease levels and the reductions of IgE-binding potency of perennial rye extracts in mixtures with these fungal extracts after storage for 1 month at refrigeration temperatures (4°C).[15] Recoveries below 50% of ryegrass control (unmixed) were found in all mixtures containing fungal extracts with protease levels at or greater than 20 units per milliliter. Glycerin stabilized grass allergens mixed with fungal extracts at moderate protease levels but did not produce a substantial improvement in ryegrass potency after mixing with the protease-rich *M canis* extract. Changes in IgE binding to ryegrass allergens that had been mixed with several fungal extracts were also observed on sodium dodecyl sulfate polyacrylamide gel electrophoresis (SDS-PAGE) immunoblots (Western blots) at levels consistent with the protease activities of the fungal products.

Kordash and colleagues[20] studied the effects of fungal (*Helminthosporium interseminatum*), insect (cockroach mix), and dust mite (*D farinae*) extracts on perennial ryegrass allergens using a combination of in vitro and in vivo analyses. Consistent with the results of the Esch study,[15] companion extracts possessing relatively high proteolytic enzyme activities (fungal, insect) produced significant (10- to 40-fold) decreases in ryegrass extract potency determined using IgE radioallergosorbent test (RAST) inhibition assays and intradermal skin test titrations. Degradation of grass allergens with *Helminthosporium* extract was more pronounced at all time points tested with both methods compared with cockroach extract. High levels of glycerin (50% volume to volume [v:v]) improved ryegrass allergen recoveries in these mixtures relative to comparable formulations in HSA-saline diluent. Mixing with dust mite extract or a hickory extract control had no apparent effect on ryegrass extract potencies after storage for up to 90 days at 2°C to 4°C.

Inclusion of skin testing in extract compatibility studies is an attractive approach but presents numerous challenges. In the study by Kordash and colleagues,[20] subjects selected for testing with specific ryegrass extract mixtures were required to exhibit negative skin puncture tests for the various companion extracts to isolate reactions to grass allergens only. In relatively simple mixtures, enrolling subjects that meet these criteria is feasible, but in mixtures of increasing complexity or compositions with airborne allergens prevalent in many geographic regions, subjects with discrete sensitivities to only target extracts become more difficult to qualify. Differences in IgE specificities to allergens or distinct epitope regions recognized by these subjects could also impact the magnitude, consistency, or significance of test results. Collaborative investigations among scientists and clinicians proficient at prick and intradermal skin test procedures are needed to incorporate these important in vivo evaluations into future studies of extract stability and compatibility.

In 1996, Nelson and colleagues[21] examined the IgE-binding reactivities of various low-protease extracts (grass pollen, weed pollen, tree pollen, dust mite, or cat) after mixing with certain high-protease products (American cockroach, *Alternaria alternata*, *Cladosporium herbarum*, or *P notatum*). Two-component extract mixtures and target extract controls were prepared through adding 5 mL of glycerinated dust mite *D farinae* extract or 1 mL of aqueous (or lyophilized, reconstituted) low-protease extract concentrates to 1 mL of high-protease extracts, followed by dilution to a total volume of 10 mL with the same aqueous diluent (HSA-saline) used for reconstitution steps. The resulting solutions contained either 25% glycerin final concentrations (*D farinae*) or no glycerin.

After storage for 3 months at 4°C, samples were analyzed with ELISA inhibition using serum pools prepared from patients exhibiting strong positive skin test reactions to the target allergens. Significant levels of allergen degradation were observed in at least one mixture for all target allergens except *D farinae* and ragweed. *Alternaria* and American cockroach affected the highest number of allergens, whereas *Penicillium* and dust mite mix (*D farinae/D pteronyssinus*) had no significant impact on any allergens tested. Timothy grass and box elder allergens were compromised by individual fungal and cockroach extracts, with others degraded by fungi only (Bermuda grass, white oak, cat) or cockroach only (Russian thistle).

Allergic reactions to birch pollen or timothy grass pollen are prevalent in northern and central Europe, and are frequently included in immunotherapy vaccines for sensitive patients residing in these regions. Hoff and coworkers[22] at the Paul Ehrlich Institute in Germany assessed the compatibilities of low-protease, aqueous birch and timothy grass allergens with a protease-rich aqueous *F culmorum* extract after storage of product mixtures and controls for up to 60 days at 6°C. The protease content of the three extracts was confirmed with zymography (gelatinase activity) and chromogenic peptide hydrolysis (tryptic, chymotryptic and pepsin-like protease or peptidase activities). Rapid and complete degradation of birch or timothy extract reactivities by *Fusarium* extract components was shown using SDS-PAGE immunoblotting with target extract-specific IgE-positive human serum pools or monoclonal IgG antibodies recognizing prominent individual birch allergens (Bet v 1, Bet v 6) or timothy allergens (Phl p 1, Phl p 5). Mediator release assays using rat basophil leukemia cells also revealed time-dependent reductions of birch or timothy allergen activities after mixing with the *Fusarium* extract, with recoveries of approximately 25% and 4% of initial or control values, respectively, after 60 days at 6°C.

In certain areas of the United States, it is not unusual for unique combinations of allergens to comprise the dominant airborne sensitivities and desired extract mix formulations for immunotherapy. Imported fire ant stings are a major cause of allergic reactions in the southern United States, and mountain cedar pollinosis is also prevalent in several of these states, including Texas. Meier and colleagues[23] investigated the allergenic compatibility of extracts from these two sources using gel electrophoresis (SDS-PAGE) methods, with visualization of component protein bands by Coomassie blue dye staining. Aqueous extract mixtures stored for up to 180 days at 4°C displayed no apparent changes in band patterns or staining intensities during this period relative to analogous aqueous control extract samples. Although one mountain cedar and three fire ant bands were detected in these samples, the IgE-binding characteristics of these bands were not determined. The lack of apparent degradation of mountain cedar proteins by a whole-body fire ant extract supports combination of these products into a single immunotherapy vaccine for appropriate patients.

The high- and low-protease extracts included in the five studies summarized earlier[15,20–23] were typically obtained from a single licensed or non-licensed commercial source per study, which varied between investigators. In these studies, the stabilizing effects of glycerin were assessed at only one concentration (25% or 50%) above those usually found in most patient mixtures. In several investigations, the laboratory methods performed were different from those recognized and regulated by FDA for lot release, stability testing, and potency labeling of United States standardized extracts, with limited or no information available on the quantitative and qualitative relationships between differing analyses of similar or identical target extracts and mixtures.

In 2007, Grier and colleagues[24] incorporated licensed product lots from multiple United States manufacturers, variable glycerin concentrations for mixtures with single-extract controls at equivalent glycerin content, and quantitative compendial FDA potency methods in combination with qualitative allergen profiles to examine the compatibilities of low-protease standardized extracts (meadow fescue grass;

dust mite *D farinae* and *D pteronyssinus*; cat; short ragweed) with protease-rich non-standardized fungal and cockroach products. The IgE-binding potencies and banding patterns of meadow fescue grass allergens were not altered significantly in mixtures with dust mite products from five different commercial sources at two concentrations (1000 and 3000 AU/mL) within practice parameter guidelines for maintenance immunotherapy after storage for up to 12 months at 2°C to 8°C. When present in similar mixtures with fungal or cockroach extracts, grass allergens were highly susceptible to protease-related degradation under most conditions examined.

Among the 13 fungal extracts (24 product lots) combined with meadow fescue extract at 10% glycerin final concentrations, more than half of these products (and 75% of fungal product lots) produced rapid (1 month) and significant levels of grass allergen degradation (>50% reduction of control extract potency) at 2°C to 8°C. The lowest recoveries were associated with products derived from three of the most prevalent, allergenic, and clinically important mold species (*Penicillium*, *Aspergillus*, *Alternaria*). Comparable mixtures and controls at 10% and 50% glycerin levels prepared with these fungal extracts from three manufacturers possessed improved grass allergen compatibilities at 50% glycerin, with recoveries closely related to the compositions and protein concentrations of the fungal products.

The compatibilities of dust mite, cat, and short ragweed allergens mixed with *Alternaria*, *Aspergillus*, *Penicillium*, American cockroach, or German cockroach extracts were also examined. Dust mite *D farinae* allergen recoveries in most of these mixtures were relatively high when measured with one human serum pool but significantly lower when tested with a second pool. Differences in the IgE specificities of the two serum pools on immunoblots were consistent with the ELISA inhibition potency reductions observed using the second pool. If these analyses had been conducted with only one of the two serum pools, a different interpretation of the experimental results would likely have been reported. The importance of defining the essential properties of key assay reagents and understanding the consequences of variations in these characteristics on study outcomes cannot be understated. *Alternaria* and *Penicillium* extracts degraded short ragweed allergen Amb a 1 in 10% glycerin after 5 months at 2°C to 8°C, but higher glycerin levels (25%, 50%) afforded near-complete protection. Short ragweed allergen was stable after mixing with *Aspergillus*, American cockroach, or German cockroach extracts and stored at 2°C to 8°C. Cat allergen Fel d 1 was compatible with all companion fungal and insect extracts at 2°C to 8°C, even at minimal (10%) glycerin concentrations.

A follow-up to the Meier study reported by Rans[25] examined the compatibilities of fire ant extracts with standardized cat, ragweed, dust mite *D pteronyssinus*, and timothy grass products. In addition to SDS-PAGE, methods of analysis included the identical cat, ragweed, dust mite, and grass allergen potency tests described in the Grier study.[24] Timothy grass allergens were degraded rapidly (within 1 month) at 4°C by fire ant extract. Cat (Fel d 1), short ragweed (Amb a 1), and multiple *D pteronyssinus* allergens remained stable when mixed with fire ant extracts and stored for up to 6 months at 4°C.

Dog allergen stabilities in extract mixtures were assessed for the first time in 2009 by Grier and coworkers.[26] Clinically important and compositionally distinct dog epithelia and dog hair/dander extracts from different commercial sources were included in this investigation to reflect current use of both product types for allergen immunotherapy. Dog extracts were combined with high-protease fungal extracts (*Alternaria*, *Aspergillus*, or *Penicillium*) or insect products (American cockroach, German cockroach, or fire ant) and evaluated after storage for up to 12 to 15 months at 2°C to 8°C. Dog allergen recoveries in these mixtures were determined with IgE ELISA inhibition and immunoblotting using test samples and assay procedures analogous to those described in previous studies from this laboratory. Dog epithelia extracts retained moderate to high levels of IgE-binding potency (67%–113% of controls) in all mixtures at 10%, 25%, or 50% glycerin concentrations after storage for up to 13 months at 2°C to 8°C, comparable to recoveries observed for cat extracts under comparable mixing and incubation conditions.

Although partial degradation of intact (66 kDa) dog albumin structures was detected on immunoblots, productive IgE and anti-albumin IgG binding interactions were retained to some degree with these fragments. Dog hair/dander extracts exhibited lower recoveries of IgE ELISA inhibition activity in mixtures with *Aspergillus, Penicillium*, or *Alternaria* extracts at 10% or 25% glycerin (28%–61% of controls) after up to 15 months at 2°C to 8°C. Fungal extracts at 50% glycerin and all three insect extracts at 10%, 25%, or 50% glycerin had no appreciable impact on dog hair/dander allergens. IgE immunoblot profiles were consistent in most cases with ELISA inhibition potencies. Can f 1 ELISA reactivities of several dog hair/dander extract mixtures varied noticeably from those determined with ELISA inhibition. The largest discrepancies were observed for mixtures containing *Aspergillus* or *Penicillium* (2.5-fold higher Can f 1 recoveries) and American cockroach (2.3-fold higher ELISA inhibition recoveries). The nature of these differences remains to be determined but is believed to be related to variations in antibody specificity, allergen presentation, or both, in the antibody-detection (ELISA inhibition) and antibody-capture (Can f 1 ELISA) immunoassay formats. These data show the potential bias or preference that methods of this type can exhibit in analyses of heterogeneous extract mixtures, and shows the importance of evaluating multiple, diverse test methodologies whenever possible to provide critical and objective assessments of target allergen activities that can be compared and correlated with clinical outcomes.

In the eight compatibility investigations summarized,[15,20–26] extracts were combined to produce final product concentrations similar to those recommended in subcutaneous immunotherapy practice parameters for maintenance vial formulations (1:10 v:v dilutions of extract concentrates in most studies). These allergen concentrations also approximate the maximum tolerated dose levels for 0.5-mL injections in sensitive patients at allergy clinics in many regions of the United States.

Antibody-capture immunoassays such as ELISA inhibition are capable of quantifying allergen activities in mixtures diluted 10- to 100-fold higher than those reported in these studies, and are under investigation to document extract compatibilities at vial strengths used during the buildup or dose escalation phase of immunotherapy. Antibody-capture immunoassays exhibit a wide range of analytical sensitivities. Radial immunodiffusion assays offer very limited application to testing of extract mixtures diluted beyond the 10-fold dilutions of concentrates in the published studies. Two-site allergen-specific ELISA methods often exhibit dose–response characteristics suitable for detecting microgram levels of allergens at 1000-fold and higher dilutions of extract concentrates.

These methods and reagents were developed primarily for semiquantitative measurements of environmental allergens, and although their usefulness for extract compatibility studies seem significant, verification of the binding site specificities of these tests in relation to IgE-specific assays of the same allergens and their ability to detect comparable modified or denatured allergen structures is essential for them to be recognized and adopted as reliable indicators of extract stability. Improved availability of rare reagents and calibrated allergen standards currently used exclusively by selected laboratories is required to facilitate these critical evaluations and method comparisons. The long-term stability of these materials under appropriate storage conditions also must be evaluated, with precise limits established for validity and reproducibility.

Based on the results from the eight published studies, and extrapolations of these data to extract combinations from the same or closely related phylogenetic sources, a chart summarizing the mixing compatibilities of allergens from the major extract categories (excluding foods) was created (**Fig. 1**). Product combinations characterized as stable (green shading) have been shown to retain near-complete levels of target allergen activities ($\geq$70% recoveries compared with control samples) under refrigerated storage conditions (2°C–8°C, 36°F–46°F) at low (10%) glycerin concentrations. Mixtures represented as risky combinations (highlighted in yellow) were those exhibiting noticeable degradation of target allergens (50%–70% recoveries vs controls) during storage at 2°C to 8°C, which was prevented or improved substantially at higher (25%) glycerin levels. In unstable allergen combinations (shaded in red), target allergen potencies were not protected or stabilized under most conditions, and were often reduced significantly (<50% recoveries relative to controls) within 3 months when stored continuously at 2°C to 8°C. Clearly, the enzymatic activities that impact allergen stability and compatibility in the most significant manner are the endogenous proteases in fungal and insect extracts.

Among commercial extracts manufactured and licensed in the United States, all other product groups seem to contain much lower levels of active proteolytic enzymes. Based on the elevated levels of proteolytic enzymes in many fungal and insect extracts, physical separation of pollen, dust mite, and animal allergens from these protease-rich products in treatment mixtures has been recommended in previous and current immunotherapy practice parameter guidelines.[27,28] Some exceptions to this designation have been observed (meadow fescue grass mixed with several fungi, mountain cedar mixed with fire ant). Mountain cedar pollen proteins seem to lack the specific amino acid sequences required for recognition and catalysis by fire ant proteases. Reduced enzyme levels or activities in certain fungal products are likely responsible for the favorable grass allergen recoveries in these mixtures.

Proteins in many fungal extracts seem to be resistant to the action of endogenous proteases in these products. By comparison, cockroach extract proteases are capable of degrading prominent IgE-binding cockroach proteins in product solutions

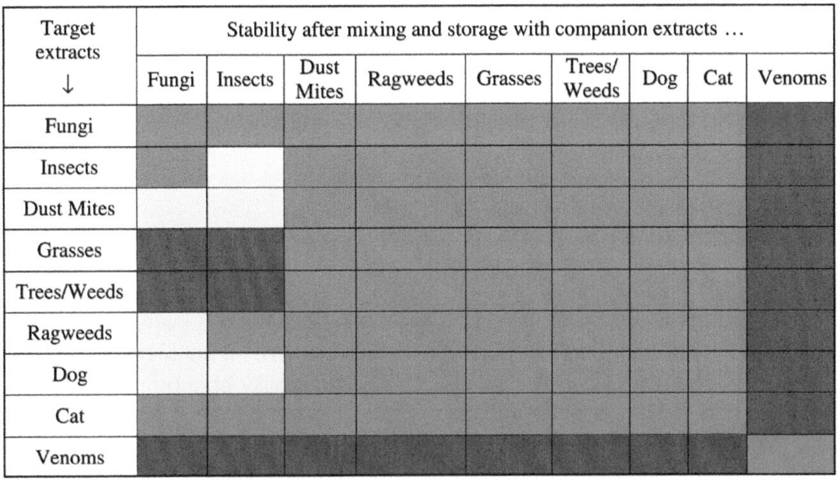

Target extracts ↓	Stability after mixing and storage with companion extracts …								
	Fungi	Insects	Dust Mites	Ragweeds	Grasses	Trees/Weeds	Dog	Cat	Venoms
Fungi									
Insects									
Dust Mites									
Grasses									
Trees/Weeds									
Ragweeds									
Dog									
Cat									
Venoms									

Fig. 1. Compatibility chart for subcutaneous allergen extract immunotherapy.

at reduced (10%–25%) glycerin levels stored at 2°C to 8°C. The compatibilities of high-protease extract mixtures (fungi with fungi, fungi with insects, insects with insects) are believed to be favorable but require further study to determine the actual recoveries of important allergens in these products when combined in specific mixtures at defined glycerin and HSA concentrations.

Regular, intermittent, or inadvertent exposures to ambient temperatures (20°C–25°C, 68°F–77°F) promote protease-catalyzed degradation events in extract mixtures, and can further reduce allergen recoveries in risky combinations to those categorized as unstable. Because glycerin typically provides concentration-dependent and time-dependent improvements in allergen stability for many risky or unstable mixtures, inclusion of higher glycerin levels or storage for shorter periods at 2°C to 8°C are options that some allergists have adopted to minimize the numbers of formulations and injections administered to certain patients. Hymenoptera venoms contain active hydrolytic enzymes, including proteases, but are usually formulated and injected separately from airborne or environmental allergens and are designated in red (not recommended) on **Fig. 1** for this reason.

SUMMARY

Considerable progress has been made over the past 20 years on the stability and mixing compatibility of allergenic extracts. Analysis of various allergens and mixtures has generated consistent results for similar or related products and established a solid foundation for future studies with new or more complex allergen combinations. Continued attention and efforts focused on improving the selectivity and robustness of immunochemical reagents and the characterization of calibrated universal standards will support validation of high-performance analytical methods. Collaborative investigations among clinicians, scientists, and extract manufacturers will ensure that appropriate extracts and methods are examined, that valid results are obtained and analyzed, and that correlations to clinical outcomes are reported. Incorporation of systematic approaches using matrix-based and higher-level (factorial) study designs will promote adoption of consistent acceptance criteria for stable, risky, and unstable allergen extract combinations in immunotherapy mixtures. Technological advances will continue to fuel development of robust immunochemical testing platforms and methodologies displaying subtle but meaningful differences in allergen-binding requirements.

REFERENCES

1. Esch RE. Allergen immunotherapy: what can and cannot be mixed? J Allergy Clin Immunol 2008;122:659–60.
2. Nelson HS. Specific immunotherapy with allergen mixes: what is the evidence? Curr Opin Allergy Clin Immunol 2009;9:549–53.
3. Arbesman CE, Eagle H. The thermolability of ragweed pollen extract and its corresponding regain. J Allergy 1939;11:18–27.
4. Hjorth N. Instability of grass pollen extracts. Acta Allergol 1958;12:316–35.
5. Center JG, Shuller N, Zelenick LD. Stability of antigen E in commercially prepared ragweed pollen extracts. J Allergy Clin Immunol 1974;54:305–10.
6. Baer H, Anderson MC, Hale R, et al. The heat stability of short ragweed pollen extract and the importance of individual allergens in skin reactivity. J Allergy Clin Immunol 1980;66:281–5.
7. Anderson MC, Baer H. Antigenic and allergenic changes during storage of a pollen extract. J Allergy Clin Immunol 1982;69:3–10.

8. Franklin RM, Baer H, Hooton ML, et al. The stability of short ragweed pollen extract as measured by skin test and antigen E. J Allergy Clin Immunol 1976;58:51–9.

9. Norman PS, Marsh DG. Human serum albumin and Tween 80 as stabilizers of allergen solutions. J Allergy Clin Immunol 1978;62:314–9.

10. Nelson HS. The effect of preservatives and dilution on the deterioration of Russian thistle (Salsola pestifer), a pollen extract. J Allergy Clin Immunol 1979;63:417–25.

11. Nelson HS. Effect of preservatives and conditions of storage on the potency of allergy extracts. J Allergy Clin Immunol 1981;67:64–9.

12. Hiatt CW, Baer H, Hooton ML. Kinetics of thermal decay of antigen E from short ragweed pollen. J Biol Stand 1977;5:39–44.

13. Baranuik JN, Esch RE, Buckley CE. Pollen grain chromatography: quantitation and biochemical analysis of ragweed pollen solutes. J Allergy Clin Immunol 1988;81:1126–34.

14. Bousquet J, Guerin B, Hewitt B, et al. Analysis of commercial pollen extracts by enzyme determination I. comparison of RAST-inhibition assay and enzyme titration for orchard grass, rye grass and short ragweed pollen extracts. Ann Allergy 1980;45:310–5.

15. Esch RE. Role of proteases on the stability of allergenic extracts. Arb Paul Ehrlich Inst Bundesamt Sera Impfstoffe Frankf A M 1992;85:171–9.

16. Esch RE. Evaluation of allergen vaccine potency. Curr Allergy Asthma Rep 2006; 6:402–6.

17. Grier TJ. Laboratory methods for allergen extract analysis and quality control. Clin Rev Allergy Immunol 2001;21:111–40.

18. Grier TJ, Hazelhurst DM, Duncan EA, et al. Major allergen measurements: sources of variability, validation, quality assurance, and utility for laboratories, manufacturers, and clinics. Allergy Asthma Proc 2002;23:125–31.

19. Morrow KS, Slater JE. Regulatory aspects of allergen vaccines in the US. Clin Rev Allergy Immunol 2001;21:141–52.

20. Kordash TR, Amend MJ, Williamson SL, et al. Effect of mixing allergenic extracts containing Helminthosporium, *D. farinae*, and cockroach with perennial ryegrass. Ann Allergy 1993;71:240–6.

21. Nelson HS, Ikle D, Buchmeier A. Studies on allergen extract stability: the effects of dilution and mixing. J Allergy Clin Immunol 1996;98:382–8.

22. Hoff M, Krail M, Kastner M, et al. *Fusarium culmorum* causes strong degradation of pollen allergens in extract mixtures. J Allergy Clin Immunol 2002;109:96–101.

23. Meier EA, Whisman BA, Rathkopf MM. Effect of imported fire ant extract on the degradation of mountain cedar pollen allergen. Ann Allergy Asthma Immunol 2006;96:30–2.

24. Grier TJ, LeFevre DM, Duncan EA, et al. Stability of standardized grass, dust mite, cat, and short ragweed allergens after mixing with mold or cockroach extracts. Ann Allergy Asthma Immunol 2007;99:151–60.

25. Rans TS, Hrabak TM, Whisman BA, et al. Compatibility of imported fire ant whole body extract with cat, ragweed, Dermatophagoides pteronyssinus, and timothy grass allergens. Ann Allergy Asthma Immunol 2009;102:57–61.

26. Grier TJ, LeFevre DM, Duncan EA, et al. Stability and mixing compatibility of dog epithelia and dog dander allergens. Ann Allergy Asthma Immunol 2009;103: 411–7.

27. Li JT, Lockey RF, Bernstein IL, et al. Allergen immunotherapy: a practice parameter. Ann Allergy Asthma Immunol 2003;90:1–40.

28. Cox LS, Li JT, Nelson HS, et al. Allergen immunotherapy: a practice parameter second update. J Allergy Clin Immunol 2007;120:S25–83.

Systemic Reactions to Subcutaneous Allergen Immunotherapy

David I. Bernstein, MD*, Tolly Epstein, MD, MS

KEYWORDS

- Subcutaneous immunotherapy • Systemic reactions
- Anaphylaxis

The prevalence of asthma and allergic rhinitis associated with aeroallergen sensitization have increased over the past 40 years, especially in "westernized" developed countries. Thus, much attention has been focused on treatment modalities that may prevent or mitigate clinical expression of severe allergic disorders including asthma.[1] One such therapy, subcutaneous allergen immunotherapy (SCIT), has been practiced for 100 years.[2] Placebo-controlled trials of seasonal allergic rhinitis (SAR) with single pollen allergens have demonstrated that SCIT is effective in reducing symptoms of SAR and in preventing seasonal allergic asthma in children with SAR.[3] Placebo-controlled trials with single allergens (ie, grass pollen, cat, and house dust mite) have also established the efficacy of SCIT in reducing symptoms of asthma due to aeroallergens.[4] SCIT with purified Hymenoptera venoms is effective in preventing anaphylaxis in patients with previous life-threatening systemic allergic reactions.[5] However, the clinical benefits of SCIT are tempered by risks of injection-related systemic reactions and life-threatening anaphylaxis.

In 1916, Robert Cooke reported that 3.5% of subcutaneous grass pollen injections were followed by systemic reactions. As early as 1932, 9 fatal reactions (FRs) after SCIT injections were reported in the United States, including one who failed to respond to epinephrine.[6] A review of fatal reactions to SCIT injections conducted in the United Kingdom identified 26 anaphylactic deaths occurring from 1957 to 1986, all of which occurred among allergic patients with asthma.[7] This report resulted in the institution of a mandatory 2-hour postinjection waiting period in Great Britain, virtually creating a moratorium on administration of SCIT for many years.

The authors have nothing to disclose.

Division of Immunology, Allergy and Rheumatology, University of Cincinnati College of Medicine, 231 Albert Sabin Way, Cincinnati, OH 45267-0563, USA

* Corresponding author.

E-mail address: bernstdd@uc.edu

Immunol Allergy Clin N Am 31 (2011) 241–249

doi:10.1016/j.iac.2011.02.007   immunology.theclinics.com

In the last 40 years, a series of surveys and descriptive studies have been conducted to define the incidence, prevalence, and factors contributing to injection-related fatal anaphylactic and near-fatal systemic reactions (SRs) in North America. Nearly all such information has been collected from retrospective surveys with the cooperation of practicing allergists in the United States, or reports from individual clinics.[8–10] Limitations of these retrospective studies include the potential for recall bias, lack of comparator populations, and low participation rates among groups of surveyed physicians. Therefore, data collected in this manner may underestimate the true incidence of fatal and near-fatal injection related to SRs and obviate the ability to define risk factors for severe SRs. Nevertheless, a national reporting program designed to capture adverse events related to SCIT does not exist and, if it did, would rely entirely on non-solicited voluntary reporting of events.

Three retrospective surveys have been performed to identify FRs, and one of these evaluated near-fatal reactions (NFRs) associated with SCIT injections.[11] In the first 2 surveys capturing FRs occurring between 1973 and 1989, members of the American Academy of Allergy Asthma and Immunology (AAAAI) were contacted to report FRs occurring after SCIT or skin testing in their practices as well as FRs in other clinical practices in their communities.[9,10] A third survey was conducted to capture events between 1990 and 2001.[8] Here, short surveys were sent to all physician members of the AAAAI to inquire about NFRs and FRs associated with either SCIT or skin testing. Physicians were contacted by email, fax, and phone to optimize response rates. Those who reported NFRs (n = 273) or FRs (n = 41) on the brief survey were contacted again to provide further details about the events in a longer itemized questionnaire. Completed questionnaires were returned for 68 NFRs and 17 FRs.[11] Subsequently, a longitudinal annual surveillance study of FRs and all SCIT-related SRs, cosponsored by the AAAAI and American College of Allergy Asthma and Immunology (ACAAI), was initiated in 2008.[12]

In this article, the authors review data derived from the aforementioned retrospective surveys and recently initiated longitudinal surveillance studies of SCIT reactions in clinical allergy practices.

FREQUENCIES OF FATAL SCIT REACTIONS IN NORTH AMERICA

There were 76 direct or indirect reports of FRs after SCIT injections occurring between 1973 and 2001.[13] In the survey conducted between 1985 and 1989, it was estimated that a FR occurred once in every 2 million injection visits and once in every 2.5 million injection visits from 1990 to 2001.[8,10] From 1985 to 2001, this averaged to 3 to 3.4 reported deaths per year. Of interest, these incidences were quite similar between surveys despite different methods used for estimating total numbers of injections administered. Subsequently, an additional 6 FRs were identified that had transpired during 2001 to 2007.[12] Based on data collected from the aforementioned longitudinal surveillance study of SRs, no additional FRs related to SCIT occurred between 2008 and 2010.

CLINICAL MANIFESTATIONS OF SCIT-ASSOCIATED FATAL AND NEAR-FATAL ANAPHYLACTIC REACTIONS

Amin and colleagues[11] reported results from a long questionnaire regarding details of NFRs and compared these findings with detailed reports of FRs occurring between 1990 and 2001. In this study, one NFR was estimated to occur in every million injections, or 4.7 NFRs per year. Long survey responses were available for 68 of 273 NFRs and 17 of 41 FRs. The clinical manifestations of FRs and NFRs reported in this survey are summarized in **Figs. 1** and **2**. A NFR was defined as respiratory compromise,

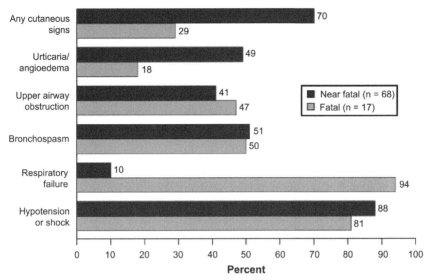

Fig. 1. Comparison of clinical features during FRs and NFRs. "Any cutaneous signs" refers to hives, angioedema, and/or pruritus. "Hypotension" refers to either transient or sustained decrease in blood pressure, and shock refers to cardiovascular collapse. (*From* Amin HS, Liss GM, Bernstein DI, et al. Evaluation of near-fatal reactions to allergen immunotherapy injections. J Allergy Clin Immunol 2006;117(1):169–75; with permission.)

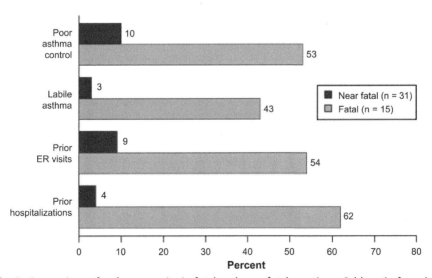

Fig. 2. Comparison of asthma severity in fatal and near-fatal reactions. Odds ratio for prior ER visits = 12.1 (95% confidence interval, 2.6–61.0; *P*<.001); odds ratio for prior hospitalizations = 34.7 (95% confidence interval, 5.7–251.1; *P*<.001). ER, emergency department. (*From* Amin HS, Liss GM, Bernstein DI, et al. Evaluation of near-fatal reactions to allergen immunotherapy injections. J Allergy Clin Immunol 2006;117(1):169–75; with permission.)

hypotension, or both, requiring emergency epinephrine treatment. Cutaneous manifestations were more frequently noted in patients experiencing NFRs than in patients succumbing to fatal SCIT reactions. It is possible that absence of skin eruptions in these cases delayed recognition and appropriate treatment of anaphylaxis. Hypotension or shock was reported in greater than 80% of FRs and NFRs. Respiratory failure occurred in 94% of FRs but in only 10% of NFRs. Compared with FRs, only a small minority of patients experiencing NFRs had severe or uncontrolled asthma (see **Fig. 2**).

FACTORS ASSOCIATED AND POTENTIALLY CONTRIBUTING TO FATAL AND NEAR-FATAL REACTIONS

In a review of 34 FRs from 1985 to 2001, associated and possible contributing factors included: uncontrolled asthma in 62% of cases; a prior history of SRs in 53%; administration of SCIT injections during peak pollen season in 47%; and delay in administration of epinephrine in 43%.[8,10] In the most recent retrospective survey, Bernstein and colleagues[8] reported that 15 of 17 fatal reactors had been previously diagnosed with asthma, whereas only 46% of nonfatal reactors had a previous diagnosis of asthma. Epinephrine was not administered to 3 patients with FRs. As shown in **Fig. 1**, features indicating uncontrolled asthma included a physician's report of labile asthma (43%), poor asthma control (53%), prior emergency department visits for acute asthma (54%), and prior asthma hospitalizations (62%). Other contributing factors identified were failure to observe the recommended postinjection waiting period and administration of injections in suboptimal settings for treatment of severe anaphylaxis (eg, at home). Bernstein and colleagues[8] reported that the majority of 17 FRs (59%) occurred after injections given from maintenance allergen vials, whereas the majority of FRs reported by Reid and colleagues[10] occurred after injections from buildup vials. Concurrent treatment with β-blockers was observed in 2% of fatal SCIT reactions, although the actual contribution of these drugs to fatal outcomes is unknown. No putative factor contributing to SCIT fatalities could be identified in 17% of the 34 FRs.

In the survey of NFRs occurring between 1990 and 2001, major contributing factors were administration of injections during a peak pollen season in 46% of respondents, and errors in dosing or administration of therapeutic allergens in 25%.[11] Other less commonly reported factors associated with NFRs included uncontrolled asthma, prior SRs to SCIT, and delay in administration of epinephrine. In a separate survey evaluating administration errors associated with SCIT, 58% of physicians reported incidents where patients received injections meant for another patient and 74% reported incorrect dosing errors.[14]

Recent anecdotal case reports suggest that coadministration of angiotensin-converting enzyme (ACE) inhibitors may enhance the severity of SRs after venom injections.[15] There is no evidence that concomitant ACE inhibitor treatment increases the overall risk for SRs to SCIT, however. Similarly, concomitant treatment with β-adrenergic blockers does not increase the risk for SRs to SCIT[16–18] β-Blockade is considered a risk factor for more protracted and difficult-to-treat postinjection anaphylaxis. This concern is based on descriptive studies showing that β-blockade enhances the risk for severe and difficult-to-treat anaphylactoid reactions after intravenous contrast media.[19] In other studies, use of rush immunotherapy or some cluster SCIT schedules are associated with a higher frequency of SRs when compared with a slower buildup protocols.[4]

Uncertainty exists about the potential risk posed by large local reactions. In general, large local reactions have not been shown to predict SRs, nor does adjustment of treatment allergen doses after large local reactions prevent subsequent SRs.[20] On the other hand, in a large retrospective study of patients receiving SCIT, patients experiencing SRs had a threefold greater likelihood of having experienced prior large local reactions when compared with patients without prior SRs.[21]

OVERALL INCIDENCE AND PREVALENCE OF SYSTEMIC REACTIONS AFTER SCIT INJECTIONS

There are reasonably good data defining national incidence and characteristics of fatal and life-threatening reactions with SCIT injections. In a recent review of the published literature, the prevalence of SRs was estimated at 2 in 1000 injections (0.2%) or 5% to 7% of treated patients.[4] Although initially thought to have a lower risk profile, SRs may be no less frequent with modified polymerized allergen extracts than with standard aqueous allergens.[22,23] As mentioned, cluster and rush schedules have been reported to result in greater frequencies of systemic reactions compared with slow buildup protocols.[24,25]

The aforementioned ACAAI/AAAAI Surveillance Study investigated the national annual prevalence of SRs of varying severity among practicing allergists. In a Web-based survey, practitioners administering SCIT were asked to report the numbers of nonfatal SRs in their entire practice during the previous 12 months and to assess severity based on a 3-grade classification system (**Box 1**). In this survey, SRs were categorized as: mild (Grade 1: cutaneous or upper respiratory symptoms); moderate (Grade 2: asthma with reduced lung function); or severe (Grade 3: life-threatening airway compromise or hypotension).

In year 1 of the surveillance program, 806 physicians (representing 1922 SCIT prescribers) reported on their experiences with SRs. SRs were reported in 82% of participating practices, for a total of 8502 SRs, which translated to an overall rate of 10.2 SRs per 10,000 injection visits or 0.1% of all injection visits.[12] By far, the vast majority were mild Grade 1 SRs (74%), whereas 23% were identified as Grade 2 SRs. Only 3% (n = 265) of all SRs were serious Grade 3 events. Although Grade 3 reactions occurred in only 3 out of every 100,000 injection visits or 0.003% of injection visits, 18% of practices reported experiencing at least one Grade 3 event between 2008 and 2009. It is remarkable that the relative proportions of Grade 1, 2, and 3 reactions in year 1 of the study were nearly identical to those subsequently reported in year 2 (data unpublished at the time of writing).

Box 1
North American Surveillance Study: classification system of SRs associated with SCIT

Grade 1—Mild systemic reactions: generalized urticaria or upper respiratory symptoms (eg, itching of the palate and throat, sneezing)

Grade 2—Moderate systemic reactions: asthma (eg, peak expiratory flow rate falls 20%–40%) with or without generalized urticaria, upper respiratory symptoms, or abdominal symptoms (nausea, cramping)

Grade 3—Severe, life-threatening anaphylaxis: severe airway compromise due to severe bronchospasm (eg, peak expiratory flow rate falls >40%), or upper airway obstruction with stridor or hypotension (with or without loss of consciousness)

From Bernstein DI, Epstein T, Murphy-Berendts K, et al. Surveillance of systemic reactions to subcutaneous immunotherapy injections: year 1 outcomes of the ACAAI and AAAAI collaborative study. Ann Allergy Asthma Immunol 2010;104(6):530–5; with permission.

A follow-up Web-based questionnaire survey was conducted in a subset of physician respondents to investigate possible differences in standard SCIT practices between clinics reporting severe Grade 3 reactions and clinics reporting exclusively mild Grade 1 SRs.[26] The questionnaire evaluated: criteria for selection of asthmatic patients for SCIT; adjustment of SCIT during peak allergy seasons; adjustment of treatment allergen doses after large local reactions or SRs; customary postinjection observation periods; routine preinjection screening of asthmatics for level of asthma control; use of prediluted patient-specific vials versus sharing of common vials for multiple patients; routine premedication with antihistamines; and routine prescription of self-administered epinephrine in patients on SCIT.

Significant differences in clinical practices related to SCIT between 35 clinics with Grade 3 SRs and 39 clinics reporting only Grade 1 SRs are shown in **Table 1**. Physicians working in clinics experiencing a Grade 3 reaction within the past year were more likely to prescribe patients receiving SCIT epinephrine kits for self-administration, check patient identifiers prior to injection to prevent injection errors via misidentification, and prescribe routine preinjection treatment with H1 blockers. It is probable that practices who had previously experienced severe SRs adopted these strategies to minimize the risk of future severe reactions. In addition, those practices experiencing Grade 3 anaphylactic reactions were more frequently prescribed higher maintenance doses of house dust mite than those clinics reporting Grade 1 SRs.

Table 1
Summary of survey questions showing significant differences in responses (always, often, sometimes, or never) between a subset of allergy practices reporting severe grade 3 SRs and a subset reporting only mild grade 1 SRs after SCIT injections during 2007 and 2008 (n, percentage given in parentheses)

Question	Severity of Reported SRs	Always	Often	Sometimes	Never	P Value
Are patients asked to provide identifiers prior to immunotherapy?	Grade 1	22 (56.4)	0	2 (5.1)	15 (38.5)	.0094
	Grade 3	22 (62.9)	4 (11.4)	5 (14.3)	4 (11.4)	—
Are asthmatics prescribed epinephrine for self-administration?	Grade 1	5 (12.8)	2 (5.1)	20 (51.3)	12 (30.8)	.0062
	Grade 3	12 (34.3)	1 (2.9)	21 (60)	1 (2.9)	—
Are patients routinely instructed to premedicate with antihistamines and/or antiallergic drugs prior to immunotherapy?	Grade 1	3 (7.7)	5 (12.8)	22 (56.4)	9 (23.1)	.011
	Grade 3	8 (22.9)	10 (28.6)	16 (45.7)	1 (2.9)	—
Are patients on SCIT prescribed epinephrine and instructed on self-administration?	Grade 1	5 (12.8)	2 (5.1)	21 (53.9)	11 (28.2)	.0258
	Grade 3	12 (34.3)	1 (2.9)	20 (57.1)	2 (5.7)	—
Are patients with prior SCIT systemic reactions prescribed epinephrine and instructed on self-administration?	Grade 1	14 (35.9)	8 (20.5)	10 (25.6)	7 (18.0)	.042
	Grade 3	20 (57.1)	6 (17.1)	9 (25.7)	0	—

Data from Liss GM, Murphy-Berendts K, Epstein T, et al. Factors associated with severe versus mild immunotherapy-related systemic reactions: a case-referent study. J Allergy Clin Immunol 2011. [Epub ahead of print].

TIME OF ONSET OF SYSTEMIC REACTIONS AND DELAYED-ONSET REACTIONS

Delayed-onset FRs have been documented in the aforementioned retrospective SCIT fatality surveys. Combined data from 58 fatal SCIT reactions from 1983 to 2001, indicate that 10% of FRs began 30 to 60 minutes after administration of SCIT injections.[8–10] By contrast, only 4% of NFRs were reported to begin later than 30 minutes after injections.[11]

Previous estimates of delayed-onset injection–related SRs (later than 30 minutes) of all severity grades range between 27–50%,[18,27–31] and most are described as mild and non–life-threatening. These high estimates of delayed-onset reactions do not match the experience of many practicing allergists. In year 2 of the North American Surveillance Study, time of onset of SRs following injections was assessed, as was administration of epinephrine.[32] Of the 35% of respondents providing data regarding the time of onset of reactions, 2117 reported SRs; 71% were mild Grade 1, 25% Grade 2, and only 3% were classified as Grade 3 SRs. Of all reported SRs, 14% began at least 30 minutes after injections. Of note, 13% of severe Grade 3 reactions were delayed-onset SRs. Epinephrine was administered to most (77%) but not all SRs beginning within the recommended 30-minute postinjection waiting period, including 71% of Grade 1, 93% of Grade 2, and 94% of Grade 3 SRs. As expected, epinephrine was not administered for delayed-onset SRs as frequently as for more immediate-onset SRs. For delayed-onset SRs, epinephrine was given for only 60% of all reported delayed-onset SRs (N = 289) including 56% of Grade 1 LRs and 67% of Grade 2 LRs, and in 9 of 9 (100%) Grade 3 LRs.

SUMMARY: LESSONS LEARNED

Despite the descriptive nature of the data collected, much has been learned from the retrospective surveys of fatal and near-fatal SCIT reactions. Recent data from the ACAAI/AAAAI Surveillance Study indicates that the overall incidence of delayed-onset SRs is much less frequent than previously reported (ie, 14%), that most are not severe, and that nearly all anaphylactic reactions occur within the first 30 minutes after injections. Retrospective surveys conducted in the United States have identified consistent risk factors for postinjection anaphylaxis. This information has directly shaped recently published practice guidelines. Such recommendations have been updated in 3 iterations of the Allergen Immunotherapy Practice Parameters, the most recent third update of this document being published in 2011 (following 2003 and 2007).[33–35] With regard to improving safety of SCIT, these parameters provide specific guidance for:

1. Identifying and monitoring high-risk patients (eg, uncontrolled asthmatics) receiving allergen immunotherapy
2. Considering individual patient risk factors in the decision to recommend allergen immunotherapy
3. Preventing errors in administration
4. Assuring optimal management of anaphylaxis including postinjection observation for at least 30 minutes and epinephrine treatment
5. Considering risk/benefit of concomitant use of β-blockers in patients receiving allergen immunotherapy
6. Managing patients experiencing late-onset SRs and biphasic reactions.

Based on data collected over the previous 2 years from the ACAAI/AAAAI Surveillance Study, no new FRs have been reported. This favorable trend may be attributable in part to heightened awareness of clinical allergists of risk factors for life-threatening

SRs combined with recent implementation of risk management strategies surrounding administration of SCIT.

REFERENCES

1. Abramson MJ, Puy RM, Weiner JM, et al. Injection allergen immunotherapy for asthma. Cochrane Database Syst Rev 2010;(8):CD001186.
2. Durham SR, Leung DY. One hundred years of allergen immunotherapy: time to ring the changes. J Allergy Clin Immunol 2011;127(1):3–7.
3. Moller C, Dreborg S, Ferdousi HA, et al. Pollen immunotherapy reduces the development of asthma in children with seasonal rhinoconjunctivitis (the PAT-study). J Allergy Clin Immunol 2002;109(2):251–6.
4. Cox L, Nelson H, Calabria C, et al. Allergen immunotherapy: a practice parameter third update. J Allergy Clin Immunol 2011;127(Suppl 1):S1–55.
5. Moffitt JE, Golden DB, Reisman RE, et al. Stinging insect hypersensitivity: a practice parameter update. J Allergy Clin Immunol 2004;114(4):869–86.
6. Rezvani M, Bernstein DI. Anaphylactic reactions during immunotherapy. Immunol Allergy Clin North Am 2007;27(2):295–307, viii.
7. Frew AJ. Injection immunotherapy. British Society for Allergy and Clinical Immunology Working Party. BMJ 1993;307(6909):919–23.
8. Bernstein DI, Wanner M, Borish L, et al. Twelve-year survey of fatal reactions to allergen injections and skin testing: 1990-2001. J Allergy Clin Immunol 2004; 113(6):1129–36.
9. Lockey RF, Benedict LM, Turkeltaub PC, et al. Fatalities from immunotherapy (IT) and skin testing (ST). J Allergy Clin Immunol 1987;79(4):660–77.
10. Reid MJ, Lockey RF, Turkeltaub PC, et al. Survey of fatalities from skin testing and immunotherapy 1985-1989. J Allergy Clin Immunol 1993;92(1 Pt 1):6–15.
11. Amin HS, Liss GM, Bernstein DI, et al. Evaluation of near-fatal reactions to allergen immunotherapy injections. J Allergy Clin Immunol 2006;117(1):169–75.
12. Bernstein DI, Epstein T, Murphy-Berendts K, et al. Surveillance of systemic reactions to subcutaneous immunotherapy injections: year 1 outcomes of the ACAAI and AAAAI collaborative study. Ann Allergy Asthma Immunol 2010;104(6):530–5.
13. Lockey RF, Nicoara-Kasti GL, Theodoropoulos DS, et al. Systemic reactions and fatalities associated with allergen immunotherapy. Ann Allergy Asthma Immunol 2001;87(1 Suppl 1):47–55.
14. Aaronson DW, Gandhi TK. Incorrect allergy injections: allergists' experiences and recommendations for prevention. J Allergy Clin Immunol 2004;113(6):1117–21.
15. Stumpf JL, Shehab N, Patel AC, et al. Safety of Angiotensin-converting enzyme inhibitors in patients with insect venom allergies. Ann Pharmacother 2006; 40(4):699–703.
16. Hepner MJ, Ownby DR, Anderson JA, et al. Risk of systemic reactions in patients taking beta-blocker drugs receiving allergen immunotherapy injections. J Allergy Clin Immunol 1990;86(3 Pt 1):407–11.
17. Muller UR, Haeberli G. Use of beta-blockers during immunotherapy for Hymenoptera venom allergy. J Allergy Clin Immunol 2005;115(3):606–10.
18. Rank MA, Oslie CL, Krogman JL, et al. Allergen immunotherapy safety: characterizing systemic reactions and identifying risk factors. Allergy Asthma Proc 2008; 29(4):400–5.
19. Lang DM, Alpern MB, Visintainer PF, et al. Elevated risk of anaphylactoid reaction from radiographic contrast media is associated with both beta-blocker exposure and cardiovascular disorders. Arch Intern Med 1993;153(17):2033–40.

20. Tankersley MS, Butler KK, Butler WK, et al. Local reactions during allergen immunotherapy do not require dose adjustment. J Allergy Clin Immunol 2000;106(5): 840–3.
21. Roy SR, Sigmon JR, Olivier J, et al. Increased frequency of large local reactions among systemic reactors during subcutaneous allergen immunotherapy. Ann Allergy Asthma Immunol 2007;99(1):82–6.
22. Casanovas M, Martin R, Jiménez C, et al. Safety of immunotherapy with therapeutic vaccines containing depigmented and polymerized allergen extracts. Clin Exp Allergy 2007;37(3):434–40.
23. Grammer LC, Shaughnessy MA, Finkle SM, et al. A double-blind histamine placebo-controlled trial of polymerized whole grass for immunotherapy of grass allergy. J Allergy Clin Immunol 1983;72(5 Pt 1):448–53.
24. Cox L. Allergen immunotherapy: immunomodulatory treatment for allergic diseases. Expert Rev Clin Immunol 2006;2(4):533–46.
25. Dursun AB, Sin BA, Oner F, et al. The safety of allergen immunotherapy (IT) in Turkey. J Investig Allergol Clin Immunol 2006;16(2):123–8.
26. Liss GM, Murphy-Berendts K, Epstein T, et al. Factors associated with severe versus mild immunotherapy-related systemic reactions: a case-referent study. J Allergy Clin Immunol 2011. [Epub ahead of print].
27. Matloff SM, Bailit IW, Parks P, et al. Systemic reactions to immunotherapy. Allergy Proc 1993;14:347–50.
28. Ragusa VF, Massolo A. Non-fatal systemic reactions to subcutaneous immunotherapy: a 20-year experience comparison of two 10-year periods. Eur Ann Allergy Clin Immunol 2004;36:52–5.
29. Winther L, Arnved J, Malling HJ, et al. Side-effects of allergen-specific immunotherapy: a prospective multi-centre study. Clin Exp Allergy 2006;36:254–60.
30. Gastaminza G, Algorta J, Audicana M, et al. Systemic reactions to immunotherapy: influence of composition and manufacturer. Clin Exp Allergy 2003;33: 470–4.
31. Lin MS, Tanner E, Lynn J, et al. Nonfatal systemic allergic reactions induced by skin testing and immunotherapy. Ann Allergy 1993;71:557–62.
32. Epstein T, Bernstein DI, Murphy K, et al. AAAAI/ACAAI Surveillance Study of subcutaneousimmunotherapy (SCIT) injections (year 2): time of onset and treatment of systemicreactions (SRs) [abstract]. J Allergy Clin Immunol 2011;127(2 Suppl): AB218.
33. Joint Task Force on Practice Parameters. Allergen immunotherapy: a practice parameter. American Academy of Allergy, Asthma and Immunology. American College of Allergy, Asthma and Immunology. Ann Allergy Asthma Immunol 2003;90(1 Suppl 1):1–40.
34. Joint Task Force on Practice Parameters; American Academy of Allergy, Asthma and Immunology; American College of Allergy, Asthma and Immunology; et al. Allergen immunotherapy: a practice parameter, second update. J Allergy Clin Immunol 2007;120(Suppl 3):S25–85.
35. Cox L, Nelson H, Lockey R, et al. Allergen immunotherapy: a practice parameter, third update. J Allergy Clin Immunol 2011;127:51–5.

Accelerated Immunotherapy Schedules and Premedication

Christopher W. Calabria, MD[a],*, Linda Cox, MD[b]

KEYWORDS

- Accelerated immunotherapy • Subcutaneous immunotherapy
- Schedule • Premedication

Subcutaneous immunotherapy is divided into 2 phases: a buildup and a maintenance phase. With conventional immunotherapy schedules, the buildup phase generally involves 1 to 2 injections per week with a single injection given each visit. The duration of the buildup phase varies but typically ranges from 3 to 8 months.

Accelerated immunotherapy buildup schedules allow the patient to achieve the benefits of immunotherapy more rapidly, because the maintenance dose is reached in a shorter time period. It has the advantage of a reduced number of office visits, saving the patient time and increasing convenience. Rush and cluster immunotherapy schedules are the 2 most common accelerated schedules used in the United States. A cluster immunotherapy schedule involves the patient receiving several allergen injections (generally 2–4) sequentially in a single day of treatment on nonconsecutive days. The maintenance dose is generally reached in 4 to 8 weeks. In rush immunotherapy (RIT) protocols, higher doses are administered at intervals of 15 to 60 minutes in a period of 1 to 3 days until the maintenance dose is achieved.

CLUSTER SCHEDULES
Efficacy and Safety

Controlled studies have shown symptomatic improvement and immunologic changes shortly after reaching maintenance doses by using cluster schedules.[1–4] Although several studies have found similar systemic reaction (SR) rates between cluster and conventional immunotherapy schedules,[1–6] others have noted an increased frequency of SR.[7–9] A randomized, double-blind, placebo-controlled study of cat-allergic subjects showed symptomatic improvement in as little as 5 weeks (on reaching

[a] ENTAA Care, PA, 203 Hospital Drive Suite 200, Glen Burnie, MD 21061, USA
[b] 5333 North Dixie Highway, Suite 210, Fort Lauderdale, FL 33334, USA
* Corresponding author.
E-mail address: chriscalabs@aol.com

Immunol Allergy Clin N Am 31 (2011) 251–263
doi:10.1016/j.iac.2011.02.001   **immunology.theclinics.com**

maintenance) using an 8-visit cluster schedule for a 4-week period.[1] Response to titrated nasal challenge, skin prick testing, and allergen-specific immunoglobulin G4 (IgG4) at 5 weeks was predictive of the response at 1 year. Although not specifically designed as a safety study, there was 1 mild SR (pruritus) among the 26 subjects (4%).

A controlled study of 239 dust mite–allergic patients with or without asthma compared the safety and efficacy of a 6-week cluster schedule compared with a 12-week conventional schedule.[2] They showed improved clinical and objective parameters in the sixth week using the cluster schedule, 6 weeks earlier than the conventional schedule. There were no differences in SRs between the treatment groups (0.15% of injections in cluster group vs 0.31% of injections in conventional). A prospective randomized study involving 96 patients with dust mite allergy randomized subjects to receive either cluster or conventional immunotherapy.[5] The 6-week cluster schedule reduced the time to reach maintenance by 57% and had similar SR rates (1.0% of injections, 6.7% of patients) to the conventional schedule.

Similarly, a randomized, double-blind, placebo-controlled trial of 18 grass-allergic subjects showed that immunologic changes seem to occur early and at low doses in the active treatment group, with an increase in interleukin-10 at 2 to 4 weeks that was associated with inhibition of the late-phase skin test response.[3]

In a retrospective observational multicenter study of 1147 patients undergoing cluster immunotherapy to a variety of inhalant allergens; 39 patients (3.4%) experienced 42 SRs (0.6% of injections). Most SRs were grade 0, 1, and 2; there were no cases of shock. Higher starting doses were associated with a higher risk of SR. The investigators concluded that cluster SR rates were similar to conventional SR rates.[4]

A retrospective evaluation of 94 children receiving *Alternaria alternata* immunotherapy by either a cluster (55%) or conventional (45%) schedule revealed similar SR rates between the 2 regimens (5.8% of cluster patients vs 4.8% conventional).[6]

In contrast, several studies using cluster schedules have noted higher SRs.[7–9] Nielsen and colleagues[7] and Winther and colleagues[8] both noted higher SR rates in cluster regimens in birch and grass-allergic patients. Nielsen and colleagues[7] noted that 33% of patients (7/21) experienced SR in the antihistamine premedication group versus 79% of patients in the placebo premedicated group. Winther and colleagues[8] observed an increased SR rate during birch and grass cluster immunotherapy with the highest rates in the grass-allergic subjects. Overall, SR occurred after 0.7% of birch injections and 3.3% of grass injections (P<.0001), with more episodes of urticaria and asthma in the grass-allergic subjects. Mellerup and colleagues[9] noted a 4.4% SR rate per injection (39.1% of patients) among 657 subjects (10,369 injections) undergoing cluster to a variety of allergens; 93% of SR were mild, with cat and dust mite having the highest frequency of severe side effects.

Overall, cluster SR rates have ranged from 0.15% to 3.3% of injections and 3% to 50% of patients.[10] To provide perspective, a review of 38 studies using conventional buildup schedules found the SR rate to be between 0.05% and 3.2% of injections and 0.8% and 46.7% of patients (mean 12.92%).[11] In a review of cluster immunotherapy analyzing 29 studies, the investigators concluded that it was difficult to compare many aspects of the studies because 20 were not designed to specifically study cluster safety.[12] This review suggested that the optimal tolerance of cluster schedules was associated with[1] use of premedication (antihistamine),[2] use of depot preparation,[3] no more than 4 injections per cluster,[4] use of 4 to 6 clusters,[5] 1 to 2 clusters per week. The investigators suggested the twice-a-week cluster might be associated with less adverse effects based on 2 separate grass pollen cluster studies with virtually identical protocols except for the cluster frequency. The SR rate was 18% of premedicated patients in the twice-a-week cluster[13] and 33% with premedication/79%

without premedication in the once-a-week cluster.[7] No other studies have compared the safety of 1 versus multiple clusters per week.

Overall, cluster schedules show earlier onset of symptomatic improvement with similar or slightly increased risk of generally mild SR compared with conventional schedules, and may provide a balance between convenience and safety.

RUSH SCHEDULES

Rush schedules are more rapid than cluster immunotherapy. The inherent advantage is that the maintenance dose is achieved with fewer visits in a shorter time period, with the disadvantage being an increased risk of local and SRs, particularly for inhalant allergens. The most accelerated schedule for inhalant allergens entails the administration of 7 injections in 4 hours. Ultrarush stinging insect protocols achieve the maintenance dose in 2.5 to 4 hours.

The SR rates with RIT schedules range from 15% to 100% of patients without premedication to 3% to 79% of patients with premedication, as reported in a recent review.[10] Most reactions are not severe, with flushing being the most common systemic symptom.[14] SRs may occur up to 2 hours after the final injection, necessitating a longer waiting period than the usual 30 minutes for conventional schedules (ie, 1.5–3 hours).

Although SR rates are high in inhalant allergy protocols and seem to be decreased with premedication,[15] flying Hymenoptera rush protocols have generally not been associated with a high SR incidence.[16–19] There have been conflicting data on the frequency of SR in imported fire ant (IFR) rush protocols.[20,21] Selected RIT studies are detailed in this article by type of allergen.

Dust Mite

A study of 125 dust mite–allergic asthmatics aged 4 to 57 years (mean 25.3 ± 11.2 years) using a 3-day RIT protocol with a target dose of 4 μg of Der p 1 (3000 BU) in patients older than 10 years and 2 μg Der p 1 (1500 BU) in those younger than 10 years resulted in an overall SR rate of 4.16% per injection.[22] All SR occurred within 45 minutes after the last injection. Forty-three patients (34.4%) had severe SRs that required epinephrine or asthma treatment. Most asthmatic reactions occurred at 1200 and 1800 BU, whereas anaphylaxis occurred between 600 and 2400 BU. The 2 predictors for SRs were skin prick test end point titration ($P<.15$) and FEV_1 before RIT ($P<.001$). If patients with an FEV_1 of less than 80% had been excluded from the study, the SR rate would have decreased to 19.7% of patients (from 34.4%). Asthmatic reactions occurred in 73.3% of patients with an FEV_1 less than 80%, but only 12.6% of patients with an FEV_1 greater than 80% ($P<.0001$).

Pollen

Several pollen RIT studies have been published to include olive,[23] plane tree,[23] Parietaria,[23] Bermuda grass,[24] orchard grass,[25,26] mixed grasses,[25,26] timothy grass,[27] and ragweed.[28] These studies have used standardized extracts,[23–29] allergoids,[25,26,30] and depot preparations.[31,32] SR rates have ranged from 2.6% to 36.8% (allergoid group) of patients.

In an open, longitudinal study of 30 patients investigating the efficacy of a 1-week (3 injections per day) RIT protocol with standardized birch pollen or timothy pollen extracts without premedication, 13% (4/30) experienced SRs (3 urticaria, 1 asthma symptoms).[27] Specific immunoglobulin G (IgG) and IgG4 increased continuously after the first week, and the RIT group had improved symptom and medication scores during the first pollen season compared with the control group. In a double-blind, placebo-controlled study comparing the safety of standardized orchard grass extract with a grass pollen allergoid, 20% of patients receiving the standardized extract experienced an SR versus 36.8% of patients treated with allergoid. However, the SRs with the standardized extract were more severe.[26]

Mold

There has been 1 double-blind, placebo-controlled RIT study with an *Alternaria* extract standardized by skin tests, laboratory assays, and major allergen Alt a 1.[33] Twenty-four patients aged 5 to 56 years were administered a 7-injection, 2-day RIT protocol without premedication in the hospital. All patients reached the target maintenance dose of 1.6 μg Alt a 1 (2000 BU). Fifteen percent (2/13) of actively treated patients had an SR on the first day (asthma symptoms). At 1 year, the actively treated group had improvement in global symptom scores ($P<.001$), titrated skin prick tests ($P<.005$), nasal challenge ($P<.005$), and specific IgG ($P<.05$) compared with the placebo group.

Animal

Several RIT protocols have been published to treat patients allergic to cat and dog.[34–37] In a double-blind, placebo-controlled study, 39 children and adults allergic to cat and/or dog were treated with an RIT protocol of 1 to 2 weeks and followed for 24 months.[37] The target maintenance dose was 80,000 subcutaneously (43 pg Fel d 1). After reaching maintenance they were switched to a depot extract (Alutard SQ). All children developed mild SR during RIT at doses ranging from 1000 to 10,000 subcutaneously. The overall RIT SR rate was 7.7% per injection (44/557). The adult SR was 4% per injection during buildup and maintenance combined (18/443). The treatment group had significant changes compared with placebo after 12 and 24 months in skin prick end point titration ($P<.001$), cat allergen bronchoprovocation ($P<.001$), histamine provocation ($P<.01$), and specific immunoglobulin E and IgG4 ($P<.001$).

Inhalant Allergen Mixtures

A series of RIT studies reported the experience at a university hospital-based pediatric clinic with a 1-day and 2-day RIT protocol with and without premedication using mixtures of allergens.[15,38,39] In the initial study, 11 patients aged 5 to 18 years (4 of whom had steroid-dependent asthma) underwent a 9-injection, 2-day RIT protocol without premedication.[38] The target dose was 0.1 mL of 1:100 wt/vol (maintenance concentrate) of a nonstandardized mixture and 1500 to 2400 AU/mL for dust mites. All patients completed the RIT except 1 who experienced hypotension and respiratory distress. Fifty-five percent (6/11) of patients had SRs. Three patients had grade 3 reactions (generalized pruritus, sneezing, and mouth itchiness), 3 patients had grade 4 reactions (wheezing and shortness of breath), and 1 had anaphylaxis. The severity of SR correlated with number of positive skin tests ($r = 0.60$, $P<.01$) and cumulative size of skin test reactions ($r = 0.75$, $P<.01$). Subsequent RIT studies by the same group showed lower SR rates using premedication and are detailed later.[15,39]

Flying Hymenoptera

Many venom RIT studies have been published, and most have shown efficacy and safety comparable with or superior to conventional schedules. Venom extract package inserts provide a cluster schedule as an example of a recommended schedule. In a 3-day RIT protocol of 9 patients at high-risk who had prior SRs during conventional buildup, 6 were able to reach maintenance in 3 days (despite mild cutaneous SRs), 2 reached maintenance in 5 days, and 1 patient had anaphylaxis and discontinued treatment.[18] The patients had intravenous lines, and it was unclear whether they received premedication. In a study of 101 venom-allergic patients at high-risk treated with a 4-day RIT protocol, 99% were able to reach the maintenance dose with an SR rate of 6.9% (8 SRs in 7 patients).[40] The patients were hospitalized and premedicated with dimethindene maleate (first-generation H1-receptor antagonist). Fifty-seven patients underwent an ultrarush desensitization in 2.5 hours reaching a cumulative dose of 101.1 µg of Hymenoptera venom.[19] Four patients (4/57, 7%) had mild SRs that were treated with antihistamines and corticosteroids. Only 1 patient did not complete the protocol because of an unrelated hypertensive crisis. Venom-specific IgG4 increased significantly after 15 days ($P<.01$) and remained higher at 1 year ($P<.001$).

IFA

An initial prospective controlled 2-day rush protocol suggested no significant difference between the premedicated and placebo-treated patients (3.6% vs 6.7%),[20] whereas a more recent prospective 1-day rush protocol at the same center found a higher SR rate (24%) without premedication.[21]

PREMEDICATION
Weekly Conventional Immunotherapy

There has been theoretic concern that antihistamines may mask the early signs or symptoms of an SR if taken before a conventional buildup immunotherapy injection. However, in a post hoc analysis of the effect of omalizumab on the tolerability of cluster immunotherapy in patients with moderate-to-severe asthma, there was a similar incidence of SRs in those who received antihistamine premedication and those who did not; however, antihistamine use was based on physician discretion and was not randomized.[41] In addition, 1 randomized controlled study showed that antihistamine premedication reduced the frequency of severe systemic reactions (0% fexofenadine group vs 9% control group) caused by conventional immunotherapy and increased the proportion of patients who achieved the maintenance dose in the cedar pollen group (97% vs 83%).[42] The effect of oral antihistamines on large local reactions (LLRs) in this study was not reported.

No other study has reported the effect of antihistamines on LLRs or SRs during conventional buildup or maintenance injections with inhalant allergens. For conventional venom immunotherapy (VIT), pretreatment with antihistamines did not reduce LLR rates during conventional monthly maintenance injections after they decreased LLRs during the initial rush portion of the protocol.[43]

Because many immunotherapy patients take antihistamines as part of their overall allergy management, it is important to determine whether they have taken it on the day of their allergy injection. It might also be reasonable to recommend that they either consistently take their antihistamine or avoid it on the days of their immunotherapy.

Premedication and accelerated immunotherapy schedules
Oral antihistamines for VIT Oral antihistamines have been effective in decreasing local and systemic reactions during rush VIT protocols.[43] Although rush VIT SRs are generally low, some rush VIT studies have shown that antihistamines decrease the SR frequency compared with placebo.[44] Antihistamines also decreased the LLR frequency during the first 4 weeks compared with placebo, although the addition of ranitidine to terfenadine did not provide additional benefit compared with terfenadine alone.[44] Two additional rush VIT studies showed that antihistamine pretreatment

decreased LLRs and cutaneous systemic symptoms of pruritus, urticaria, and angioedema but did not decrease the frequency of respiratory, cardiovascular, or gastrointestinal reactions.[43,45]

A retrospective study reported that terfenadine premedication during rush VIT might improve efficacy because the terfenadine group had fewer SRs to sting challenges and field stings during an average of 3 years.[46] However, this finding was not confirmed by prospective study by the same group.[47]

Oral antihistamines for inhalant immunotherapy Most studies of premedication for accelerated inhalant schedules used combination premedication (**Table 1**). However, several cluster immunotherapy studies with antihistamines alone have been performed. A controlled study showed that premedication with a nonsedating antihistamine (loratadine) was shown to reduce the number and frequency of SRs during cluster immunotherapy with grass or birch pollen extract when taken 2 hours before the first injection of each visit (33% of patients in loratadine group, 79% of patients in placebo group).[7] A cat cluster immunotherapy study using loratadine pretreatment of all 28 subjects (no placebo premedication) showed no SRs.[48] A grass cluster immunotherapy study using loratadine pretreatment of all subjects resulted in no immediate large local or SRs during grass cluster immunotherapy, but 18% (4/22) of patients experienced a delayed SR during the 4-week cluster period.[13]

Leukotriene antagonists A pilot study showed that montelukast premedication taken 2 hours before the injection decreases the size, and delays the onset, of local reactions during rush VIT.[49] No controlled studies have investigated the effect of leukotriene antagonists on the incidence of SRs.

Combination pretreatment Two separate studies showed that combination pretreatment with ketotifen, methylprednisolone, and theophylline used during a 3-day rush treatment with either pollen[23] or dust mite immunotherapy[50] decreased the frequency of SR.

A study of 1152 dust mite–allergic subjects (3–63 years old) examined the effects of 4 different RIT regimens with the same maintenance dose and found a significant reduction in the SR rate with preventive measures and premedication.[50] Preventive measures included modifying the schedule for LLR greater than 10 cm and excluding patients with an FEV_1 less than 70%. Premedication with methylprednisolone, ketotifen, and long-acting theophylline reduced the SR rate from 36% to 16.2% of patients ($P<.015$), and premedication plus preventive measures reduced the rate further to 7.3% ($P<.005$).

The same group found similar results in a study of 454 pollen-allergic subjects (olive, *Parietaria*, plane tree, orchard grass).[23] Premedication reduced the risk of SR from 31.3% to 14.7% ($P<.015$), and premedication plus preventive measures reduced the SR to 7.5% ($P<.005$).

After an initial RIT study without premedication resulted in a 55% SR rate (6/11),[38] a university-based pediatric group investigated the effect of premedication on RIT with allergen mixtures in subsequent studies. The first of these 2 studies was a double-blind, placebo-controlled, 9-injection, 2-day RIT study of 22 children (5–18 years old).[15] Premedication with astemizole, ranitidine, and prednisone or placebo was begun the day before RIT and continued through the 2-day rush. Premedication reduced the SR rate to 27% compared with 73% in the placebo premedication group ($P = .047$). The number of local reactions was also decreased, as was the size of the erythema, but not the wheal.

In a subsequent study, the schedule was modified into an 8-injection, 1-day RIT (cumulative dose 0.2 mL maintenance concentrate) with similar premedication with

Table 1
Selected studies investigating the effect of premedication on accelerated immunotherapy schedules

Study	Allergen	Protocol	Target Dose	Premedication Regimen	Results (SR are % of Patients)
Cluster Studies					
Walker et al[13]	Grass	7 visits, 4 wk	20 µg Phl p 5	Loratadine 10 mg >15 min before cluster OR placebo	All SR delayed; SR rate 18 loratadine vs 22 placebo
Ewbank et al[48]	Cat	8 visits, 4 wk	0.6, 3.0, and 15 µg of Fel d 1	Loratadine 10 mg 2 h before, no placebo group	No SR
Nielsen et al[7]	Timothy and birch	7 weekly visits	23 µg Bet v 1 25 µg Phl p 5	Loratadine 10 mg 2 h before OR placebo	Fewer SR in loratadine group (33) vs placebo (79.2)
Nanda et al[1]	Cat	8 visits, 4 wk	0.6, 3.0 and 15 µg of Fel d 1	Zafirlukast and loratadine, no placebo group	1/26 SR
Rush Studies					
Heijaoui et al[50]	Dust mite	1-d rush	3000 BU (4 µg Der p 1) if >10 y old; 1500 BU if <10 y old	Methylprednisolone, ketotifen, theophylline vs historical control from earlier trials	36 nonpremedicated group vs 16 premedicated group vs 7.3 if excluding FEV$_1$<70 and modifying for LLR
Portnoy et al[15] Sharkey and Portnoy[39]	Multiple inhalant allergens	1-d and 2-d rush	0.1 mL maint concentrate (1:100–1:400 wt/vol)	Astemizole, ranitidine, prednisone	55–73 nonpremedicated group vs 23–27 premedicated group
Casale et al[28]	Ragweed	Rush	4 µg initially then 2 µg Amb a 1	Fexofenadine and omalizumab for 9 wk before rush	Any SR: 56.4 placebo vs 33.3 omalizumab Anaphylaxis: 25.6 placebo group vs 5.6 omalizumab
Brockow et al[44]	Venom	Rush	100 µg of venom	Terfenadine 120 mg ± ranitidine 300 mg	SR causing immunotherapy discontinuation: 15 placebo vs 2 premedication

astemizole, ranitidine, and prednisone.[39] SR occurred in 23% (5/22) of patients: 1 patient had urticaria, 3 had wheezing or respiratory symptoms, and 1 had hypotension plus respiratory symptoms. All SRs occurred at doses of 0.3 mL of 1:1,000 wt/vol or higher.

In 1 of the few cluster protocols using combination premedication, a cat cluster immunotherapy regimen using loratadine 10 mg and zafirlukast 20 mg taken 2 hours before dosing resulted in SR rates in 3.8% of patients (1/26).[1]

A retrospective review of 65 patients undergoing RIT to a mixture of inhalant allergens reported that 38% (25/65) of patients had an SR.[14] They used a modification of the 1-day protocol noted earlier and gave 7 injections in 4 hours, reaching a dose of 0.05 mL of the undiluted concentrate. All patients were premedicated with prednisone, cetirizine, ranitidine, and zafirlukast or montelukast. Most SRs (72%) occurred after the final dose of the protocol. Nineteen (76%) were mild, 5 (20%) were moderate, and 1 (4%) was severe. SRs were associated with a higher degree of skin test sensitivity and the presence of weed or dog allergen in the extract.

Two IFR studies have yielded conflicting results. During a 2-day IFR rush protocol evaluating the effect of combination therapy with antihistamines and steroids, there were no statistically significant differences in SR rates between the premedication group (3.6%) and the placebo group (6.7%).[20] However, a recent 1-day IFR rush protocol involving 37 patients performed without premedication (no premedication group) reported higher systemic reaction rates (24.3%) than the 2-day regimen, with most reactions involving urticaria and pruritus.[21]

Omalizumab in combination with immunotherapy Omalizumab used in combination with immunotherapy 2 weeks before and during the grass season was compared with immunotherapy alone. Combination therapy improved symptom load and asthma control, with more patients reporting good or excellent efficacy.[51] Omalizumab added to standard maintenance doses of birch and grass immunotherapy resulted in fewer symptomatic days and rescue medication use compared with immunotherapy or omalizumab alone.[52]

In addition to symptomatic improvement, omalizumab has been shown to reduce SRs to rush immunotherapy. The use of omalizumab 9 weeks before and in conjunction with ragweed rush immunotherapy improved symptom severity scores during the ragweed season compared with immunotherapy alone. Furthermore, omalizumab pretreatment resulted in a fivefold decrease in the risk of anaphylaxis during rush immunotherapy.[28] A prospective study examined the effect of 16 weeks of treatment with omalizumab or placebo on the incidence of SRs during cluster immunotherapy in 248 asthmatic subjects.[41] Eligible subjects were required to have perennial asthma not well controlled despite inhaled corticosteroids and to be sensitive to at least 1 of 3 perennial aeroallergens (dust mite, cat, or dog). After 13 weeks of pretreatment with omalizumab or placebo, subjects received immunotherapy to 1, 2, or 3 allergens (dust mite, cat, and dog) through a 4-week cluster regimen, which overlapped with continued omalizumab/placebo treatment of 3 weeks. Compared with placebo, omalizumab pretreatment reduced the rate of SRs from 26.2% to 13.5% of subjects. The cluster regimen was followed by 7 weeks of maintenance injections during which omalizumab or placebo were not given; there were no SRs during this phase of treatment.

World Allergy Organization Subcutaneous Systemic Reaction Grading System

A new SR grading system was recently created by the World Allergy Organization in an effort to standardize SR definitions and to allow better comparisons of SRs between different immunotherapy formulations and practice patterns (**Table 2**).[53] The grading

Table 2
World Allergy Organization Subcutaneous Immunotherapy Systemic Reaction Grading System (endorsed by the American Academy of Allergy Asthma and Immunology and American College of Allergy, Asthma and Immunology)

Grade 1	Grade 2	Grade 3	Grade 4	Grade 5
Symptom(s)/sign(s) of 1 organ system present[a] *Cutaneous* Generalized pruritus, urticaria, flushing, or sensation of heat or warmth[b] or Angioedema (not laryngeal, tongue, or uvular) or *Upper respiratory* Rhinitis (eg, sneezing, rhinorrhea, nasal pruritus, and/or nasal congestion) or Throat clearing (itchy throat) or Cough perceived to originate in the upper airway, not the lung, larynx, or trachea or *Conjunctival* Conjunctival erythema, pruritus, or tearing *Other* Nausea, metallic taste, or headache	*Symptom(s)/sign(s) of more than 1 organ system present* or *Lower respiratory* Asthma: cough, wheezing, shortness of breath (eg, less than 40% PEF or FEV_1 reduction, responding to an inhaled bronchodilator) or *Gastrointestinal* Abdominal cramps, vomiting, or diarrhea or *Other* Uterine cramps	*Lower respiratory* Asthma (eg, 40% PEF or FEV_1 reduction NOT responding to an inhaled bronchodilator) or *Upper respiratory* Laryngeal, uvula, or tongue edema with or without stridor	*Lower or upper respiratory* Respiratory failure with or without loss of consciousness or *Cardiovascular* Hypotension with or without loss of consciousness	Death

Patients may also have a feeling of impending doom, especially in grades 2, 3, or 4

Note: children with anaphylaxis seldom convey a sense of impending doom and their behavior changes may be a sign of anaphylaxis (eg, becoming quiet or irritable)

Scoring includes a suffix that denotes whether and when epinephrine is administered in relation to symptom(s)/sign(s) of the SR: a, ≤5 minutes; b, >5 minutes to ≤10 minutes; c, >10 to ≤20 minutes; d, >20 minutes; z, epinephrine not administered

The final grade of the reaction will not be determined until the event has ended, regardless of the medication administered. The final report should include the first symptom(s)/sign(s) and the time of onset after the subcutaneous allergen immunotherapy injection[c] and a suffix reflecting whether and when epinephrine was administered (eg, grade 2a; rhinitis: 10 minutes)

(*continued on next page*)

Table 2 (continued)				
Grade 1	**Grade 2**	**Grade 3**	**Grade 4**	**Grade 5**
Final report: Grade a–d, or z ——————————— First symptom ———————————				
Time of onset of first symptom ———————————				
Comments[d]				

[a] Each grade is based on organ system involved and severity. Organ systems are defined as cutaneous, conjunctival, upper respiratory, lower respiratory, gastrointestinal, cardiovascular, and other. A reaction from a single organ system such as cutaneous, conjunctival, or upper respiratory, but not asthma, gastrointestinal, or cardiovascular is classified as a grade 1. Symptom(s)/sign(s) from more than 1 organ system or asthma, gastrointestinal, or cardiovascular are classified as grades 2 or 3. Respiratory failure or hypotension, with or without loss of consciousness, defines grade 4 and death grade 5. The grade is determined by the physician's clinical judgment.
[b] This constellation of symptoms may rapidly progress to a more severe reaction.
[c] Symptoms occurring within the first minutes after the injection may be a sign of severe anaphylaxis. Mild symptoms may progress rapidly to severe anaphylaxis and death.
[d] If signs or symptoms are not included in the table or the differentiation between an SR and vasovagal (vasodepressor) reaction, which may occur with any medical intervention, is difficult, please include comment, as appropriate.
Reprinted from Cox L, Larenas-Linnemann D, Lockey RF, et al. Speaking the same language: the World Allergy Organization subcutaneous immunotherapy systemic reaction grading system. J Allergy Clin Immunol 2010;125(3):571; with permission from Elsevier.

system applies specifically to situations in which a known allergen has been administered. A reaction from a single organ system, such as cutaneous, upper respiratory, or gastrointestinal, but not asthma, gastrointestinal, or cardiovascular, is classified as grade 1. Signs/symptoms from more than 1 organ system or asthma, gastrointestinal, or cardiovascular are classified as grades 2 or 3. Respiratory failure or hypotension, with or without syncope, defines grade 4, whereas death is grade 5. Grades are determined after the event has ended. Consistent use of this grading system in future studies may help determine the best approach to treating subcutaneous SRs, including when to give epinephrine.

REFERENCES

1. Nanda A, O'Connor M, Anand M, et al. Dose dependence and time course of the immunologic response to administration of standardized cat allergen extract. J Allergy Clin Immunol 2004;114:1339–44.
2. Tabar AI, Echechipia S, Garcia BE, et al. Double-blind comparative study of cluster and conventional immunotherapy schedules with *Dermatophagoides pteronyssinus*. J Allergy Clin Immunol 2005;116:109–18.
3. Francis JN, James LK, Paraskevopoulos G, et al. Grass pollen immunotherapy: IL-10 induction and suppression of late responses precedes IgG4 inhibitory antibody activity. J Allergy Clin Immunol 2008;121:1120–5.
4. Serrano P, Justicia JL, Sanchez C, et al. Systemic tolerability of specific subcutaneous immunotherapy with index-of-reactivity-standardized allergen extracts administered using clustered regimens: a retrospective, observational, multicenter study. Ann Allergy Asthma Immunol 2009;102:247–52.
5. Zhang L, Wang C, Han D, et al. Comparative study of cluster and conventional immunotherapy schedules with *Dermatophagoides pteronyssinus* in the treatment of persistent allergic rhinitis. Int Arch Allergy Immunol 2009;148:161–9.

6. Martinez-Canavate A, Eseverri JL, Rodenas R, et al. Evaluation of paediatric tolerance to an extract of *Alternaria alternata* under two treatment regimes. A multicentre study. Allergol Immunopathol (Madr) 2005;33(3):138–41.
7. Nielsen L, Johnsen CR, Mosbech H, et al. Antihistamine premedication in specific cluster immunotherapy: a double-blind, placebo-controlled study. J Allergy Clin Immunol 1996;97:1207–13.
8. Winther L, Malling HJ, Mosbech H. Allergen-specific immunotherapy in birch- and grass-pollen-allergic rhinitis, II: side-effects. Allergy 2000;55:327–35.
9. Mellerup MT, Hahn GW, Poulsen LK, et al. Safety of allergen-specific immunotherapy. Relation between dosage regimen, allergen extract, disease and systemic side-effects during induction treatment. Clin Exp Allergy 2000;30:1423–9.
10. Cox L. Accelerated immunotherapy schedules: review of efficacy and safety. Ann Allergy Asthma Immunol 2006;97:126–38.
11. Stewart GE, Lockey RF. Systemic reactions from allergen immunotherapy. J Allergy Clin Immunol 1992;90:567–78.
12. Parmiani S, Fernandez Tavora L, Moreno C, et al. Clustered schedules in allergen-specific immunotherapy. Allergol Immunopathol (Madr) 2002;30(5):283–91.
13. Walker SM, Pajno GB, Lima MT, et al. Grass pollen immunotherapy for seasonal rhinitis and asthma: a randomized, controlled trial. J Allergy Clin Immunol 2001; 107:87–93.
14. Harvey SM. Safety of rush immunotherapy to multiple aeroallergens in an adult population. Ann Allergy Asthma Immunol 2004;92:414–9.
15. Portnoy J, Bagstad K, Kanarek H, et al. Premedication reduces the incidence of systemic reactions during inhalant rush immunotherapy with mixtures of allergenic extracts. Ann Allergy Asthma Immunol 1994;73:409–18.
16. Bernstein JA, Kagen SL, Bernstein DI, et al. Rapid venom immunotherapy is safe for routine use in the treatment of patients with Hymenoptera anaphylaxis. Ann Allergy 1994;73:423–8.
17. Roll A, Hofbauer G, Ballmer-Weber BK, et al. Safety of specific immunotherapy using a four-hour ultra-rush induction scheme in bee and wasp allergy. J Investig Allergol Clin Immunol 2006;16:79–85.
18. Goldberg A, Confino-Cohen R. Rush venom immunotherapy in patients experiencing recurrent systemic reactions to conventional venom immunotherapy. Ann Allergy Asthma Immunol 2003;91:405–10.
19. Schiavino D, Nucera E, Pollastrini E, et al. Specific ultrarush desensitization in Hymenoptera venom-allergic patients. Ann Allergy Asthma Immunol 2004;92:409–13.
20. Tankersley MS, Walker RL, Butler WK, et al. Safety and efficacy of an imported fire ant rush immunotherapy protocol with and without prophylactic treatment. J Allergy Clin Immunol 2002;109:556–62.
21. Dietrich JJ, Moore LM, Nguyen S, et al. Imported fire ant hypersensitivity: a 1-day rush immunotherapy schedule without premedication. Ann Allergy Asthma Immunol 2009;103:535–6.
22. Bousquet J, Hejjaoui A, Dhivert H, et al. Immunotherapy with a standardized *Dermatophagoides pteronyssinus* extract. III. Systemic reactions during the rush protocol in patients suffering from asthma. J Allergy Clin Immunol 1989;83:797–802.
23. Heijaioui A, Ferrando R, Dhivert H, et al. Systemic reactions occurring during immunotherapy with standardized pollen extracts. J Allergy Clin Immunol 1992; 89:925–33.
24. Armentia-Medina A, Blanco-Quiros A, Martin-Santos JM, et al. Rush immunotherapy with a standardized Bermuda grass pollen extract. Ann Allergy Asthma Immunol 1989;63:127–35.

25. Bousquet J, Braquemond P, Feinberg J, et al. Specific IgE response before and after rush immunotherapy with a standardized allergen or allergoid in grass pollen allergy. Ann Allergy Asthma Immunol 1986;56:456–9.

26. Bousquet J, Hejjaoui A, Skassa-Brociek W, et al. Double-blind, placebo-controlled immunotherapy with mixed grass-pollen allergoids, I: rush immunotherapy with allergoids and standardized orchard grass-pollen extract. J Allergy Clin Immunol 1987;80:591–8.

27. Moverare R, Vesterinen E, Metso T, et al. Pollen-specific rush immunotherapy: clinical efficacy and effects on antibody concentrations. Ann Allergy Asthma Immunol 2001;86:337–42.

28. Casale TB, Busse WW, Kline JN, et al. Omalizumab pretreatment decreases acute reactions after rush immunotherapy for ragweed-induced seasonal allergic rhinitis. J Allergy Clin Immunol 2006;117:134–40.

29. Bousquet J, Becker WM, Hejjaoui A, et al. Differences in clinical and immunologic reactivity of patients allergic to grass pollens and to multiple-pollen species, II: efficacy of a double-blind, placebo-controlled, specific immunotherapy with standardized extracts. J Allergy Clin Immunol 1991;88:43–53.

30. Bousquet J, Maasch HJ, Hejjaoui A, et al. Double-blind, placebo-controlled immunotherapy with mixed grass-pollen allergoids, III: efficacy and safety of unfractionated and high-molecular-weight preparations in rhinoconjunctivitis and asthma. J Allergy Clin Immunol 1989;84:546–56.

31. Bousquet J, Guerin B, Dotte A, et al. Comparison between rush immunotherapy with a standardized allergen and an alum adjuved pyridine extracted material in grass pollen allergy. Clin Allergy 1985;15:179–93.

32. Dolz I, Martinez-Cocera C, Bartolome JM, et al. A double-blind, placebo-controlled study of immunotherapy with grass-pollen extract Alutard SQ during a 3-year period with initial rush immunotherapy. Allergy 1996;51:489–500.

33. Horst M, Hejjaoui A, Horst V, et al. Double-blind, placebo-controlled rush immunotherapy with a standardized *Alternaria* extract. J Allergy Clin Immunol 1990; 85:460–72.

34. Hedlin G, Graff-Lonnevig V, Heilborn H, et al. Immunotherapy with cat- and dog-dander extracts, V: effects of 3 years of treatment. J Allergy Clin Immunol 1991; 87:955–64.

35. Hedlin G, Braff-Lonnevig V, Heilborn H, et al. Immunotherapy with cat- and dog-dander extracts, II: in vivo and in vitro immunologic effects observed in a 1-year double-blind placebo study. J Allergy Clin Immunol 1986;77:488–96.

36. Hedlin G, Heilborn H, Lilja G, et al. Long-term follow-up of patients treated with a three-year course of cat or dog immunotherapy. J Allergy Clin Immunol 1995; 96:879–85.

37. Lilja G, Sundin B, Graff-Lonnevig V, et al. Immunotherapy with cat- and dog-dander extracts, IV: effects of 2 years of treatment. J Allergy Clin Immunol 1989;83:37–44.

38. Portnoy J, King K, Kanarek H, et al. Incidence of systemic reactions during rush immunotherapy. Ann Allergy Asthma Immunol 1992;68:493–8.

39. Sharkey P, Portnoy J. Rush immunotherapy: experience with a one-day schedule. Ann Allergy Asthma Immunol 1996;76:175–80.

40. Sturm G, Kranke B, Rudolph C, et al. Rush Hymenoptera venom immunotherapy: a safe and practical protocol for high-risk patients. J Allergy Clin Immunol 2002; 110:928–33.

41. Massanari M, Nelson H, Casale T, et al. Effect of pretreatment with omalizumab on the tolerability of specific immunotherapy in allergic asthma. J Allergy Clin Immunol 2010;125:383–9.

42. Ohashi Y, Nakai Y, Murata K. Effect of pretreatment with fexofenadine on the safety of immunotherapy in patients with allergic rhinitis. Ann Allergy Asthma Immunol 2006;96:600–5.

43. Reimers A, Hari Y, Muller U. Reduction of side-effects from ultrarush immunotherapy with honeybee venom by pretreatment with fexofenadine: a double-blind, placebo-controlled trial. Allergy 2000;55:484–8.

44. Brockow K, Kiehn M, Riethmuller C, et al. Efficacy of antihistamine pretreatment in the prevention of adverse reactions to Hymenoptera immunotherapy: a prospective, randomized, placebo-controlled trial. J Allergy Clin Immunol 1997; 100:458–63.

45. Berchtold E, Maibach R, Muller U. Reduction of side effect from rush-immunotherapy with honey bee venom by pretreatment with terfenadine. Clin Exp Allergy 1992;22:59–65.

46. Muller U, Hari Y, Berchtold E. Premedication with antihistamines may enhance efficacy of specific-allergen immunotherapy. J Allergy Clin Immunol 2001;107:81–6.

47. Muller U, Jutel M, Reimers A, et al. Clinical and immunologic effects of H1 antihistamine preventive medication during honeybee venom immunotherapy. J Allergy Clin Immunol 2008;122:1001–7.

48. Ewbank PA, Murray J, Sanders K, et al. A double-blind, placebo-controlled immunotherapy dose-response study with standardized cat extract. J Allergy Clin Immunol 2003;111:155–61.

49. Wohrl S, Gamper S, Hemmer W, et al. Premedication with montelukast reduces local reactions of allergen immunotherapy. Int Arch Allergy Immunol 2007;144: 137–42.

50. Heijaioui A, Dhivert H, Michel FB, et al. Immunotherapy with a standardized *Dermatophagoides pteronyssinus* extract. IV. Systemic reactions according to the immunotherapy schedule. J Allergy Clin Immunol 1990;85:473–9.

51. Kopp MV, Brauburger J, Riedinger F, et al. The effect of anti-IgE treatment on in vitro leukotriene release in children with seasonal allergic rhinitis. J Allergy Clin Immunol 2002;110:728–35.

52. Kuehr J, Brauburger J, Zielen S, et al. Efficacy of combination treatment with anti-IgE plus specific immunotherapy in polysensitized children and adolescents with seasonal allergic rhinitis. J Allergy Clin Immunol 2002;109:274–80.

53. Cox L, Larenas-Linnemann D, Lockey RF, et al. Speaking the same language: the World Allergy Organization subcutaneous immunotherapy systemic reaction grading system. J Allergy Clin Immunol 2010;125:569–74.

Sublingual Immunotherapy for Allergic Respiratory Diseases: Efficacy and Safety

Giovanni Passalacqua, MD*, Giorgio Walter Canonica, MD

KEYWORDS
- Sublingual immunotherapy • Asthma • Rhinitis • Efficacy
- Safety

The subcutaneous modality of immunotherapy (SCIT) is effective and safe when properly prescribed and administered. However, a certain risk of severe side effects exists, even when the adverse reaction is managed correctly. The potential adverse effects associated with SCIT stimulated the search for new administration routes (nasal, bronchial, oral, sublingual), which were expected to be safer. Not all of these alternative routes provided an improved benefit–safety profile compared with SCIT. The bronchial administration route provoked significant adverse reactions, and the pure oral route required very high amounts of allergen to be effective. The nasal route was effective and safe in terms of systemic side effects, but associated local adverse effects likely contributed to its progressively reduced use.[1] However, since its first description in 1986, the sublingual route (SLIT) seemed to be a good candidate for the clinical practice because of its satisfactory safety profile. For this reason, SLIT was investigated extensively and is now considered an acceptable alternative to SCIT[2,3] in adults and children. The evidence supporting SLIT for the treatment of respiratory allergy (rhinitis/asthma) is now remarkable, and some of the unmet needs have been effectively addressed recently.

CLINICAL EFFICACY
An Overview on Clinical Trials

In the official document, the World Allergy Organization (WAO) position paper on sublingual immunotherapy, 60 randomized, double-blind, placebo-controlled trials

Funding and conflict of interest: none to declare.
Allergy and Respiratory Diseases, Department of Internal Medicine, University of Genoa, Padiglione Maragliano, Largo Rosanna Benzio 10, 16132 Genoa, Italy
* Corresponding author.
E-mail address: passalacqua@unige.it

(RDBPC) performed with SLIT were reviewed.[4] Of these, 26 trials were performed with grass extracts, 15 with mite, 5 with *Parietaria*, 3 with cat, and the remaining 11 with other pollen extracts. The duration of the trials ranged between 4 months and 4 years, with 19 of them being of 6 months or less. Most studies was conducted in patients with rhinitis or rhinitis plus asthma, and only a few studies were specifically designed to evaluate the efficacy in asthma. One single trial was performed in allergic conjunctivitis. Of the 60 RDBPC trials, 18 enrolled more than 100 patients,[4] but only 10 had a formal sample size calculation; 20 trials were performed in children. As an overall evaluation, most trials provided positive results for one or all of the parameters investigated. However, 4 studies were totally negative[5–8] and 8 reported only partial or negligible clinical efficacy.

After the WAO position paper was published, two new RDBPC trials appeared. One with ragweed extract involved 115 patients and reported a 15% overall symptom reduction versus placebo during the entire season, which is slightly inferior to that described with grasses.[9] The other trial used *Alternaria* extract[10] and showed a 30% reduction in symptom scores in the SLIT group compared with the placebo group.

The most important problem in evaluating the literature is the heterogeneity of the trials in terms of doses used, regimen, type and concentration of extracts, duration, inclusion criteria, and measurements. Most trials used the 0 to 3 clinical scores, with a score of 3 representing the worse symptoms. Positive results were consistent across the variable aspects, especially in rhinitis symptoms. The methodological problems were partially solved in the past 5 years by the so-called big trials, which included hundreds of patients and rigorous experimental methodology.

THE BIG TRIALS

The recent "big trials" were all conducted with grass pollen extracts (**Table 1**), and enrolled several patients (between 250 and 850).[11–16] All these trials followed well-established methodological criteria, had a power calculation, and clearly defined outcomes and statistical analyses.[17] These large trials represent the best evidence available on the efficacy of SLIT. Only one study with a similar number of patients exists for SCIT.[18] The big trials invariably showed an effect of SLIT compared with placebo ranging from 25% to more than 50% improvement in clinical outcomes. The cutoff of 20% is considered the threshold for a significant, clinically relevant effect.[17] In addition, two of those trials had a dose-ranging design, which identified the optimal maintenance dose range for grass pollen SLIT: approximately 600 μg major allergen administered monthly (roughly 50 times the monthly dose of SCIT). These trials clearly established that the efficacy of SLIT was clearly dose-dependent, and provided robust proof of the efficacy according to Grades of Recommendation Assessment Development and Evaluation (GRADE) rules.[19] One of the trials showed that a preseasonal period of treatment of 8 weeks should be recommended to achieve significant clinical efficacy in the first treatment season.[11,20]

META-ANALYSES

The large number of RDBPC SLIT trials available allowed for some meta-analyses to be conducted (**Table 2**). The inclusion criteria in these meta-analyses varied, including rhinitis only,[21] asthma only,[22] asthma in children,[23] and rhinitis in children.[24] In all of the meta-analyses comparing SLIT with placebo, SLIT provided a significant effect,[25] at least for clinical symptoms and rescue medication consumption.

Table 1
The "big trials" with grass extracts

Author (Year)	Age Range (y)	Patients A/P	Allergen	Duration	Dose Preparation	Main Positive Results Over Placebo
Durham et al,[11] 2006	18–66	569/286	Grass, 3 doses	6 m	15 µg (136 pts) 150 µg (139 pts) 450 µg (294 pts) Phl p 5/month Tablets	Drug score, 28% (.012) Symptoms, 21% (.002) Only with the highest dose QoL improved No clinical change with the 2 low doses
Dahl et al,[12] 2006	23–35	316/318	Grass	6 m	450 µg Phl p 5/month Cumulative, 2.7 mg Tablets	RC symptoms, −30% (.001) RC drugs, −38% (.001) Well days, −52% (.004)
Didier et al,[13] 2007	25–47	472/156	Grass, 3 doses	6 m	240 µg/mo (157 pts) 750 µg/mo (155 pts) 1.2 mg/mo (160 pts) Tablets	For 300 and 500IR Total and individual symptom and drug scores (<.001) RQLQ improved
Wahn et al,[14] 2009	4–17	139/139	Grass	8 m	600 µg/mo major allergen Tablets	Rhinitis score, −28% (.01) Medications, −24% (.006) Medication-free days (.01)
Ott et al,[15] 2009	20–50	142/67	Grass	5 y 4 seasons	Cumulative 1.5 mg major allergen/season	Combined score and symptom score significantly reduced since first season Symptoms decrease from −33% to 47% (third season) No change med scores
Bufe et al,[16] 2009	5–16	126/127	Grass	6 m	450 µg Phl p 5/month	Significant reduction in RC symptom score (−24%), asthma score (−64%), RC medications (−34%), and well days (+28%) All $P<.03$

Abbreviations: A/P, active/placebo; Pts, patients; QoL, quality of life; RC, rhinoconjunctivitis; RQLQ, Rhinitis Quality of Life Questionnaire.

Table 2
Meta-analyses on SLIT

Author	Patients	Disease	Trials	Effect Size on Symptoms	Comment
Calamita et al,[22] 2006	303 adults + children	Asthma	5 pollens 4 mite	−0.38 (P = .07)	No change in symptom score Significant reduction medication score
Wilson et al,[21] 2005	959 adults + children	Rhinitis	16 pollens 6 mite	−0.42 (P = .002)	Decreased symptoms and medications for rhinitis Asthma not evaluable
Penagos et al,[24] 2006	484 children	Rhinitis	5 pollens 4 mite	−0.56 (P = .02)	Decreased symptoms and medications for rhinitis No subanalysis feasible
Penagos et al,[23] 2008	441 children	Asthma	3 pollen 3 mite	−1.42 (P = .02)	Decreased symptoms and medications for asthma
Compalati et al,[28] 2009	858 adults + children	Rhinitis Asthma	Mite 8 rhinitis 9 asthma	Rhinitis, −0.95 Asthma, −0.95 (P = .02)	Significant effect on symptoms and drug intake for both rhinitis and asthma
Di Bona et al,[29] 2010	2791 adults + children	Rhinitis	19 grass	−0.32 (P<.0001)	Decreased symptoms and medications for rhinitis Greater effect in adults

The reliability of the meta-analyses was recently questioned.[26] The main concerns expressed by the authors were possible publication biases, some incorrect reporting of the data for meta-analyses, and the high heterogeneity of the trials included. However, even considering the reporting errors in these meta-analyses, the overall results would have not changed. The statistical evaluation of the publication biases was itself poorly reliable in this context.[27]

The problem of heterogeneity has been repeatedly highlighted as a drawback of meta-analyses. However, the meta-analyses are intended to summarize results of studies that are not directly comparable with each other, and are the only instruments currently available that can do this.

Finally, these meta-analyses pooled together the studies with all allergenic extracts, although differences may exist among allergens. This aspect was recently addressed by two further analyses, one restricted to mite extracts[28] and one to grass extracts.[29] Both articles confirmed the significant clinical effect of SLIT over placebo for these two allergens.

Special Aspects: SLIT in Asthma

The effect of SLIT in asthma is still a matter of debate, because some studies reported marginal or no effect on asthma symptoms.[30,31] However, in these studies, all the patients (active and controls) had no symptoms of asthma at baseline or during the trial, and therefore no effect could be seen. When patients have measurable asthma symptoms, the effect of SLIT is apparent, which was clearly shown in an early study involving 85 patients with mite-induced asthma.[32] In this study, an increase in functional spirometric parameters was seen in addition to the improvement in clinical parameters. In another study, Pajno and colleagues[33] reported a significant clinical improvement of asthma symptoms in mite-allergic children, although no functional parameter was evaluated. Similar results were reported by Lue and colleagues[34] and Niu and colleagues,[35] who evaluated nighttime and daytime symptoms and also the FEV_1. The most recent pediatric trial specifically designed for asthma also reported a significant improvement in clinical parameters.[36] Finally an RDBPC trial showed that SLIT is capable of reducing the degree of nonspecific bronchial hyperresponsiveness in children.[37]

Another important aspect regarding asthma and SLIT, compared with SCIT, is that the treatment seems to be able to reduce the risk of developing asthma in children with rhinitis (see later discussion). This fact, if confirmed in rigorous trials, is expected to result not only in an enhanced clinical benefit but also in relevant socioeconomic savings.[38]

Special Aspects: Comparison with SCIT and Drugs

When comparing two different routes of administration, the gold standard methodology is the double-blind, double-dummy design. This design is difficult to apply in the case of immunotherapy, in which long-term treatments are needed and a large number of dropouts typically occur. In one early double-dummy study in patients allergic to grass pollen, conducted with no placebo group, the clinical scores showed that the clinical efficacy of SLIT was equivalent to that of SCIT.[39] Five other comparative studies are available,[40–44] but although they reported an overall equivalence between the routes, they were all conducted in an open fashion and therefore their value for recommendations remains limited. The most recent of these studies[44] compared (in open controlled fashion) the clinical efficacy and immunologic effects of SLIT and SCIT in mite-allergic children with asthma/rhinitis. This study failed to detect a difference in clinical and immunologic effects between the routes, showing that both were significantly more effective than medications alone.

The only rigorous double-blind, double-dummy, placebo-controlled study comparing SLIT and SCIT was conducted in patients allergic to birch pollen.[45] Symptoms and medication use were reduced by approximately one-third in the SLIT group and by one-half in the SCIT group. However, no statistically significant differences were evident between treatment groups, possibly because of the small patient numbers at the end of the 3-year study. In terms of systemic reactions, five grade 3 and one grade 4 reactions were seen in the SCIT group and none in the SLIT group (according the European Academy of Allergy and Clinical Immunology 1993 systemic reaction grading system).

Comparing efficacy between SLIT and medications can be problematic because the effects of immunotherapy may be appreciated only in the long-term (months). A trial conducted in asthmatic children showed that the clinical efficacy of SLIT plus fluticasone is equal to that of fluticasone alone, but that the addition of SLIT also resulted in improvement of nonbronchial symptoms.[46] One open randomized trial of grass-allergic asthmatic patients comparing continuous SLIT treatment with inhaled budesonide add-on therapy during grass-pollen season showed that immunotherapy was overall superior in the long-term because it provided an improvement both in nasal symptoms and nasal inflammation, in addition to improved functional parameters, which was seen in both treatment groups.[47] In this open trial, the measurements were obtained after 3 and 5 years of SLIT.

Special Aspects: Disease-Modifying Effects

Allergic rhinitis and allergic asthma are considered two different clinical pictures of a single immunologic disorder of the airways (united airways disease). The link between upper and lower airways is supported by epidemiologic, mechanistic, and clinical data.[48] It is well established that rhinitis is an independent risk factor for the development of asthma. It is also known that immunotherapy can interfere with the natural history of the disease (ie, reducing the risk of asthma onset) because it may alter the immune response to allergens overall, inducing sustained immune tolerance. The preventive effect on asthma onset was previously shown with SCIT in the Preventative Allergy Treatment study.[49] Recently, the disease-modifying effect was also shown for SLIT. In an open controlled study,[50] 113 children aged 5 to 14 years experiencing seasonal rhinitis from grass pollen were randomly assigned to medications plus SLIT or medications only. After 3 years, 8 of 45 children treated with SLIT and 18 of 44 controls had developed asthma, with a relative risk of 3.8 for untreated patients developing asthma. In another randomized, open, controlled trial, 216 children aged 5 to 17 years experiencing rhinitis with/without intermittent asthma were randomly allocated 2:1 to drugs plus SLIT or drugs only, and followed up for 3 years for the presence of persistent asthma.[51] The prevalence of persistent asthma was 2 of 130 (1.5%) in the SLIT group and 19 of 66 (30%) in the control group. Overall, four patients would have had to be treated with SLIT to prevent the onset of asthma in one. This latter study also showed that SLIT prevented the onset of new allergen sensitizations, as determined using skin prick test.

Another beneficial effect of SIT, similar to SCIT, is the long-lasting or carry-over effect. This effect was shown in an early open controlled study in children in which the beneficial clinical effect of SLIT was still seen for 4 to 5 years after discontinuation.[52] One 15-year prospective controlled study in patients allergic to mites showed that the effects of a 4-year course of SLIT persisted for more than 5 years after discontinution.[53] In a 6-year randomized prospective trial, Tahamiler and colleagues[54] showed that the improvement achieved with SLIT was maintained for 3 years after discontinuation. More recently, follow-up of a large and methodologically rigorous trial conducted with grass allergen tablets confirmed the existence of a carry-over effect of SLIT.[55]

SAFETY
Clinical Trials, Surveys, and Case Reports

The safety of SLIT is overall superior to that of SCIT.[56] No fatality has been reported with SLIT in 23 years of trials and extensive clinical use. Systemic adverse events, such as rhinitis, asthma, urticaria, angioedema, and hypotension, make up only a minority of all adverse events, and represent fewer than 5% of adverse events reported in clinical trials. However, local reactions (oropharyngeal or gastrointestinal), such as oral itching/swelling/burning, throat pruritus, altered taste, and uvular oedema, are frequently reported and may be experienced by more than 50% of patients. A minority of patients also report lower gastrointestinal complaints (nausea, vomiting, diarrhea, or abdominal pain), which are also considered to be local. According to recent data, similar to SCIT, the number of side effects seems to be dose-dependent.[57] Most adverse events in postmarketing studies are reported as local, mild, and self limiting, and the rate is fewer than 10 per 1000 doses.[4]

The safety of SLIT in randomized controlled trials is extensively reviewed in the WAO position paper[4] and some other reviews.[56,58,59] One of the most detailed reviews examined the available studies on SLIT at the time the paper was written.[56] Among a total of 386,149 doses, 1047 adverse reactions occurred, which is 2.7 per 1000 doses in 41 studies with sufficient information to analyze. The occurrence of severe reactions was 0.56 per 1000 doses in studies that specified the severity of the reaction. Overall, 14 serious adverse events were considered most likely treatment-related. Gastrointestinal complaints (nausea, upper abdominal pain, and vomiting) occurred more frequently with higher doses.

Six cases of anaphylaxis with SLIT have been reported in literature.[60–64] Because two anaphylactic reactions occurred with the first grass tablet, experts recommend the first dose be given under medical supervision.[4]

Great attention has been paid to the safety of SCIT in children. In fact, ages younger than 5 years have generally been considered too young for SCIT, primarily because systemic reactions may be more difficult to treat in young children, who may have difficulty communicating early signs/symptoms of a systemic reaction. Some of the SLIT postmarketing surveys that involved children aged 3 to 5 years confirmed that the safety risk is not greater in younger ages.[65–67] Finally, in two postmarketing surveys of adults and children, the use of multiple allergens (2 or 3) for SLIT did not increase the rate of side effects.[68,69]

The Difficultly of Grading Side Effects

One of the most important problems in evaluating the safety of SLIT is that no universal system exists for reporting and grading its side effects. As a result, the rate of SLIT adverse events reported is largely variable across the studies. In addition, the rate of adverse events is lower in postmarketing surveys than in RDBPC trials, especially for local (oropharyngeal) adverse events. Most adverse events in postmarketing studies are reported as local, mild, and self-limiting, and the rate is fewer than 10 per 1000 doses and occur in fewer than 15% of patients, whereas in RDBPC trials adverse events occur in approximately 50% of patients. This discrepancy is probably because many of the events are judged by patients to be mild and therefore are not self-reported in the postmarketing surveillance studies. The manner of describing SLIT adverse reactions can be extremely variable, making results among different studies difficult to compare, thereby making it difficult to identify risk factors and determine proper actions to take to treat these adverse reactions. The WAO recently approved a grading system for adverse reactions to SCIT.[70]

Local adverse events with SCIT are common, expected, and usually not mentioned or included in the WAO systemic reaction grading system. In contrast, with SLIT, local reactions represent most adverse events, sometimes leading to treatment discontinuation, necessitating a separate grading system for SCIT-induced systemic reactions. Therefore, a uniform grading system for adverse events associated with SLIT is necessary. To accomplish this goal, a panel of experts from WAO, in cooperation with regional societies, is currently working on a grading system for local SLIT-induced adverse events. In this system, all of the adverse events occurring at the site of administration (**Table 3**) were considered local. For practical purposes, the lower gastrointestinal signs are considered local adverse events, unless they occur with other systemic manifestations, in which case they would be considered systemic reactions. The Medical Dictionary for Regulatory Activities (MeDRA) terms are recommended for reporting adverse events (see **Table 3**).[71]

A certain degree of subjectivity is unavoidable in grading local adverse events. In general, the severity of local side effects depends on the signs and symptoms and their duration, keeping in mind that local side effects of SLIT tend to disappear after the initial doses. Another aspect to consider is whether a local side effect is sufficiently severe to cause discontinuation of SLIT, either because of single-event severity or

Table 3
Description of the local side effects related to SLIT

	Local Side Effect	MeDRA Preferred Term	MeDRA Code
Mouth/ear	Altered taste perception	Dysgeusia	10013911
	Itching of lips	Oral pruritus	10052894
	Swelling of lips	Lip swelling	10024570
	Itching of the oral mucosa	Oral pruritus	10052894
	Swelling of the oral mucosa	Mucosal oedema	10030111
	Itching of the ears	Ear pruritus	10052138
	Swelling of the tongue	Swollen tongue	10042727
	Glossodynia	Glossodynia	10018388
	Mouth ulcer	Mouth ulceration	10028034
	Tongue ulcer	Tongue ulceration	10043991
	Throat irritation	Throat irritation	10043521
	Uvular oedema	Pharyngeal oedema	10034829
Upper gastrointestinal	Nausea	Nausea	10028813
	Stomachache	Abdominal pain upper	10000087
	Vomiting	Vomiting	10047700
Lower gastrointestinal	Abdominal pain	Abdominal pain	10000081
	Diarrhea	Diarrhea	10012735

duration, or persistence of local reactions with repeated dosing that ultimately become intolerable. A grading system based on this consideration is currently under construction. Concerning the systemic side effects, the WAO grading system for systemic reactions caused by SCIT is also considered adequate for SLIT.

Unmet Needs?

One of the most critical aspects in evaluating the efficacy of SLIT in respiratory allergy is the large variability of doses used in clinical trials. Both positive and negative results were obtained with low and high doses of allergens, and the dose range for efficacy is reported to be between 2 and 375 times the amount given with SCIT. A clear dose–response relationship has been formally shown only for grass-pollen extracts, for which the optimal dosage of major allergen has been identified to be between 15 and 25 μg/d. Thus, dose–response trials and the identification of the optimal maintenance dose are needed for many more of the relevant allergens. This problem is also linked to the variability in standardization methods among manufacturers[72]

The variability of the study design, patient selection, duration, and regimen among the trials is another major problem impacting interpretation of the meta-analyses. This challenge reinforces the need for standardization of the methodology so that trials can be compared and more clear information can be provided to clinicians.[73] Finally, the reporting of clinical trials for SCIT and SLIT is far from satisfactory, potentially introducing further problems in the interpretation of results.[74]

From a practical standpoint, no consensus exists on the best administration regimen among the preseasonal, coseasonal, precoseasonal, or continuous schedules, although for pollen allergens, most of the trials use a precoseasonal regimen.[75] Similarly, the usefulness of a buildup phase is still debated because some of the big trials have used a no-updosing regimen. In addition the optimal maintenance dosing (eg, once daily, alternate days, once weekly) has not yet been defined, nor has the optimal duration of a SLIT been established. Concerning safety, it would be crucial to identify risk factors for systemic side effects, if any exist. The safety in subjects with previous reactions to injections has not been well studied, nor has the risk for adverse events after a temporary suspension of SLIT. Well-designed controlled studies should help answer these unmet needs concerning the optimal regimen for SLIT efficacy and safety.

REFERENCES

1. Canonica GW, Passalacqua G. Non injection routes for immunotherapy. J Allergy Clin Immunol 2003;111(3):437–48.
2. Bousquet J, Lockey R, Malling HJ. Allergen immunotherapy: therapeutical vaccines for allergic diseases. WHO position paper. Allergy 1998;53(Suppl): 1–33.
3. Bousquet J, Van Cauwenberge P. Allergic rhinitis and its impact on asthma. J Allergy Clin Immunol 2001;108(Suppl 5):S146–50.
4. Canonica GW. World Allergy Organization position paper on sublingual immunotherapy. Allergy 2009;64(Suppl 91):1–59.
5. Nelson H, Oppenheimer J, Vatsia GA, et al. A double-blind, placebo-controlled evaluation of sublingual immunotherapy with standardized cat extract. J Allergy Clin Immunol 1993;92:229–36.
6. Guez S, Vatrinet C, Fadel R, et al. House dust mite sublingual swallow immunotherapy in perennial rhinitis: a double-blind placebo controlled study. Allergy 2000;55:369–75.
7. Roder E, Berger MY, Hop WC, et al. Sublingual immunotherapy with grass pollen is not effective in symptomatic youngsters in primary care. J Allergy Clin Immunol 2007;119:892–8.
8. Okubo K, Gotoh M, Fujieda S, et al. A Randomized double-blind comparative study of sublingual immunotherapy for cedar pollinosis. Allergol Int 2008;57: 265–75.
9. Skoner D, Gentile D, Bush R, et al. Sublingual immunotherapy in patients with allergic rhinoconjunctivitis caused by ragweed pollen. J Allergy Clin Immunol 2010;125:660–6.
10. Cortellini G, Spadolini I, Patella V, et al. Sublingual immunotherapy is effective in alternaria induced allergic rhinitis. A randomized placebo controlled trial. Ann Allergy Asthma Immunol 2010;101:382–6.
11. Durham SR, Yang WH, Pedersen MR, et al. Sublingual immunotherapy with once-daily grass-allergen tablets: a randomised controlled trial in seasonal allergic rhinoconjunctivitis. J Allergy Clin Immunol 2006;117:802–9.
12. Dahl R, Kapp A, Colombo G, et al. Efficacy and safety of sublingual immunotherapy with grass allergen tablets for seasonal allergic rhinoconjunctivitis. J Allergy Clin Immunol 2006;118:434–40.
13. Didier A, Malling HJ, Worm M, et al. Optimal dose, efficacy, and safety of once-daily sublingual immunotherapy with a 5-grass pollen tablet for seasonal allergic rhinitis. J Allergy Clin Immunol 2007;120:1338–45.
14. Wahn U, Tabar A, Kuna P, et al. Efficacy and safety of 5 grass pollen sublingual immunotherapy in pediatric allergic rhinoconjunctivitis. J Allergy Clin Immunol 2009;123:160–6.
15. Ott H, Sieber J, Brehler R, et al. Efficacy of grass pollen sublingual immunotherapy for three consecutive seasons and after cessation of treatment: the ECRIT study. Allergy 2009;64:179–86.
16. Bufe A, Eberle P, Franke-Beckmann E, et al. Safety and efficacy in children of an SQ-standardized grass allergen tablet for sublingual immunotherapy. J Allergy Clin Immunol 2009;123:167–73.

17. Canonica GW, Baena Cagnani C, Bousquet J, et al. Recommendations for standardization of clinical trials with allergen specific immunotherapy for respiratory allergy. A statement of a World Allergy Organization (WAO) taskforce. Allergy 2007;62:317–24.

18. Frew A, Powell JL, Corrigan CJ, et al. Efficacy and safety of specific immunotherapy with SQ allergen extract in treatment-resistant seasonal allergic rhinoconjunctivitis. J Allergy Clin Immunol 2006;117:319–25.

19. Brozek JL, Baena Cagnani C, Canonica GW, et al. Methodology for development of the allergic rhinitis and its impact on asthma guideline 2008 update. Allergy 2008;63:38–46.

20. Calderon MA, Birk AO, Andersen JS, et al. Prolonged preseasonal treatment phase with Grazax sublingual immunotherapy increases clinical efficacy. Allergy 2007;62:958–61.

21. Wilson DR, Torres L, Durham SR. Sublingual immunotherapy for allergic rhinitis. Allergy 2005;60:3–8.

22. Calamita Z, Saconato H, Bronhara Pelà A, et al. Efficacy of Sublingual immunotherapy in asthma. Systematic review of randomized clinical trials. Allergy 2006;61:1162–72.

23. Penagos M, Passalacqua G, Compalati E, et al. Metaanalysis of the efficacy of sublingual immunotherapy in the treatment of allergic asthma in pediatric patients, 3 to 18 years of age. Chest 2008;133:599–609.

24. Penagos M, Compalati E, Tarantini F, et al. Efficacy of sublingual immunotherapy in the treatment of allergic rhinitis in children. Meta analysis of randomized controlled trials. Ann Allergy Asthma Immunol 2006;97:141–8.

25. Compalati E, Penagos M, Tarantini F, et al. Specific immunotherapy for respiratory allergy: state of the art according to current meta-analyses. Ann Allergy Asthma Immunol 2009;102:22–8.

26. Nieto A, Mazon A, Pamies R, et al. Sublingual immunotherapy for allergic respiratory diseases: an evaluation of meta-analyses. J Allergy Clin Immunol 2009; 124:157–61.

27. Compalati E, Canonica GW, Passalacqua G, et al. Considerations about the evaluation of the SLIT meta-analyses. J Allergy Clin Immunol 2010;125(2):509.

28. Compalati E, Passalacqua G, Bonini M, et al. The efficacy of sublingual immunotherapy for house dust mites respiratory allergy: results of a GA2LEN meta-analysis. Allergy 2009;64:1570–9.

29. Di Bona D, Plaia A, Scafidi V, et al. Efficacy of sublingual immunotherapy with grass allergens for seasonal allergic rhinitis: a systematic review and meta-analysis. J Allergy Clin Immunol 2010;126(3):558–66.

30. Dahl R, Stender A, Rak S. Specific immunotherapy with SQ standardized grass allergen tablets in asthmatics with rhinoconjunctivitis. Allergy 2006;61: 185–90.

31. Pham-Thi N, Scheinmann P, Fadel R, et al. Assessment of sublingual immunotherapy efficacy in children with house dust mite-induced allergic asthma optimally controlled by pharmacologic treatment and mite-avoidance measures. Pediatr Allergy Immunol 2007;8:47–57.

32. Bousquet J, Scheinmann P, Guinnepain MT, et al. Sublingual swallow immunotherapy (SLIT) in patients with asthma due to house dust mites: a double-blind placebo-controlled study. Allergy 1999;54:249–60.

33. Pajno GB, Morabito L, Barberio G, et al. Clinical and immunological effects of long-term sublingual immunotherapy in asthmatic children sensitized to mite: a double-blind study. Allergy 2000;55:842–9.

34. Lue KH, Lin YH, Sun HL, et al. Clinical and immunologic effects of sublingual immunotherapy in asthmatic children sensitized to mites: a double-blind, randomized, placebo-controlled study. Pediatr Allergy Immunol 2006;17:408–15.
35. Niu CK, Chen WY, Huang JL, et al. Efficacy of sublingual immunotherapy with high-dose mite extracts in asthma: a multi-center, double-blind, randomized, and placebo-controlled study in Taiwan. Respir Med 2006;100:1374–83.
36. Stelmach I, Kaczmarek-Woźniak J, Majak P, et al. Efficacy and safety of high-doses sublingual immunotherapy in ultra-rush scheme in children allergic to grass pollen. Clin Exp Allergy 2009;39:401–8.
37. Pajno G, Passalacqua G, Vita D, et al. Sublingual immunotherapy abrogates seasonal bronchial hyperresponsiveness in children with parietaria-induced respiratory allergy: a randomized controlled trial. Allergy 2004;59:883–7.
38. Canonica GW, Passalacqua G. Disease modifying effect and economic implications of Sublingual immunotherapy. J Allergy Clin Immunol 2011;127:44–5.
39. Quirino T, Iemoli E, Siciliani E, et al. Sublingual vs injective immunotherapy in grass pollen allergic patients: a double-blind double-dummy study. Clin Exp Allergy 1996;26:1253–61.
40. Bernardis P, Agnoletto M, Puccinelli P, et al. Injective VS sublingual immunotherapy in Alternaria tenuis allergic patients. J Investig Allergol Clin Immunol 1996;6:55–62.
41. Piazza I, Bizzarro N. Humoral response to subcutaneous, oral and nasal immunotherapy for allergic rhinitis due to dermatophagoides pteronyssinus. Ann Allergy 1993;71:461–9.
42. Mungan D, Misirligil Z, Gurbuz L. Comparison of the efficacy of subcutaneous and sublingual immunotherapy in mite sensitive patients with rhinitis and asthma: a placebo-controlled study. Ann Allergy Asthma Immunol 1999;82:485–90.
43. Mauro M, Russello M, Incorvaia C, et al. Comparison of efficacy, safety and immunologic effects of subcutaneous and sublingual immunotherapy in birch pollinosis: a randomized study. Eur Ann Allergy Clin Immunol 2007;39:119–22.
44. Eifan AO, Akkoc T, Yildiz A, et al. Clinical efficacy and immunological mechanisms of sublingual and subcutaneous immunotherapy in asthmatic/rhinitis children sensitized to house dust mite: an open randomized controlled trial. Clin Exp Allergy 2010;40:922–32.
45. Khinchi S, Poulsen LK, Carat F, et al. Clinical efficacy of sublingual and subcutaneous birch pollen allergen-specific immunotherapy: a randomized, placebo-controlled, double-blind, double-dummy study. Allergy 2004;59:45–53.
46. Pajno GB, Vita D, Parmiani S, et al. Impact of sublingual immunotherapy on seasonal asthma and skin reactivity in children allergic to Parietaria pollen treated with inhaled fluticasone propionate. Clin Exp Allergy 2003;33:1641–7.
47. Marogna M, Spadolini I, Massolo A, et al. Long-term comparison of sublingual immunotherapy vs inhaled budesonide in patients with mild persistent asthma due to grass pollen. Ann Allergy Asthma Immunol 2009;102:69–75.
48. Cruz AA, Popov T, Pawankar R, et al. Common characteristics of upper and lower airways in rhinitis and asthma: ARIA update, in collaboration with GA(2)LEN. Allergy 2007;62(Suppl 84):1–41.
49. Möller C, Dreborg S, Ferdousi HA, et al. Pollen immunotherapy reduces the development of asthma in children with seasonal rhinoconjunctivitis (the PAT-study). J Allergy Clin Immunol 2002;109:251–6.
50. Novembre E, Galli E, Landi F, et al. Coseasonal sublingual immunotherapy reduces the development of asthma in children with allergic rhinoconjunctivitis. J Allergy Clin Immunol 2004;114:851–7.

51. Marogna M, Tomassetti D, Bernasconi A, et al. Preventive effects of sublingual immunotherapy in childhood: an open randomized controlled study. Ann Allergy Asthma Immunol 2008;101:206–11.

52. Di Rienzo V, Marcucci F, Puccinelli P, et al. Long-lasting effect of sublingual immunotherapy in children with asthma due to house dust mite: a 10-year prospective study. Clin Exp Allergy 2003;33:206–10.

53. Marogna M, Spadolini I, Massolo A, et al. Long-lasting effects of sublingual immunotherapy according to its duration: a 15-year prospective study. J Allergy Clin Immunol 2010;126:969–75.

54. Tahamiler R, Saritzali G, Canakcioglu S. Long-term efficacy of sublingual immunotherapy in patients with perennial rhinitis. Laryngoscope 2007;117:965–9.

55. Durham SR, Emminger W, Kapp A, et al. Long-term clinical efficacy in grass pollen-induced rhinoconjunctivitis after treatment with SQ-standardized grass allergy immunotherapy tablet. J Allergy Clin Immunol 2010;125:131–8.

56. Cox LS, Linnemann DL, Nolte H, et al. Sublingual immunotherapy: a comprehensive review. J Allergy Clin Immunol 2006;117:1021–35.

57. Kleine-Tebbe J, Ribel M, Herold DA. Safety of a SQ-standardised grass allergen tablet for sublingual immunotherapy: a randomized, placebo-controlled trial. Allergy 2006;61:181–4.

58. André C, Vatrinet C, Galvain S, et al. Safety of sublingual swallow immunotherapy in children and adults. Int Arch Allergy Immunol 2000;121:229–34.

59. Gidaro GB, Frati F, Sensi L, et al. The safety of sublingual-swallow immunotherapy: an analysis of published studies. Clin Exp Allergy 2005;35:565–71.

60. Dunsky E, Goldstein MF, Dvorin MJ, et al. Anaphylaxis due to sublingual immunotherapy. Allergy 2006;61:1235.

61. Antico A, Pagani M, Crema A. Anaphylaxis by latex sublingual immunotherapy. Allergy 2006;61:1236.

62. Eifan AO, Keles S, Bahceciler NN, et al. Anaphylaxis to multiple pollen allergen sublingual immunotherapy. Allergy 2007;62:567–8.

63. Blazowski L. Anaphylactic shock because of sublingual immunotherapy overdose during third year of maintenance dose. Allergy 2008;63:374.

64. de Groot H, Bijl A. Anaphylactic reaction after the first dose of sublingual immunotherapy with grass pollen tablet. Allergy 2009;64:963–4.

65. Agostinis F, Tellarini L, Falagiani P, et al. Safety of SLIT in very young children. Allergy 2005;60:133.

66. Fiocchi A, Pajno G, La Grutta S, et al. Safety of sublingual-swallow immunotherapy in children aged 3 to 7 years. Ann Allergy Asthma Immunol 2005;95:254–8.

67. Di Rienzo V, Minelli M, Musarra A, et al. Post-marketing survey on the safety of sublingual immunotherapy in children below the age of 5 years. Clin Exp Allergy 2005;35:560–4.

68. Agostinis F, Foglia C, Landi M, et al. The safety of sublingual immunotherapy with one or multiple pollen allergens in children. Allergy 2008;63:1637–9.

69. Lombardi C, Gargioni S, Cottini M, et al. The safety of sublingual immunotherapy with one or more allergens in adults. Allergy 2008;63:375–6.

70. Cox L, Larenas-Linnemann D, Lockey RF, et al. Speaking the same language: the World Allergy Organization subcutaneous immunotherapy systemic reaction grading system. J Allergy Clin Immunol 2010;125:569–74.

71. Medical dictionary for regulatory activities. Maintenance support services and organization. Available at: http://www.meddramsso.com/. Accessed September, 2010.

72. Sander I, Fleischer C, Meurer U, et al. Allergen content of grass pollen preparations for skin prick testing and sublingual immunotherapy. Allergy 2009;64: 1486–92.
73. Casale TB, Canonica GW, Bousquet J, et al. Recommendations for appropriate sublingual immunotherapy clinical trials. J Allergy Clin Immunol 2009;124: 665–70.
74. Bousquet PJ, Calderon MA, Demoly P, et al. The Consolidated Standards of Reporting Trials (CONSORT) statement applied to allergen-specific immunotherapy with inhalant allergens: a Global Allergy and Asthma European Network (GA(2)LEN) article. J Allergy Clin Immunol 2011;127:49–56.
75. Lombardi C, Braga M, Incorvaia C, et al. Administration regimens for sublingual immunotherapy. What do we know? Allergy 2009;64:849–54.

Sublingual Immunotherapy: Other Indications

Giovanni Passalacqua, MD*, Enrico Compalati, MD,
Giorgio Walter Canonica, MD

KEYWORDS

- Sublingual immunotherapy • Atopic dermatitis • Food allergy
- Latex allergy • Hymenoptera venom

Subcutaneous immunotherapy (SCIT) has been the only available and accepted route of administration for several decades. It still represents the standard immunotherapy route for the treatment of respiratory allergy and hymenoptera venom hypersensitivity. SCIT is effective and safe when properly prescribed and administered, although there is a potential risk of severe side effects, such as life-threatening anaphylaxis. The SCIT risk/benefit ratio has prompted the search for safer administration routes such as nasal, bronchial, oral, and sublingual.[1] Among those noninjection routes, sublingual immunotherapy (SLIT) is the most recent, but it was immediately recognized as a promising approach. In less than 20 years, an impressive amount of clinical data has conferred credibility to SLIT, such that it was introduced in the literature as a viable alternative to the standard SCIT.[2,3] To date, SLIT is commercialized and routinely used in almost all European countries and in many other parts of the world. However, in the United States, no SLIT product has been approved by the Food and Drug Administration for clinical use to date, although several large studies are ongoing.

THE RATIONALE FOR EXPANDING THE INDICATIONS

During the last 20 years, more than 60 randomized clinical trials of SLIT in respiratory allergy have been published.[4] Despite considerable design heterogeneity, the clinical results in these studies were generally favorable, confirming the efficacy of SLIT. This efficacy is further supported by several meta-analyses performed in rhinitis only,[5–7] asthma only,[8] and asthma and rhinitis in children.[9,10] The other relevant aspect of SLIT is the favorable safety profile, which seems to be superior to that of SCIT.[4,11] Mild local side effects (oral itching/swelling, altered taste perception, itching of the

Funding and conflict of interest: none to declare.
Allergy and Respiratory Diseases, Department of Internal Medicine, University of Genoa, Padiglione Maragliano, Largo R. Benzi 10, Genoa 16132, Italy
* Corresponding author.
E-mail address: passalacqua@unige.it

tongue, nausea) account for most of the adverse events associated with SLIT. In most cases, these side effects are usually self-limiting and require no medical intervention In the published literature, there have been no reported fatalities associated with SLIT in more than 20 years, although 6 cases of SLIT-associated anaphylactic reactions have been described.[4] The tolerability of SLIT is good even in children less than the 5 years of age.[12–14] SLIT also exerts a systemic immunologic effect that seems to be similar to that of SCIT; a reduction in symptoms or reactivity on organ-provocation challenge has been shown in multiple organ systems, such as the nose, eye, and bronchi.[15,16] Recent studies suggest that the mechanisms of action of SLIT are similar to those of SCIT, involving the Th1/Th2 balance and the activation of T regulatory cells.[17–22]

Safety, systemic effects, and immunologic mechanisms represent the main rationale for exploring the use of SLIT in allergic disease other than respiratory allergy. The clinical effect of specific immunotherapy in allergic diseases is expected to correlate with the immunoglobulin E (IgE)–mediated component of the disease (as in food allergy or hymenoptera venom allergy; **Fig. 1**).

SLIT IN FOOD ALLERGY

IgE-mediated food allergy reactions (eg, nut anaphylaxis), for which dietary avoidance is the standard treatment, represents an target for specific allergen immunotherapy. In the past, attempts to vaccinate peanut-allergic patients subcutaneously have been made. In a preliminary study investigating the efficacy of SCIT with an aqueous extract of peanut, there was a reduction of symptoms during oral challenge, which ranged from 60% to 100%.[23] In a subsequent study of 12 peanut-allergic subjects, the clinical benefits of peanut SCIT were found to be incomplete, and the treatment induced an unacceptably high rate of systemic reactions.[24] For this reasons, the SCIT approach was virtually abandoned.

Enrique and colleagues[25] performed a randomized, double-blind, placebo-controlled trial with SLIT in 23 hazelnut-allergic subjects, evaluating the oral threshold dose before and after treatment, which was administered in a 4-day rush buildup. A significant increase of the oral threshold dose was seen only in the active group, paralleled by an increase in hazelnut-specific immunoglobulin G4 (IgG4). The rate of systemic reactions was 0.2% of administered doses. A similar study was conducted in 49 peach-allergic subjects, with a purified extract standardized for Pru p 3 content.[26] In this study, a significant increase in the oral challenge threshold dose was seen, along with a reduction of the skin test response to the Pru p 3 extract. There were 16 systemic reactions in more than 1500 adverse events, all mild and spontaneously resolving. Other studies have been performed with a peanut extract. In these

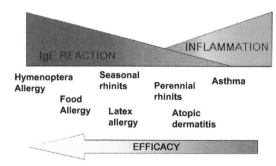

Fig. 1. Where immunotherapy works in allergic diseases.

studies, the treatment was administered orally and not sublingually. The results were similar to those reported with peach or hazelnut SLIT, with a significant reduction of the threshold provocative dose and an increase of specific IgG4.[27] Follow-up of the patients during the home maintenance dose phase confirmed the clinical efficacy and safety profile of this treatment.[28] Blumchen and colleagues[29] treated 23 children with severe peanut allergy by a rush protocol and found that, after 7 to 8 months of maintenance, more than 50% of patients had reached clinical protection. At the end of the study, the oral provocation dose at the food challenge had increased tenfold compared with baseline. Mild to moderate side effects were observed in 2.6% of doses and the treatment was discontinued in 4/22 patients because of adverse events. In this study there was also a significant increase in peanut-specific serum IgG4 and a decrease interleukin (IL)-5 and IL-4 production.

SLIT IN HYMENOPTERA VENOM ALLERGY

Specific immunotherapy with hymenoptera venom (venom immunotherapy [VIT]) is the cornerstone of the management of hymenoptera venom allergy, and results in an almost complete protection against severe allergic reactions from stings in the most patients. Although no fatal events have been described with VIT, its potential risks require administration in a medical facility with appropriate staff and resuscitation/emergency equipment. A safer route of immunotherapy, which allows for home administration, may increase the convenience, and possibly the adherence, to this highly effective, protective treatment. Because of its excellent safety profile, SLIT was considered a potential candidate for VIT. To date, there has been a single randomized controlled trial with honeybee venom (maintenance dose 525 μg/month) conducted in 30 subjects with a history of large local reactions only. The diameter of the local reaction was assessed before and after 6 months of SLIT by means of a sting challenge.[30] In the active group, the median of the peak large local reaction maximum diameter significantly decreased, from 20.5 to 8.5 cm ($P = .014$), whereas no change was seen in the placebo group. The diameter was reduced by more than 50% in 57% of patients. A similar clinical effect (reduction of local reactions) has also been shown for SCIT.[31] Although appealing, this was only a proof-of-concept study, and SLIT cannot yet be recommended for the treatment of hymenoptera venom allergy.[32,33]

SLIT IN LATEX ALLERGY

Although its incidence has been decreasing with time, latex allergy remains an important clinical problem, probably because it is often an occupational disease. In these cases, total latex avoidance may only be achieved by changing the occupation. However, specific immunotherapy is expected to reduce or prevent symptoms when individuals are exposed to the offending allergen. Several attempts to vaccinate against latex have been made with SCIT. Three randomized trials investigating the efficacy and safety of latex SCIT have been conducted.[34–36] The first, which included 20 patients, showed a significant reduction in symptom scores and medication usage along with an increase in the latex conjunctival provocative dose. Nonetheless, all patients displayed local reactions after injections and 50% also experienced systemic reactions. In the second trial, which included 24 patients, there was no change in symptom scores, and systemic reaction (including severe reactions) occurred in 67% of patients. In the third trial, no clinical effect could be shown, but the rate of systemic reactions was reported to be as high as 50% of patients. Based on these results, the subcutaneous approach for latex allergy was abandoned.

There have been at least 5 clinical trials with SLIT for latex allergy.[37-41] The trials had different experimental designs and durations (**Table 1**), but all were in agreement in showing significant clinical efficacy in the measured parameters. Four of the trials used a 5-day rush buildup regimen. Unlike the latex SCIT studies, all of these latex SLIT trials showed good safety profiles. In 2 trials no side effect was reported,[37,40] 1 trial reported only local side effects in 11% of patients,[39] and the remaining trial reported that 10% of the reactions (local) were reported as requiring a medical intervention.[38]

A new ultrarush protocol has recently been described.[41] It lasted only 3 days and therefore can be administered under medical supervision in a convenient way for patients. In this ultrarush trial of 21 patients, which only evaluated safety, there was 1 local reaction (8%) in the active group and 3 (33%) nonspecific reactions in the placebo group.

The case reports of SLIT anaphylaxis were reported with a latex extract during the rush buildup phase.[42] This suggests that, if used, SLIT for latex should be administered under direct medical supervision during the induction phase.

In the pediatric SLIT latex trial, children who received active treatment[40] subsequently received latex SLIT for a further 2 years.[43] In those children, the glove test became completely negative at the third year of treatment, suggesting that a sufficiently prolonged SLIT can virtually abrogate the specific reactivity.

SLIT FOR ATOPIC DERMATITIS

Atopic dermatitis (AD) may be easy to diagnose from a clinical point of view, but it still represents a mystery from the pathogenic and immunologic points of view.[44] The prevalence of atopy in AD is largely variable and the reported prevalence may differ between population-based and physician-based studies.[45] Nevertheless, it is generally agreed that there may be a link between some forms of AD and allergic sensitization (eg, dust mite of foods). Based on these clinical consideration, it was hypothesized that specific immunotherapy could beneficially affect the disease by acting on the allergic component. The first trial of SCIT in AD was published about 20 years ago[46] and, despite the equivocal results, stimulated new research in this field. Several trials of SCIT in AD have been conducted, most have used with house dust mite extracts (for review see Refs.[47,48]), and many of them reported a measurable and significant improvement of cutaneous symptoms after immunotheray.[49,50]

Table 1
SLIT for latex allergy: controlled studies

Author	Patients	Build	Duration	Results
Patriarca et al,[37] 1999	12+12	4d rush	6 mo	All active tolerated the glove. No side effects
Cistero et al,[38] 2001	26	4d rush	3 mo	Improvement in glove test, 21% side effects, 10% needing treatment
Nettis et al,[39] 2006	18+17	4d rush	1 y	Improvement in glove test, symptoms, and medication, 11 % local reactions
Bernardini et al,[40] 2006	12+8 children	4d rush	1 y	Improvement in glove test and symptoms. No side effects

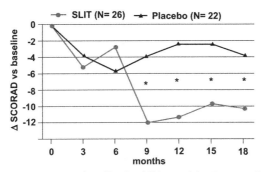

Fig. 2. Reduction in SCORAD versus baseline in children with AD treated for 18 months with mite SLIT. (*From* Pajno GB, Caminiti L, Vita D, et al. Sublingual immunotherapy in mite-sensitized children with atopic dermatitis: a randomized, double-blind, placebo-controlled study. J Allergy Clin Immunol 2007;120:167; with permission.)

Some trials in AD were also performed with SLIT.[51–53] Mastrandrea and colleagues[52] evaluated the efficacy of SLIT in an open, prospective, uncontrolled study of 53 patients with AD only or AD plus respiratory allergy, and found that, after 2 years, about 70% of subjects had a complete disappearance of cutaneous lesions. Another open, noncontrolled, nonrandomized pilot trial investigated the efficacy of dust mite SLIT in 86 patients with AD.[51] After 1 year of treatment, there was a mean reduction in Scoring Atopic Dermatitis (SCORAD) score of about 50%, and that only 6% of patients had no change. These results are of interest, but the open, uncontrolled design strongly limits their validity. However, there has been a single randomized, double-blind, placebo-controlled trial that investigated the efficacy of SLIT in AD.[53] Fifty-six children with AD, monosensitized to mite and without asthma or food allergy, were randomized to receive dust mite SLIT or placebo for 18 months. Starting from the ninth month of treatment, a clear-cut decrease in the SCORAD was observed in the active group, and this improvement was maintained until the end of the study (**Fig. 2**). Nonetheless, a subanalysis showed that the clinical improvement was limited to the mild and moderate patients, whereas, in the more severe subjects, the improvement was only marginal.

SUMMARY

SLIT represents a significant advance because of its efficacy, safety, and convenience, and it seems particularly suitable in pediatric patients, for whom an optimal safety profile is required.[54] The clinical efficacy and safety in respiratory allergy, along with the systemic immunologic effect, suggest that SLIT can be used in other allergic conditions.[55] There are favorable results for food allergy in controlled trials. Nonetheless, many aspects of food allergy need to be clarified, such as the optimal induction regimen, the maintenance dose, and the duration. The investigators who researched peanut desensitization caution that the treatment is still not ready for clinical use.[56] For latex allergy, the results of several controlled trials are encouraging. Latex allergy is not considered an indication to SLIT in the World Allergy Organization position paper on sublingual immunotherapt.[4] Nonetheless, commercial, standardized extracts are available and may be considered, providing they are administered in the appropriate medical setting to selected patients with occupational allergy who cannot avoid latex.[57] For AD, previous experience with SCIT and the results of a few trials suggest the possible application of SLIT. Demonstrated efficacy with SLIT in AD suggests limiting it to children with mild to moderate forms and ascertained sensitization to dust mite, but this recommendation is not considered to be sufficiently evidence based. In hymenoptera allergy, the only trial available is a proof-of-concept study in the treatment of large local reactions that needs to be confirmed in well-controlled studies.

REFERENCES

1. Passalacqua G, Canonica GW. Sublingual immunotherapy: update 2006. Curr Opin Allergy Clin Immunol 2006;6:449–54.
2. Bousquet J, Lockey R, Malling HJ, et al. Allergen immunotherapy: therapeutical vaccines for allergic diseases. World Health Organization position paper. Allergy 1998;53(Suppl 43):1–33.
3. Bousquet J, Van Cauwenberge P. Allergic rhinitis and its impact on asthma. J Allergy Clin Immunol 2001;108(Suppl 5):S146–50.
4. Canonica GW. WAO Position Paper on Sublingual immunotherapy. Allergy 2009; 66(Suppl 82):1–15.
5. Wilson DR, Torres L, Durham SR. Sublingual immunotherapy for allergic rhinitis. Allergy 2005;60:3–8.
6. Compalati E, Passalacqua G, Bonini M, et al. The efficacy of sublingual immunotherapy for house dust mites respiratory allergy: results of a GA2LEN meta-analysis. Allergy 2009;64(11):1570–9.
7. Di Bona D, Plaia A, Scafidi V, et al. Efficacy of sublingual immunotherapy with grass allergens for seasonal allergic rhinitis: a systematic review and meta-analysis. J Allergy Clin Immunol 2010;126(3):558–66.
8. Penagos M, Compalati E, Tarantini F, et al. Efficacy of sublingual immunotherapy in the treatment of allergic rhinitis in children. Meta analysis of randomized controlled trials. Ann Allergy Asthma Immunol 2006;97:141–8.
9. Calamita Z, Saconato H, Bronhara Pelà A, et al. Efficacy of sublingual immunotherapy in asthma. Systematic review of randomized clinical trials. Allergy 2006;61:1162–72.
10. Penagos M, Passalacqua G, Compalati E, et al. Metaanalysis of the efficacy of sublingual immunotherapy in the treatment of allergic asthma in pediatric patients, 3 to 18 years of age. Chest 2008;133:599–609.
11. Cox LS, Linnemann DL, Nolte H, et al. Sublingual immunotherapy: a comprehensive review. J Allergy Clin Immunol 2006;117:1021–35.
12. Agostinis F, Tellarini L, Falagiani P, et al. Safety of SLIT in very young children. Allergy 2005;60:133.
13. Fiocchi A, Pajno G, La Grutta S, et al. Safety of sublingual-swallow immunotherapy in children aged 3 to 7 years. Ann Allergy Asthma Immunol 2005;95:254–8.
14. Di Rienzo V, Minelli M, Musarra A, et al. Post-marketing survey on the safety of sublingual immunotherapy in children below the age of 5 years. Clin Exp Allergy 2005;35:560–4.
15. Stelmach I, Kaczmarek-Woźniak J, Majak P, et al. Efficacy and safety of high-doses sublingual immunotherapy in ultra-rush scheme in children allergic to grass pollen. Clin Exp Allergy 2009;39:401–8.
16. Mortemousque B, Bertel F, De Casamayor J, et al. House-dust mite sublingual-swallow immunotherapy in perennial conjunctivitis: a double-blind, placebo-controlled study. Clin Exp Allergy 2003;33:464–9.
17. Cosmi L, Santarlasci V, Angeli R, et al. Sublingual immunotherapy with *Dermatophagoides* monomeric allergoid down-regulates allergen-specific

immunoglobulin E and increases both interferon-gamma- and interleukin-10-production. Clin Exp Allergy 2006;36:261–72.

18. Ciprandi G, Fenoglio D, Cirillo I, et al. Induction of interleukin 10 by sublingual immunotherapy for house dust mites: a preliminary report. Ann Allergy Asthma Immunol 2005;95:38–44.

19. Bohle B, Kinaciyan T, Gerstmayr M, et al. Sublingual immunotherapy induces IL-10-producing T regulatory cells, allergen-specific T-cell tolerance, and immune deviation. J Allergy Clin Immunol 2007;120:707–13.

20. Ippoliti F, De Sanctis W, Volterrani A, et al. Immunomodulation during sublingual therapy in allergic children. Pediatr Allergy Immunol 2003;14:216–21.

21. Savolainen J, Jacobsen L, Valovirta E. Sublingual immunotherapy in children modulates allergen induced in vitro expression of cytokine mRNA in PBMC. Allergy 2006;61:1184–90.

22. Scadding GW, Shamji MH, Jacobson MR, et al. Sublingual grass pollen immunotherapy is associated with increases in sublingual Foxp3-expressing cells and elevated allergen-specific immunoglobulin G4, immunoglobulin A and serum inhibitory activity for immunoglobulin E-facilitated allergen binding to B cells. Clin Exp Allergy 2010;40:598–606.

23. Oppenheimer JJ, Nelson HS, Bock SA, et al. Treatment of peanut allergy with rush immunotherapy. J Allergy Clin Immunol 1992;90:256–62.

24. Nelson HS, Lahr J, Rule R, et al. Treatment of anaphylactic sensitivity to peanuts by immunotherapy with injections of aqueous peanut extract. J Allergy Clin Immunol 1997;99:744–51.

25. Enrique E, Pineda F, Malek T, et al. Sublingual immunotherapy for hazelnut food allergy: a randomized, double-blind, placebo-controlled study with a standardized hazelnut extract. J Allergy Clin Immunol 2005;116:1073–9.

26. Fernández-Rivas M, Garrido Fernández S, Nadal JA, et al. Randomized double-blind, placebo-controlled trial of sublingual immunotherapy with a Pru p 3 quantified peach extract. Allergy 2009;64:876–83.

27. Jones SM, Pons L, Roberts JL, et al. Clinical efficacy and immune regulation with peanut oral immunotherapy. J Allergy Clin Immunol 2009;124:292–300.

28. Varshney P, Steele PH, Vickery BP, et al. Adverse reactions during peanut oral immunotherapy home dosing. J Allergy Clin Immunol 2009;124(6):1351–2.

29. Blumchen K, Ulbricht H, Staden U, et al. Oral peanut immunotherapy in children with peanut anaphylaxis. J Allergy Clin Immunol 2010;126:83–91.

30. Severino M, Cortellini G, Bonadonna P, et al. Sublingual immunotherapy for large local reactions due to honeybee sting. Double blind placebo controlled trial. J Allergy Clin Immunol 2008;122:44–8.

31. Golden DB, Kelly D, Hamilton RG, et al. Venom immunotherapy reduces large local reactions to insect stings. J Allergy Clin Immunol 2009;123:1371–5.

32. Ruëff F, Bilò MB, Jutel M, et al. Sublingual immunotherapy with venom is not recommended for patients with Hymenoptera venom allergy. J Allergy Clin Immunol 2009;123:272–3.

33. Severino M, Bonadonna P, Passalacqua G. Large local reactions from stinging insects: from epidemiology to management. Curr Opin Allergy Clin Immunol 2009;9:334–7.

34. Leynadier F, Herman D, Vervloet D, et al. Specific immunotherapy with a standardized latex extract versus placebo in allergic healthcare workers. J Allergy Clin Immunol 2000;106:585–90.

35. Sastre J, Fernández-Nieto M, Rico P, et al. Specific immunotherapy with a standardized latex extract in allergic workers: a double-blind, placebo-controlled study. J Allergy Clin Immunol 2003;111:985–94.
36. Tabar AI, Anda M, Bonifazi F, et al. Specific immunotherapy with standardized latex extract versus placebo in latex-allergic patients. Int Arch Allergy Immunol 2006;141:369–76.
37. Patriarca G, Nucera E, Pollastrini E, et al. Sublingual desensitization: a new approach to latex allergy problem. Anesth Analg 2002;95:956–60.
38. Cisteró Bahima A, Sastre J, Enrique E, et al. Tolerance and effects on skin reactivity to latex of sublingual rush immunotherapy with a latex extract. J Investig Allergol Clin Immunol 2004;14:17–25.
39. Nettis E, Colanardi MC, Soccio AL, et al. Double-blind, placebo-controlled study of sublingual immunotherapy in patients with latex-induced urticaria: a 12-month study. Br J Dermatol 2007;156:674–81.
40. Bernardini R, Campodonico P, Burastero S, et al. Sublingual immunotherapy with a latex extract in paediatric patients: a double-blind, placebo-controlled study. Curr Med Res Opin 2006;22:1515–22.
41. Nettis E, Di Leo E, Calogiuri G, et al. The safety of a novel sublingual rush induction phase for latex desensitization. Curr Med Res Opin 2010;26:1855–9.
42. Antico A, Pagani M, Crema A. Anaphylaxis by latex sublingual immunotherapy. Allergy 2006;61:1236.
43. Bernardini R, Pecora S, Milani M, et al. Natural rubber latex allergy in children: clinical and immunological effects of 3-years sublingual immunotherapy. Eur Ann Allergy Clin Immunol 2008;40:142–5.
44. Boguniewicz M, Leung DY. Recent insights into atopic dermatitis and implications for management of infectious complications. J Allergy Clin Immunol 2010;125: 4–13.
45. Flohr C. How atopic is atopic dermatitis? J Allergy Clin Immunol 2004;114:150–8.
46. Glover MT, Atherton DJ. A double-blind controlled trial of hyposensitization to Dermatophagoides pteronyssinus in children with atopic eczema. Clin Exp Allergy 1992;22:440–6.
47. Bussmann C, Bockenhoff A, Henke H, et al. Does allergen-specific immunotherapy represent a therapeutic option for patients with atopic dermatitis? J Allergy Clin Immunol 2006;118:1292–8.
48. Novak N. Allergen specific immunotherapy for atopic dermatitis. Curr Opin Allergy Clin Immunol 2007;7:542–6.
49. Werfel T, Breuer K, Ruéff F, et al. Usefulness of specific immunotherapy in patients with atopic dermatitis and allergic sensitization to house dust mites: a multi-centre, randomized, dose-response study. Allergy 2006;61(2):202–5.
50. Bussmann C, Maintz L, Hart J, et al. Clinical improvement and immunological changes in atopic dermatitis patients undergoing subcutaneous immunotherapy with a house dust mite allergoid: a pilot study. Clin Exp Allergy 2007;37:1277–85.
51. Cadario G, Galluccio AG, Pezza M, et al. Sublingual immunotherapy efficacy in patients with atopic dermatitis and house dust mites sensitivity: a prospective pilot study. Curr Med Res Opin 2007;23:2503–6.
52. Mastrandrea F, Serio G, Minelli M, et al. Specific sublingual immunotherapy in atopic dermatitis. Results of a 6-year follow-up of 35 consecutive patients. Allergol Immunopathol (Madr) 2000;28:54–62.
53. Pajno GB, Caminiti L, Vita D, et al. Sublingual immunotherapy in mite-sensitized children with atopic dermatitis: a randomized, double-blind, placebo-controlled study. J Allergy Clin Immunol 2007;120:164–70.

54. Passalacqua G, Pawankar R, Baena-Cagnani CE, et al. Sublingual immunotherapy: where do we stand? Present and future. Curr Opin Allergy Clin Immunol 2009;9:1–3.
55. Incorvaia C, Mauro M, Cappelletti T, et al. New applications for sublingual immunotherapy in allergy. Recent Pat Inflamm Allergy Drug Discov 2009;3:113–7.
56. Thyagarajan A, Varshney P, Jones SM, et al. Peanut oral immunotherapy is not ready for clinical use. J Allergy Clin Immunol 2010;126(1):31–2.
57. Nowak-Wegrzyn A, Sicherer SH. Immunotherapy for food and latex allergy. Clin Allergy Immunol 2008;21:429–46.

Allergen-Specific Immunotherapy: Which Outcome Measures are Useful in Monitoring Clinical Trials?

O. Pfaar, MD[a],*, J. Kleine-Tebbe, MD[b], K. Hörmann, Prof.MD[c],
L. Klimek, Prof.MD[a]

KEYWORDS

- Allergic rhinoconjunctivitis • Clinical studies
- Allergen-outcome parameters • Study end points
- Quality of life • Specific immunotherapy • Responder-analysis
- Allergen challenge

Sneezing, rhinorrhea, itching, nasal obstruction, and sleep disturbance are typical symptoms of allergic rhinitis (AR). These symptoms may impair patients' daily abilities as well as their general well-being and work productivity.[1] Current treatments of AR include allergen elimination, pharmacologic treatment, and specific immunotherapy (SIT). A revision of the Allergic Rhinitis and its Impact on Asthma (ARIA) guideline,

Financial disclosure: O. Pfaar and L. Klimek have received research grants from ALK-Abello, Denmark; Allergopharma, Germany; Stallergenes, France; HAL, The Netherlands; Artu Biologicals, The Netherlands; Allergy-Therapeutics/Bencard, UK/Germany; Hartington, Spain; Lofarma, Italy; Novartis/Leti, Germany/Spain, and Roxall, Germany. These 2 authors have also served as advisors and on the speakers' bureaus for the above-mentioned pharmaceutical companies. J. Kleine-Tebbe has received lecture fees from Allergopharma, ALK-Abelló, AstraZeneca, Bencard, Essex, HAL Allergy, Leti, Novartis, Phadia, Roxall, Stallergenes, and has received grants for industry-sponsored research projects from Allergopharma, ALK-Abelló, Dr Fooke, HAL Allergy, Phadia, and was consultant for ALK-Abelló, Bencard, HAL Allergy, Novartis, Parexel International, Paul-Ehrlich-Institut, European Medicines Agency (EMA).
[a] Center for Rhinology and Allergology Wiesbaden, Department of Otorhinolaryngology, Head and Neck Surgery, University Hospital Mannheim, An den Quellen 10, 65183 Wiesbaden, Germany
[b] Outpatient Clinic and Associated Research Center Hanf, Herold & Kleine-Tebbe, Allergy & Asthma Center Westend, 14050 Berlin, Germany
[c] Department of Otorhinolaryngology, Head and Neck Surgery, University Hospital Mannheim, 68167 Mannheim, Germany
* Corresponding author.
E-mail address: oliver.pfaar@allergiezentrum.org

Immunol Allergy Clin N Am 31 (2011) 289–309
doi:10.1016/j.iac.2011.02.004
0889-8561/11/$ – see front matter © 2011 Elsevier Inc. All rights reserved.

aimed at providing systematically and transparently developed recommendations about the 3 therapeutic options in AR, has been published.[2] Specific subcutaneous immunotherapy (SCIT) and specific sublingual immunotherapy (SLIT) represent the only immune-modifying and causal treatments available for allergic patients.[1,3] The evidence for the effects of SIT is based on controlled and randomized clinical trials using specific primary and secondary outcome measures (end points).[4,5]

Primary end points for evaluating clinical outcome are the severity of symptoms and the need for concomitant medication, and are usually obtained on a daily basis by keeping diaries.[6] Secondary end points may include the specific and general (generic) quality of life (QoL)[7] or impact on work-related abilities,[8] and are usually obtained by questionnaires at follow-up. Some trials have also included allergen provocation tests, allergen chambers, or other surrogate markers such as allergen-specific IgG_4, the ratio of IgE to IgG_4, the IgE-binding capacity of the patient's serum, cytokine analysis, cell-activation markers, the number or differentiation of immune cells, and cell proliferation assays, but these are not considered to be suitable parameters for primary assessment. However, they might be used for investigating the immunologic mechanisms of SIT.[9,10]

This article gives an overview of approved and widely used methods of monitoring the clinical outcome of SCIT and SLIT in both clinical trials and daily routine. In 2000, a draft guidance document on outcome parameters was provided by the US Department of Health and Human Services Food and Drug Administration (FDA).[11] More recently, the European Medicines Agency (EMA) Committee for Medicinal Products for Human Use (CHMP) guideline on the clinical development of products for SIT has outlined recommendations in assessing outcome variables in clinical trials.[12] It must be noted, however, that universally accepted and authoritative national and international guidelines are still lacking with respect to the assessment of the therapeutic effects of SIT.[6]

PATIENTS' SELF-RATED DIARIES: VALUABLE TOOLS IN ASSESSING PRIMARY END POINTS

Successful SIT results in a decrease in both symptom severity and the need for concomitant medication, which can be monitored by daily entries in patients' diaries. In 2007, a task force of the World Allergy Organization (WAO) proposed a model for standardization of SIT clinical trials stipulating that patient-rated scores should be preferred as primary outcome parameters.[6] The individual scores can be recorded instantaneously (ie, an evaluation of symptom severity immediately before the next dose) and reflectively (predefined time period such as 12 hours).

However, this requires a compliant and motivated patient. The design of the diary depends very much on the experience of the allergologist concerned. According to the authors' experience, some practical aspects recommended for a diary to be a reliable and reproducible source of data can be summarized thus[5,13]:

1. Clear and easy to understand instructions
2. Small and handy size to be carried around easily
3. Only one page for each day
4. Large print for elderly patients
5. Waterproofed bindings
6. Multiple-choice questions as well as some space for free text.

As an alternative to paper diaries, electronic tools (eg, handheld computer or Internet-based devices) might be used in clinical trials, with the advantage that timely and appropriate entries by the patients can be verified. On the other hand, electronic diaries require well-trained and experienced patients and additional logistic expenditures.

PRIMARY END POINTS IN CLINICAL TRIALS: SYMPTOMS AND CONCOMITANT MEDICATION

Following the guidance in *Good Clinical Practice: Consolidated Guideline* (ICH E6) adopted by the ICH, May 1, 1996, clinical trials should include primary parameters "capable of providing the most clinically relevant and convincing evidence directly related to the primary objective of the trial."[14] However, in the 2008 *Guideline on the Clinical Development of Products for Specific Immunotherapy for the Treatment of Allergic Diseases* the European Medicines Agency (EMA) states that to date, there are no symptoms scores thoroughly validated for clinical trials on SIT.[12] However, for the evaluation of AR the 4 individual nasal symptoms "congestion," "sneezing," "itching," and "secretion," and 2 conjunctival symptoms "itching of eyes" and "ocular secretions," are generally accepted. These symptoms are scored by patients on the diary card using a 4-point rating scale between 0 (no symptoms) and 3 (severe symptoms) so that the (combined) sum of the 6 individual symptom scores for a given day results in a rhinoconjunctivitis total symptom score (RTSS) ranging between 0 and 18 points (**Table 1**).[12]

The average RTSS (ARTSS) is then defined as the average of the daily RTSS during the observation period, for example, the peak pollen season.[15] The RTSS was included in several recent trials on both SCIT[16] and SLIT.[17–19]

Shortness of breath, cough, wheezing, and chest tightness may also be considered in patients with concomitant lower airway symptoms.[6] Hence, in other studies a total of 9 types of symptoms were rated in a combined symptom score of 3 nasal symptoms (running, blockage, sneeze), 3 ocular symptoms (itching, redness, tearing), and 3 bronchial symptoms (cough, wheezing, asthma/dyspnoe). Each symptom was scored on a scale of 0 to 3 and totaled daily, allowing a maximum score of 27 points.[20,21] Another trial on SLIT included 4 nasal symptoms together with 3 conjunctival and 3 bronchial symptoms, resulting in a maximum score of 30 points[22,23] and in trials on SLIT with tablets on both grass pollen allergic children/adolescents[24,25] and adults[26,27] 4 nasal together with 2 conjunctival symptoms (maximum: 18 points) and separately 4 bronchial symptoms (maximum: 12 points) were analyzed.

Fig. 1 displays examples of 6 different scoring systems that are used at present by some European allergen manufacturers.

Table 1 Evaluation of nasal symptoms using a 4-digit score	
0	*No sign/symptom evident*
1	Mild symptoms (*sign/symptom clearly present, but minimal awareness; easily tolerated*)
2	Moderate symptoms (*definite awareness of sign/symptom that is bothersome but tolerable*)
3	Severe symptoms (*sign/symptom that is hard to tolerate; causes interference with activities of daily living and/or sleeping*)

Data from Committee for Medicinal Products for Human Use (CHMP). Guideline on the clinical development of products for specific immunotherapy for the treatment of allergic diseases.CHMP/EWP/18504/2006. London; 2008; and Guidance for Industry. Allergic rhinitis: clinical development programs for drug products. Draft guidance. U.S. Department of Health and Human Services, Food and Drug Administration. Center for Drug Evaluation and Research; 2000.

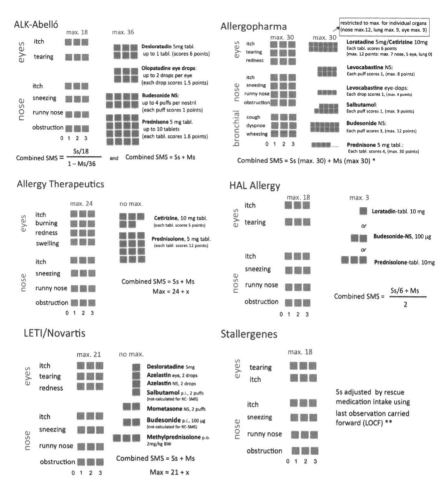

Fig. 1. Examples of currently applied symptom and medication score systems from different European allergen manufacturers. Allergic symptoms (*orange box* = 1 score point) and rescue medication scoring (*green box* = 1 score point) are given as well as the way symptom score (Ss) and medication score (Ms) are weighted for a combined symptom-medication score (SMS). Some medication scores do not restrict the entry in the case of multiple drug doses leaving the score open for extraordinarily high values (no max.). top, topical; NS, nasal spray; RC, rhinoconjunctivitis. * Based on this combined SMS the "Allergy-Control-Score (ACS)" has recently been validated.[29] ** The "average Adjusted Symptom Score" (AdSS) is derived from the RTSS using "last-observation-carried-forward" (LOCF).[30]

In SIT clinical trials, symptom and medication scores are often assessed independently, with defining symptom scores regarded as primary efficacy end points (eg, RTSS) while use of concomitant medication defined as a secondary outcome parameter.[15] However, there is a complex and multifactorial interaction between symptom scores and the use of concomitant medication. First, the use of concomitant antiallergic medication results in reduction of clinical symptoms of AR, and thereby alleviates the daily symptom scores in both active and placebo-treated patients. Second, placebo-treated patients are expected to use concomitant medication in a higher extent that patients in the active group. Hence, if the assessment of efficacy is estimated on the symptom scores alone, the use of rescue medication will alleviate the superiority of active over placebo treatment.[15]

Because of these interdependences, a task force of the WAO suggested a model for standardization of clinical trials on SIT. The task force recommended that symptom scores always be combined with the concomitant medication scores to provide clinically more relevant information on SIT than assessing each of these two outcome parameters separately[6]; this is achievable by a combined score (weighted sum scores of symptoms and rescue medications)[28] or a symptom score adjusted for the use of medication, using a predefined algorithm.[4] However, to date no standardized method for combined scores has been accepted.[6,15]

Following the WAO guidelines, nasal, conjunctival, and oral antihistamines should be weighted with a score of 1, inhalative or nasal corticosteroids with a score of 2, and the daily administration of oral corticosteroids with a score of 3 points. The "symptom load" of each day is then evaluated by equally adding the sum of the symptom score to the medication score, aiming to reproduce a weighted balance between use of concomitant medication and the extent of symptoms.[6] However, there is a high variability between studies on SIT of how concomitant medication is scored, as topically and systemically applied rescue medication is differently weighted (see **Fig. 1**). Comparison of these studies suggests that the symptom and medication scores currently used in clinical trials as primary outcome parameters are not standardized and give variable results.

Recently, a novel combined symptom-medication score (Allergy-Control-SCORE [ACS] [TM]) has been formally validated for the first time in a clinical trial on 81 patients with allergic rhino-conjunctivitis and/or asthma and 40 healthy controls by comparing this score to global allergy severity, quality of life, and allergy-related medical consultations.[29] Moreover, the average Adjusted Symptom Score (AdSS) has been calculated in a post-hoc analysis of a Phase IIb/III trial on 628 grass pollen allergic adults[17] and a Phase III trial on 278 paediatric patients[18] and has been recently published giving extensive formula for exact calculation of this score.[30] It adjusts the symptom for the use of medication by calculating the "last observation carried forward", which has been frequently applied to handle missing data in clinical trials.[15] In the case that the patient is taking concomitant medication, the last (most recent) RTSS score of the day before medication has been started is calculated for further analysis. This AdSS-score is carried forward until the day the patient stops antiallergic medication again.

It is obvious that the clinical outcome should be taken into account for the final interpretation of the clinical efficacy of SIT ("nonresponder" vs "responder"), that is, the decrease in symptom scores should be high enough to clearly reduce allergy-related morbidity under "real life" conditions.[31] In some clinical trials, more emphasis is placed on the statistical significance of changes rather than their clinical relevance, but this does not always illustrate the clinical benefit of a therapy in practice. For example, a 15% reduction in combined symptom-medication scores might reveal statistical significance, but this does not necessarily mean a clinical benefit for the patient per se. Therefore, ranges of improvements of symptom or medication scores for discriminating between effective and noneffective therapy in SIT have been proposed by Malling.[32]

1. No effect, improvement of <30%
2. Little effect, improvement of 30%–44%
3. Moderate effect, improvement of 45%–59%
4. Strong effect, improvement of $\geq$60%.

Although this classification seems arbitrary, it has served as a simplified "rule of thumb" in assessing "relevant" effects of therapy in SIT trials.

Assessing the Relevant (Pollen-)Allergen Exposition

In pollen allergies, it is standard to measure pollen concentrations in a defined volume of air (eg, using Burkard volumetric spore traps). Pollen counts are usually expressed as the mean daily number of pollen grains per cubic meter of filtered air. Usually a limited time interval is defined as the time frame for the evaluations. This interval may be the "time of peak pollen season" or the "relevant pollen season," or others. An exact definition is still lacking.[6] In one approach, a certain number of pollen grains per cubic meter is predefined and the "peak pollen season" or "relevant pollen season" and starts per definition when this number is reached, for example, once or on more than 3 consecutive days. The season ends, vice versa, if the pollen count falls below this value in the same way. However, there is the question of the "relevant" pollen exposure and defining threshold values for this. In a double-blind, placebo-controlled (DBPC) trial on 184 tree pollen–allergic patients receiving SCIT with a depigmented polymerized tree pollen extract, Pfaar and colleagues[33] analyzed symptom and medication scores on days above a series of different threshold values for pollen exposure ($\geq$250, $\geq$300, $\geq$400, $\geq$500 grains/m^3 per 24 hours). A clear relationship between pollen exposure and the magnitude of combined symptom and medication score caused by this exposure, as well as differences for the size of response to treatment for different thresholds, were demonstrated. Further studies are necessary to define more precisely the optimal threshold value for pollen exposure and, therefore, the "relevant" time frame for evaluation.

A different approach is to retrospectively evaluate the time with the maximum pollen count over a certain time frame, for example, 4 weeks. Rarely, a complete analysis of the entire pollen season will be performed. However, the latter approach would more likely reflect the expectations of the patient in real life, who would like to achieve relief during the entire pollen season and not only during an arbitrarily defined peak period.

Analyzing Different Pollen Counts in Different Areas

In multicenter trials it is necessary to take into account the different pollen counts in different areas. One model is to choose several pollen traps nearest to the study centers, possibly within the same area. However, it is well known that the "real" allergen exposition of the individual patient cannot be detected in this way. The duration and intensity of the pollen season is expected to be variable and, therefore, pollen counts are conducted at least 3 times each week in the vicinity of each center. However, as each study center could recruit subjects from a wide area, this approach may not necessarily identify the most appropriate peak weeks of the pollen season for individual subjects. A previous study investigating the allergic response to birch pollen highlighted that some subjects report severe symptoms even on days with low birch pollen levels.[34,35]

While a recent analysis by Buters and colleagues[36] demonstrated that although, in general, pollen count and allergen levels overlapped, in some cases the difference between estimated allergen exposure based on pollen counts and determination of allergen levels by immunoassay could vary by as much as a factor of 10. The investigators explained this variance by demonstrating a large increase in expression of the birch pollen allergen Bet v 1 just before pollination. Consequently, the day the pollen is released during ripening will affect its potency. These results suggest that even in locations close to the pollen trap, pollen counting may not be the most appropriate measure of allergen exposure.

The same applies for indoor allergens such as house dust mites and cat allergens. Here, assessments of allergen exposure by measuring major allergens in reservoir dust samples (bed, carpet, soft furnishings, and so forth) using monoclonal antibody-based enzyme-linked immunosorbent assays might provide levels of individual exposure. The World Health Organization/International Union of Immunological Societies Allergen Standardization Committee has initiated a multicenter project to develop international standards for purified allergens. This program had been coordinated through the European Union CREATE project (Certified Reference Materials for Allergenic Products).[37,38]

Individual pollen samplers are an alternative that has been used to assess pollen, mites, and cat allergens.[39,40]

Peak Placebo Symptom Days

Another approach to evaluating the relevant pollen exposure in allergic individuals is to identify the peak symptom days for the 4 weeks with the highest symptom medication score (SMS) during the pollen season, based on the findings in the placebo group.[41] These "peak placebo symptom days" are not necessarily consecutive and vary between centers. It is assumed that the period when the SMS in the placebo group of the specific study center is at its highest indicates the heaviest pollen load. This novel approach allows the local allergy burden to be determined at different centers. However, representing a postrandomization variable, leading to a post hoc analysis, this attempt would not be valid for the design of a controlled prospective study.

Responder Analysis and Baseline Year

The current European Union regulatory bodies (EMA) recommend that a responder analysis should be performed in addition to assessing efficacy on the basis of SMS scores alone.[12] In this guideline "responders" are defined as "patients with a combined score below a pre-specified level indicating a clinical benefit for the patient." However, for this analysis a "baseline period" assessing the patient's symptom load one pollen season before randomization (and treatment) is required. Due to the unpredictability and variability of allergen exposure to pollen exposure (see earlier discussion), baseline pollen seasons are not generally useful for this pretreatment/posttreatment analysis.[6] Moreover, this procedure is time-consuming and expensive.[6]

For this reason, a "modified responder analysis" has been recently described, setting the median value for the primary outcome using area under the curve (AUC) for SMS for the entire pollen season for the placebo group as "baseline," and analyzing numbers of responders and nonresponders at different levels of reduction in the combined scores from this baseline.[33] By the use of receiver-operator curves (ROC), the authors found a cutoff of 30% to optimally discriminate between active and placebo-treated patients during the entire season. These results are in line with the "Malling definition" of a clinically relevant treatment effect of SIT of at least 30% (see earlier discussion[32]).

Visual Analog Scales

Another self-assessment method, the visual analog scale (VAS) or visual rating scale (VRS), has been recommended for psychometric analysis.[6,12] VAS has been shown to be useful in the monitoring of the severity of symptoms, especially for long-term follow-up in the treatment of perennial AR, for example, comparison of baseline- and posttreatment conditions. Patients grade their symptoms retrospectively (eg, in the last week or in the last month) by putting a vertical line on a 10-cm line representing the severity of symptoms from 0 = "no symptoms" to 10 = "very severe symptoms."

Thereby, one advantage of the VAS is through the use of a continuous variable rather than an ordinate scale. One the other hand this narrows the spectrum of the responses, as patients tend to avoid marking the extremes of the VAS.[7] However, as secondary outcome parameters VAS have been widely used in different SIT trials and have supplemented other outcome variables such as symptom and medication scores.[16,22,42,43]

SECONDARY END POINTS IN CLINICAL TRIALS: HEALTH-RELATED QUALITY OF LIFE

The impact of AR on the patient's health status goes far beyond the organ-specific (nasal, conjunctival, and bronchial) symptoms alone.[5] Thus, the objective of a clinical trial of SIT should not simply be to monitor certain organ-related symptoms but to additionally evaluate the patient's mental and physical condition, the so-called health-related quality of life (HRQoL).[44] The impairment of allergic patient's physical fitness, school and occupational achievements, life satisfaction, and "day-to-day activities" has been clearly evaluated in many clinical trials. Moreover, reports have revealed that sleep impairment results in a noticeable reduction in general activities and diminished HRQoL of patients with AR.[45] Therefore, assessing the HRQoL is a valuable and sensitive tool for evaluating a therapeutic improvement of SIT as a secondary outcome, with symptom and medication scores as the primary outcome parameters. Two types of HRQoL questionnaires are available: generic and disease-specific (**Table 2**).

Generic QoL Questionnaires

First, there are general health-related (generic) questionnaires available, which enable patients with different diseases to be compared on the basis of their QoL from the patient's point of view. In other words, these generic QoL questionnaires compare

Table 2
Generic and disease-specific QoL questionnaires for specific immunotherapy trials

Generic (Not Disease Related)	
Medical Outcome Study Short Form-36	Stewart et al,[46] Ware and Sherbourne[47]
Medical Outcome Study Short Form-20	Carver et al[52]
Munich Life Dimension List (MLDL)	Kremer et al[54]
Work Productivity and Activity Impairment Questionnaire (WPAI)	Prasad et al[8]
Specific (Disease Related)	
Asthma Quality of Life Questionnaire	Juniper et al[98]
Mini Asthma Quality of Life Questionnaire	Juniper et al[99]
Asthma Questionnaire 30	Barley et al[100]
Asthma Questionnaire 20	Barley et al[100]
Rhinoconjunctivitis Quality of Life Questionnaire	Juniper and Guyatt[55]
Mini-Rhinoconjunctivitis Quality of Life Questionnaire	Juniper et al[56]
Pediatric Rhinoconjunctivitis Quality of Life Questionnaire	Juniper et al[58]
Rhinasthma	Baiardini et al[63]
Rhinasthma (adapted German version)	Mosges et al[64]

Data from Canonica GW, Baena-Cagnani CE, Bousquet J, et al. Recommendations for standardization of clinical trials with Allergen Specific Immunotherapy for respiratory allergy. A statement of a World Allergy Organization (WAO) taskforce. Allergy 2007;62:317–24.

the burden of the different diseases, such as asthma or rhinitis, utilizing the identical questionnaire tool.[7]

To date, the best validated and most commonly applied generic questionnaire is the Health Status Questionnaire Short Form-36 (SF-36) (**Table 3**,[46,47]). In 1994, Bousquet and colleagues[48] confirmed the SF-36 as a valuable tool in discriminating between patients with perennial AR and healthy subjects. It has also been validated by other groups.[49]

This questionnaire comprises 36 questions in 9 health domains, and renders mental component summary (MCS) scores as well as a psychometrically based physical component summary (PCS).[50,51] A modified version (SF-36 v2) has been translated into more than 120 languages in both standard 4-week and acute 1-week recall periods (detailed information on www.sf-36.org).

Other generic QoL questionnaires are the Medical Outcome Study Short Form-20 (SF-20),[52] the Satisfaction Profile (SAT-P),[53] and the Munich Life Dimension List.[54] One additional example is the Work Productivity and Activity Impairment Questionnaire (WPAI), one of the most frequently used instruments in assessing the extent of the patients' occupational impairment caused by the disease.[8]

Taken together, the generic QoL questionnaires have the advantage that the impact of illness on the individual's quality of life can be globally assessed independently from the specific, underlying disease. Consequently the questionnaires have to be broad in

Table 3
Definition of health concepts with the SF-36 questionnaire

Measure	Number of Items	Definition
Functional Status		
Physical functioning	10	Extent to which health interferes with a variety of activities (eg, sports, carrying groceries, climbing of stairs, and walking)
Social functioning	2	Extent to which health interferes with normal social activities (eg, visiting with friends during past month)
Role limitations attributed to physical problems	4	Extent to which health interferes with usual daily activities (eg, accomplished less than would like)
Role limitations attributed to emotional problems	3	Extent to which health interferes with usual daily social activities (eg, accomplished less than would like)
Well-Being		
Mental health	5	General mood or affect, including depression, anxiety, and psychological well-being during the past month
Energy/fatigue	4	Tiredness, energy level
Pain	2	Extent of bodily pain in past 4 weeks
Overall Evaluation of Health		
General perception of health	5	Overall rating of current health in general
Change of health[a]	1	Evolution of general perception of health

[a] Not included in (SF-36 v2).

Data from Ware JE Jr, Sherbourne CD. The MOS 36-item short-form health survey (SF-36). I. Conceptual framework and item selection. Med Care 1992;30(6):473–83; and Bousquet J, Bullinger M, Fayol C, et al. Assessment of quality of life in patients with perennial allergic rhinitis with the French version of the SF-36 Health Status Questionnaire. J Allergy Clin Immunol 1994;94(2 Pt 1):182–8.

their comprehensiveness, but this results in very little depth of assessment.[7] Therefore in many conditions, such as rhinitis, generic QoL questionnaires are quite insensitive and often unresponsive to changes that might be small but undoubtedly essential to the patient's QoL. This disadvantage limits the usage of generic QoL questionnaires as tools in clinical trials on SIT, where the effects of the treatment on a homogeneous group of allergic patients are measured. As a consequence, disease-specific measures are more valuable tools in finding small, but clinically relevant changes in the patients' QoL in clinical trials on SIT.[7]

Disease-Specific QoL Questionnaires for AR and Asthma

HRQoL can be assessed on the basis of specific disease-related questionnaires, such as the Rhinoconjunctivitis Quality of Life Questionnaire (RQLQ),[55] which was validated in 1991 by Juniper and Guyatt, based on how symptoms and treatment affect the patient's social, emotional, and physical well-being. The RQLQ consists of 28 questions/items divided across 7 "main factors"/domains (activity limitations, emotional function, eye symptoms, non–hay fever symptoms, nasal symptoms, practical problems, and sleep problems), all of which are scored by the patients using a 7-point Likert scale ranging from 0 (ie, not troubled/none of the time) to 6 (ie, extremely troubled/all the time).[55] The 7 domains that impair the patient's QoL with AR as assessed by the RQLQ are as follows[55]:

1. Practical problems: 3 items
2. Activities: 3 items
3. Sleep problems: 3 items
4. Emotional condition: 4 items
5. Nasal symptoms: 4 items
6. Eye symptoms: 4 items
7. Non-nasal/eye symptoms: 7 items.

For the domain "sleep problems" these items refer to "difficulty getting to sleep," "waking up during the night," and "lack of a good night's sleep." For the domain "activities" 3 items can be selected out of a list of 29 activities freely by the patient. These activities should be the 3 considered by the patient to be most affected by the disease.

The mean value for overall (global) RQLQ including all domains is calculated, as well as the mean value of each domain. The higher the score, the higher is the impairment of QoL. In controlled clinical trials a difference of 0.5 or greater in RQLQ domains between active and placebo-treated patients is regarded as clinically relevant.[55]

A shortened version of this RQLQ, the Mini Rhinoconjunctivitis Quality of Life Questionnaire (Mini RQLQ), with 14 questions spanning the 5 domains "nose symptoms," "eye symptoms," "other symptoms," "practical problems," and "activity limitations," has been recently validated by the same group.[56] Furthermore, the RQLQ has been modified and adapted to different age groups of patients, taking into account that the effect on QoL may be different in allergic children and adolescents from that in adult allergic patients.[7,57,58]

Several clinical studies have investigated the effect of antiallergic medication on QoL in allergic patients. A recent trial by Ciprandi and colleagues[59] on 123 patients with persistent AR clearly revealed a close relationship between QoL as measured by the RQLQ and clinical parameters such as nasal flow and eye symptoms, as well as immunologic parameters and functional surrogate markers. The investigators concluded that QoL is strictly related to the allergic inflammation process, and thereby might be used as a valuable leveling parameter in managing patients with AR.

Furthermore, RQLQ scores as secondary outcome measures have been assessed in several clinical trials on both SLIT[60–62] and SCIT.[16,20] In a dose-finding study with grass-allergen tablets containing timothy grass (*Phleum pratense*), overall RQLQ scores were significantly improved compared with placebo in the high-dose group (75,000 standardized quality tablet units daily), both at the first and second grass pollen season.[62] A recent study on SLIT with grass-allergen tablets containing 5 grass allergens demonstrated that the RQLQ scores were improved in active treated patients, as were both primary (RTSS) and other secondary parameters (efficacy at pollen peak, combined scores, and immunologic changes).[60] RQLQ was also measured in a recent DBPC trial on grass tablets, with significant improvements in both RQLQ overall and all-domain scores (except "emotional function") in the peak pollen seasons, not only in the 3-year course of therapy but also sustained in a follow-up year.[61] In another DBPC dose-finding SCIT trial the effectiveness of 2 doses of an unmodified grass pollen extract in patients with moderately severe seasonal AR was investigated, and a clear dose-related response was found for the primary outcome parameter, symptom and medication scores.[16] Of interest, a significantly better RQLQ as compared with placebo in 5 of the 7 RQLQ domains in the high-dose group (maintenance dose: 100,000 standardized quality units [SQ-U]) and only in 1 of the 7 RQLQ domains in the low-dose group (maintenance dose 10,000 SQ-U) was also revealed. Another SCIT trial using a mixture of 5 recombinant grass pollen allergens found that in addition to a significant improvement in combined symptom and medication scores in the first grass pollen season, SCIT resulted in a significant improvement of 5 of the RQLQ subdomains and of the global RQLQ in the second grass pollen season.[20]

The specific disease-related questionnaire RQLQ only evaluates QoL as related to AR symptoms but not to allergic asthma, although both diseases are linked and often show comorbidity (concept of "united airways"). Therefore, the "Rhinasthma" questionnaire was validated by Baiardini and colleagues[63] for assessing the functional, physical, and emotional status of adult patients as influenced by AR *and* bronchial hyperreactivity. The German adapted Rhinasthma questionnaire is composed of 42 patients' self-rated items and, more than other RQLQ questionnaires, considers the impact on AR on the social interactions of the patients.[64]

Defining "Well Days" as New Outcome-Parameters

In addition to symptom scores and the use of antiallergic medication, the EMA recommends evaluating "days with sufficient symptom control."[12] According to the EMA guidelines, these are defined as "days without intake of rescue medication and a symptom score below a pre-defined and clinically justified threshold."[12] In recent years, this parameter has been increasingly included in several clinical studies on SLIT.[24,42,65] However, the definition of the "clinically justified threshold" symptom score varies between different studies:

In a DBPC study on SLIT including 89 grass pollen–allergic patients, a 42-day period during the grass pollen season was analyzed.[65] During this 42-day period, "well days" were defined as days without any medication intake and with a symptom score of 4 or less. After 18 months of SLIT, actively treated patients reported a significantly higher median number of "well days" (52.4%) than did the placebo group (10.7%). These results corresponded well to results in the combined SMS scores.

In another DBPC study on SLIT with grass tablets, that included 253 children, aged 5 to 16 years, with grass pollen–induced rhinoconjunctivitis with or without asthma, "well days" were defined as days without any intake of concomitant medication and with a rhinoconjunctivitis symptom score of 2 or less.[24] The active group reported

53% well days whereas the placebo group reported 42% well days, with the difference being significant. Again, this result was in line with the study's other primary and secondary end points.

A large DBPC dose-finding study on SLIT with grass tablets by Didier and colleagues[17] measured "symptom-free days" (%) during the pollen season. These days were defined when "0" (absence of symptoms) was recorded for each of the 6 rhinoconjunctivitis symptoms. In accordance with the differences in RTSS scores between the active groups and the placebo group and other outcome parameters, differences in the percentage of the symptom-free days were also shown.

Provocation Tests as Surrogate Markers

In its 2008 *Guideline on the Clinical Development of Products for Specific Immunotherapy for the Treatment of Allergic Diseases* the EMA emphasized that "provocation tests (eg, conjunctival, nasal or bronchial provocation or allergen exposure in allergen challenge chambers) and/or clinical end points may be used as primary end points" in early-stage, dose-ranging (phase 2) studies.[12]

The nasal provocation test (NPT) is a diagnostic tool used to confirm the clinical relevance of inhalative allergens for AR.[66,67] This method is standardized, and provides both high sensitivity and high specificity.[68] It has been used in several clinical trials on SIT to reveal changes of the allergen-specific organ-related reactivity after treatment.[69,70] For the latter, NPT should be performed with increasing threshold concentrations and the response compared with the results at baseline. In a controlled open trial of 53 grass pollen–allergic children, SCIT with a chemically modified preparation resulted in a 10-fold higher allergen concentration required to provoke a positive test result compared with pretreatment.[71] In a SCIT-study with a short-term regimen of 7 preseasonal injections over 6 weeks, a significant increase in the dose that provoked a positive response in nasal allergen challenge was clearly demonstrated in active treated patients compared with patients on placebo.[72]

The NPT with increasing threshold concentrations of allergens was also performed in a study on intralymphatic allergen administration (ILIT) in comparison with SCIT.[73] As early as 4 months after the start of therapy, a significant increase in tolerance to nasal provocation in the ILIT-group was found as compared with baseline. By contrast, there were no significant differences in threshold concentrations compared with baseline in the SCIT-treated group at this early stage of therapy. In another DBPC "proof of concept" trial, the same group investigated the effects of transcutaneous immunotherapy using allergen-containing patches, with NPT used as primary outcome parameter.[74] Actively treated patients revealed significantly decreased scores in nasal provocation tests in the first and second year after treatment compared with baseline. However, the differences in comparison with the group with placebo patches did not reach statistical significance. Taken together, the NPT reproduces the response of the upper airways to natural allergen exposure under controlled and reproducible conditions.[68] However, this method is a time-consuming and laborious procedure.

As an alternative allergen challenging method, the conjunctival provocation test (CPT) has been performed in several studies as an inclusion criterion and as an outcome measure after pharmacotherapy or SIT.[75–77] In a DBPC study of La Rosa and colleagues,[78] 41 children allergic to *Parietaria*-induced rhinoconjunctivitis were randomized to receive sublingual standardized *Parietaria judaica* extract or placebo. As a secondary outcome parameter, CPT was performed with titrated doses. After 1 year of SLIT treatment the threshold dose in CPT increased in both groups, but to significantly greater extent in the active treatment group. CPT was also investigated in the Preventive Allergy Treatment (PAT) study, the first prospective long-term follow-up trial addressed to investigate whether SCIT has a preventive effect on the development of asthma.[43,79] In this trial 147 allergic patients, aged 16 to 25 years, have been analyzed 10 years after initiation of a 3-year course of SCIT with standardized allergen extracts of grass and/or birch or no SCIT (antiallergic medication only), respectively. In addition to a preventive long-term effect on the prevalence of asthma found in this trial, the conjunctival sensitivity in the titrated CPT was significantly reduced in the active group as compared with the control group 7 years after termination of SCIT.[43]

Riechelmann and colleagues[80] compared the value of CPT in comparison with NPT on 50 mite-allergic patients, and found a high correlation between both challenge tests with concordant results in 90% of the patients tested. Taken together, the CPT is a very sensitive test for providing information about the patient's clinical allergy status. However, one disadvantage of the CPT is that there is a lack of an objective outcome measure, as positive or negative results are only clinically assessed.

Pollen Chambers

Allergen challenge chambers (ACC) provide a promising tool for evaluating the therapeutic effects of SIT, as this method circumvents some drawbacks of conventional clinical outdoor studies such as the unpredictable levels of pollen, weather conditions during the study period, and high diversity of pollen exposure in different regions.[5,12,66,81] The exposure chamber facilitates both a controlled and reproducible pollen challenge of allergic patients, as well as the assessment of responses to that challenge, using a predefined protocol.[81] The pollen levels in the ACC can be continuously measured and adjusted to stimulate a similar allergen exposure as in ambient air during the natural pollen season.[66] Hence this method is capable of reproducing the study conditions of an outdoor allergy study with high specificity and high sensitivity.[82] Provocation chambers have been widely used to evaluate symptomatic antiallergic medications[83,84] but have been only marginally employed in allergen immunotherapy.[85–87] Single challenge tests, however, will not be able to imitate the priming effect seen in real life, which is due to repeated or continuous allergen exposures.

In a DBPC clinical trial on 89 grass-allergic patients, Horak and colleagues[88] investigated the onset of action of a 5-grass pollen sublingual tablet formulation using the "Vienna" ACC. A standardized allergen challenge with grass pollen and assessment of allergic symptoms (ARTSS) was performed at baseline, week 1, and months 1, 2, and 4 during a preseasonal treatment. SLIT tablets revealed a significant improvement in ARTSS scores versus placebo from the first month of treatment onward.

Taken together, ACCs might be valuable tools in detecting the clinical efficacy of SIT in clinical trials performed independently from the natural pollen season. ACCs have been recommended by both the FDA and the EMA guidelines as outcome parameters in phase 2 trials. However, future studies will be needed to validate ACCs more thoroughly compared to the (natural) seasonal pollen exposure.

Asthma-Specific Outcome Measures

The peak expiratory flow (PEF) and the forced expiratory volume in 1 second (FEV_1) are sufficient, practical, and objective tools for the monitoring of asthma. These tools may vary with individual performance (effort-dependent) and provide only a snapshot of pulmonary function, particularly in subjects with highly variable airway obstruction. Therefore, frequent measurements are necessary to create an appropriate data set reflecting the overall pulmonary function. Furthermore, inhalation tests with metacholine (metacholine bronchial provocation test [MBPT]) are valuable in assessing nonspecific bronchial hypersensitivity in asthma patients with nearly normal PEF and FEV_1 results despite asthmatic symptoms.

In addition to other outcome variables such as the clinical diagnosis of asthma or CPT results, MBPT has been used in the PAT study described earlier.[43,79] In contrast to other outcome variables, no significant differences regarding MBPT between the SCIT group and control group were found after 10 years in this long-term observation study.

Sting Challenges as Outcome Parameter After Hymenoptera SIT

The efficacy of Hymenoptera SIT can be estimated by a controlled sting provocation under clinical conditions performed according to international guidelines.[89] As a predictive value for tolerance to Hymenoptera venom after venom immunotherapy, the sting challenge test is superior to an accidental "field" sting.[90] However, as challenge tests are high-risk procedures, they should be only performed in specialized centers and not be executed for the diagnosis of patients who have not been treated with SIT. Furthermore, a negative challenge test does not ensure the absence of reactions after subsequent Hymenoptera stings.

IN VITRO PARAMETERS: SURROGATE MARKERS USEFUL TO SOME EXTENT

In vitro parameters such as allergen-specific IgE and specific IgG levels, cytokines such as interferon-γ, interleukins, tryptase, eosinophil cationic protein (ECP), and other inflammatory parameters are valuable additional secondary outcome measures assessing the immunologic effect of SIT in clinical trials (**Table 4**).[6] Some examples of these surrogate markers used in SIT trials are characterized below. These markers cannot substitute for the assessment of clinical parameters described earlier, but can be used to assess secondary outcomes in combination with the clinical outcomes or to analyze particular aspects of SIT, for example, immunologic mechanisms of treatment.[6,10] In its 2008 *Guideline on the Clinical Development of Products for Specific Immunotherapy for the Treatment of Allergic Diseases* the EMA[12] emphasizes

Table 4
Surrogate markers and paraclinical parameters to evaluate the therapeutic effect of specific immunotherapy

Organ-Related Provocation	Immunologic Parameters
Skin: skin prick test (SPT), favorably with titrated allergen-doses Intracutaneous test (IT): late cutaneous response	Total IgE, specific IgE and IgG subclasses
Nose and eye: allergen challenge tests, favorably with titrated allergen-doses	Mucosal IgA Mucosal IgE
Lung: spirometric results: FEV_1, peak flow variability (PEF), metacholine challenge, allergen challenge	Lymphocyte subgroups Cytokines (eg, IFNγ, IL-5, IL-10, IL-12) Local and systemic inflammatory parameters (eg, adhesion molecules, ECP, tryptase)

Abbreviations: ECP, eosinophilic cationic protein; FEV_1, forced expiratory volume in 1 second; IFNγ, interferon-γ; IL, interleukin.

Data from Canonica GW, Baena-Cagnani CE, Bousquet J, et al. Recommendations for standardization of clinical trials with Allergen Specific Immunotherapy for respiratory allergy. A statement of a World Allergy Organization (WAO) taskforce. Allergy 2007;62:317–24.

that "as long as laboratory parameters such as allergen specific antibodies, T cell reactivity or cytokines are not validated and not correlated to the clinical outcome, they can only provide supportive information."

Specific IgG Antibodies and Clinical Effects

The relevance of IgG levels for assessing the outcome in SIT remains controversial, as trials have demonstrated variable data in IgG_4 responses.[10] In the first published DBPC trial of SCIT using a cocktail of 5 recombinant grass pollen allergens, IgG_1 concentrations increased approximately 60-fold, peaking during the first 12 months of the study, and IgG_4 levels achieved an approximately 4000-fold increase by the end of treatment, indicating a high allergen-specific IgG antibody response combined with a good clinical efficacy.[20] Another 2-year SCIT trial with 2 consecutive preseasonal short-term treatments demonstrated a 48.4% difference in combined SMS after the second year combined with a 210-fold increase of allergen-specific IgG_4.[21] However, other studies on both SCIT and SLIT have revealed lower increases of IgG_4 responses although they demonstrated clear clinical efficacy.[33,91,92] Quirino and colleagues[93] performed a direct comparison of SCIT and SLIT in adults with grass pollen seasonal AR with and without asthma in a double-dummy design, and demonstrated both procedures to be equally effective in the clinical outcome. The study revealed that only in the SCIT-treated patients clinical efficacy was associated with a significant increase in specific IgG and specific IgG_4. A 2-year study on 29 grass pollen–allergic children also failed to demonstrate changes for specific IgE/specific IgG_4 ratios over time, either in the active group or between active and placebo-treated children.[94] By contrast, two well-designed studies on SLIT with grass pollen tablets in pediatric patients showed that clinical efficacy was associated with a significant increase of specific IgG_4 levels in grass pollen, although the extent of the increase was lower than in SCIT-studies.[18,24] Taken together, specific IgG, particularly IgG_4 antibodies, are produced following SIT, indicating an immunologic response to the applied allergen preparation.[10] However, their specific role in the underlying mechanism of tolerance induction as well as the extent and predictive value of the rises of these surrogate markers have to be further evaluated in future trials.

EFFECTS OF SIT ON THE NASAL MUCOSA: CELLULAR LEVEL AND INFLAMMATORY MARKERS

Taking smears or biopsies of allergen challenged mucosal sites of the nose before and after SIT has been used to investigate changes of the inflammatory process at the cellular level in several studies of SIT. In a DBPC study on SLIT in adult patients with rhinitis and asthma monosensitized to birch pollen, a nasal smear for eosinophil count revealed a significant decrease in the active group in the birch pollen season after approximately 18 months of therapy, further aggravated in the subsequent years.[95] Another study by Durham and colleagues[96] investigated the effect of grass pollen SCIT on late nasal responses and associated cellular infiltration following nasal provocation by taking nasal biopsies. These tests were performed after a 12-months DBPC trial on SCIT. SCIT was associated with a significantly decreased accumulation of eosinophils and $CD4^+$ cells as well as a significant increase in cells expressing mRNA for interferon-γ in the nasal mucosa after provocation.

In an open, randomized SCIT trial conducted by Klimek and colleagues,[97] the effect of a short-term, preseasonal immunotherapy on ECP and tryptase in nasal secretions of 48 grass pollen–allergic patients was investigated. In both groups of actively treated and placebo-treated patients, ECP and tryptase levels increased significantly during natural allergen exposure in the grass pollen season. However, the increase in the SCIT group was significantly blunted in comparison with placebo. Taken together, there are interesting experimental findings on the specific effects of SIT on the nasal mucosal level. If and to what extent these tools will be useful in interpreting the outcome of SIT has to be verified.

SUMMARY

The assessment of the clinical efficacy of SIT in clinical trials involves measurement of several clinical parameters. Primary outcome parameters include a measure of symptoms and of the usage of concomitant medication, and should ideally combine both scores in a weighted balance. Both disease-specific (RQLQ) and generic QoL and other surrogate markers are usually regarded as secondary outcome parameters. Taken together, the outcome measures described in this article are valuable parameters in assessing the efficacy of SIT in clinical trials. However, further validation of these parameters in future trials as well as stringent and transparent guidance by the regulators is mandatory.

REFERENCES

1. Bousquet J, Khaltaev N, Cruz AA, et al. Allergic Rhinitis and its Impact on Asthma (ARIA) 2008 update (in collaboration with the World Health Organization, GA(2)LEN and AllerGen). Allergy 2008;63(Suppl 86):8–160.
2. Brozek JL, Bousquet J, Baena-Cagnani CE, et al. Allergic Rhinitis and its Impact on Asthma (ARIA) guidelines: 2010 revision. J Allergy Clin Immunol 2010;126(3): 466–76.
3. Passalacqua GC, Canonica W. Sublingual immunotherapy: clinical indications in the WAO-SLIT position paper. World Allergy Organiz J 2010;3(7):4.
4. Bousquet PJ, Brozek J, Bachert C, et al. The CONSORT statement checklist in allergen-specific immunotherapy: a GA2LEN paper. Allergy 2009;64(12): 1737–45.
5. Pfaar O, Anders C, Klimek L. Clinical outcome measures of specific immunotherapy. Curr Opin Allergy Clin Immunol 2009;9(3):208–13.
6. Canonica GW, Baena-Cagnani CE, Bousquet J, et al. Recommendations for standardization of clinical trials with Allergen Specific Immunotherapy for respiratory allergy. A statement of a World Allergy Organization (WAO) taskforce. Allergy 2007;62(3):317–24.
7. Juniper EF, Stahl E, Doty RL, et al. Clinical outcomes and adverse effect monitoring in allergic rhinitis. J Allergy Clin Immunol 2005;115(3 Suppl 1):S390–413.
8. Prasad M, Wahlqvist P, Shikiar R, et al. A review of self-report instruments measuring health-related work productivity: a patient-reported outcomes perspective. Pharmacoeconomics 2004;22(4):225–44.
9. James LK, Durham SR. Update on mechanisms of allergen injection immunotherapy. Clin Exp Allergy 2008;38(7):1074–88.
10. Frew AJ. Cellular responses, serological changes, or both: what are they good for? Arb Paul Ehrlich Inst Bundesamt Sera Impfstoffe Frankf A M 2009;96:233–6 [discussion: 236].
11. US Department of Health and Human Serviced. Food and Drug Administration (FDA). Center for Drug Evaluation and Research (CDER): Guidance for Industry. Allergic rhinitis: clinical development programs for drug products. Draft guidance (2718 draft/06/14/00), 2000.

12. Commitee for medicinal products for human use (CHMP). Guideline on the clinical development of products for specific immunotherapy for the treatment of allergic diseases. London: CHMP/EWP/18504/2006; 2008.

13. Pfaar O, Klimek L. [Clinical outcome measures of specific immunotherapy]. Allergo J 2007;16:576–81 [in German].

14. ICH Harmonised Tripartite guideline. Note for guidance on statistical principles for clinical trial. CPMP/ICH/363/96; 1998.

15. Clark J, Schall R. Assessment of combined symptom and medication scores for rhinoconjunctivitis immunotherapy clinical trials. Allergy 2007;62(9):1023–8.

16. Frew AJ, Powell RJ, Corrigan CJ, et al. Efficacy and safety of specific immunotherapy with SQ allergen extract in treatment-resistant seasonal allergic rhinoconjunctivitis. J Allergy Clin Immunol 2006;117(2):319–25.

17. Didier A, Malling HJ, Worm M, et al. Optimal dose, efficacy, and safety of once-daily sublingual immunotherapy with a 5-grass pollen tablet for seasonal allergic rhinitis. J Allergy Clin Immunol 2007;120(6):1338–45.

18. Wahn U, Tabar A, Kuna P, et al. Efficacy and safety of 5-grass-pollen sublingual immunotherapy tablets in pediatric allergic rhinoconjunctivitis. J Allergy Clin Immunol 2009;123(1):160–6.e3.

19. Durham SR, Emminger W, Kapp A, et al. Long-term clinical efficacy in grass pollen-induced rhinoconjunctivitis after treatment with SQ-standardized grass allergy immunotherapy tablet. J Allergy Clin Immunol 2010;125(1):131 e1–7–138 e1–7.

20. Jutel M, Jaeger L, Suck R, et al. Allergen-specific immunotherapy with recombinant grass pollen allergens. J Allergy Clin Immunol 2005;116(3):608–13.

21. Corrigan CJ, Kettner J, Doemer C, et al. Efficacy and safety of preseasonal-specific immunotherapy with an aluminium-adsorbed six-grass pollen allergoid. Allergy 2005;60(6):801–7.

22. Pfaar O, Klimek L. Efficacy and safety of specific immunotherapy with a high-dose sublingual grass pollen preparation: a double-blind, placebo-controlled trial. Ann Allergy Asthma Immunol 2008;100(3):256–63.

23. Worm M. Efficacy and tolerability of high dose sublingual immunotherapy in patients with rhinoconjunctivitis. Eur Ann Allergy Clin Immunol 2006;38(10):355–60.

24. Bufe A, Eberle P, Franke-Beckmann E, et al. Safety and efficacy in children of an SQ-standardized grass allergen tablet for sublingual immunotherapy. J Allergy Clin Immunol 2009;123(1):167 e167–73 e167.

25. Blaiss M, Maloney J, Nolte H, et al. Efficacy and safety of timothy grass allergy immunotherapy tablets in North American children and adolescents. J Allergy Clin Immunol 2011;127(1):64–71, e1–4.

26. Dahl R, Stender A, Rak S. Specific immunotherapy with SQ standardized grass allergen tablets in asthmatics with rhinoconjunctivitis. Allergy 2006;61(2):185–90.

27. Nelson HS, Nolte H, Creticos P, et al. Efficacy and safety of timothy grass allergy immunotherapy tablet treatment in North American adults. J Allergy Clin Immunol 2011;127(1):72–80, e1–2.

28. Jacobsen L. Primary and secondary endpoints in clinical trials. Arb Paul Ehrlich Inst Bundesamt Sera Impfstoffe Frankf A M 2009;96:96–104 [discussion: 104–5].

29. Hafner D, Reich K, Matricardi PM, et al. Prospective validation of 'Allergy-Control-SCORE(TM)': a novel symptom-medication score for clinical trials. Allergy 2011. DOI:10.1111/j.1398-9995.2010.02531.x.

30. Grouin JM, Vicaut E, Jean-Alphonse S, et al. The average Adjusted Symptom Score, a new primary efficacy end-point for specific allergen immunotherapy trials. Clin Exp Allergy 2011. DOI:10.1111/j.1365-2222.2011.03700.x.

31. Malling HJ. Criteria for clinical efficacy—readout and monitoring of clinical studies. Arb Paul Ehrlich Inst Bundesamt Sera Impfstoffe Frankf A M 2003;(94):119–23 [discussion: 123–5].

32. Malling HJ. Immunotherapy as an effective tool in allergy treatment. Allergy 1998;53(5):461–72.

33. Pfaar O, Robinson DS, Sager A, et al. Immunotherapy with depigmented-polymerized mixed tree pollen extract: a clinical trial and responder analysis. Allergy 2010;65(12):1614–21.

34. Taylor PE, Flagan RC, Miguel AG, et al. Birch pollen rupture and the release of aerosols of respirable allergens. Clin Exp Allergy 2004;34(10):1591–6.

35. Taylor PE, Jonsson H. Thunderstorm asthma. Curr Allergy Asthma Rep 2004; 4(5):409–13.

36. Buters JT, Weichenmeier I, Ochs S, et al. The allergen Bet v 1 in fractions of ambient air deviates from birch pollen counts. Allergy 2010;65(7):850–8.

37. Chapman MD, Ferreira F, Villalba M, et al. CREATE consortium. The European Union CREATE project: a model for international standardization of allergy diagnostics and vaccines. J Allergy Clin Immunol 2008;122(5):882–9.e2.

38. Chapman MD, Filep S, Tsay A, et al. Allergen standardization: CREATE principles applied to other purified allergens. Arb Paul Ehrlich Inst Bundesamt Sera Impfstoffe Frankf A M. 2009;96:21–4.

39. Fiorina A. A personal sampler to monitor airborne particles of biological origin. Aerobiologia 1998;14:299–301.

40. Gore RB, Curbishley L, Truman N, et al. Intranasal air sampling in homes: relationships among reservoir allergen concentrations and asthma severity. J Allergy Clin Immunol 2006;117(3):649–55.

41. Frew A, Fischer von Weikersthal-Drachenberg K, Huber B, et al. An innovative approach to the analysis of seasonal diaries after specific immunotherapy—definition of peak season based on symptom/medication scores of the placebo group rather than on pollen counts (Abstr. 1876). Allergy 2010;65(Suppl s92): 690.

42. Dahl R, Kapp A, Colombo G, et al. Efficacy and safety of sublingual immunotherapy with grass allergen tablets for seasonal allergic rhinoconjunctivitis. J Allergy Clin Immunol 2006;118(2):434–40.

43. Jacobsen L, Niggemann B, Dreborg S, et al. Specific immunotherapy has long-term preventive effect of seasonal and perennial asthma: 10-year follow-up on the PAT study. Allergy 2007;62(8):943–8.

44. Baiardini I, Braido F, Brandi S, et al. Allergic diseases and their impact on quality of life. Ann Allergy Asthma Immunol 2006;97(4):419–28 [quiz: 429–30, 476].

45. Santos CB, Pratt EL, Hanks C, et al. Allergic rhinitis and its effect on sleep, fatigue, and daytime somnolence. Ann Allergy Asthma Immunol 2006;97(5): 579–86 [quiz: 586–9, 671].

46. Stewart AL, Hays RD, Ware JE Jr. The MOS short-form general health survey. Reliability and validity in a patient population. Med Care 1988;26(7):724–35.

47. Ware JE Jr, Sherbourne CD. The MOS 36-item short-form health survey (SF-36). I. Conceptual framework and item selection. Med Care 1992;30(6):473–83.

48. Bousquet J, Bullinger M, Fayol C, et al. Assessment of quality of life in patients with perennial allergic rhinitis with the French version of the SF-36 Health Status Questionnaire. J Allergy Clin Immunol 1994;94(2 Pt 1):182–8.

49. Brazier JE, Harper R, Jones NM, et al. Validating the SF-36 health survey questionnaire: new outcome measure for primary care. BMJ 1992;305(6846):160–4.

50. McHorney CA, Ware JE Jr, Raczek AE. The MOS 36-Item Short-Form Health Survey (SF-36): II. Psychometric and clinical tests of validity in measuring physical and mental health constructs. Med Care 1993;31(3):247–63.

51. McHorney CA, Ware JE Jr, Lu JF, et al. 36-item Short-Form Health Survey (SF-36): III. Tests of data quality, scaling assumptions, and reliability across diverse patient groups. Med Care 1994;32(1):40–66.

52. Carver DJ, Chapman CA, Thomas VS, et al. Validity and reliability of the medical outcomes study short form-20 questionnaire as a measure of quality of life in elderly people living at home. Age Ageing 1999;28(2):169–74.

53. Majani G, Baiardini I, Giardini A, et al. Health-related quality of life assessment in young adults with seasonal allergic rhinitis. Allergy 2001;56(4):313–7.

54. Kremer B, Klimek L, Bullinger M, et al. Generic or disease-specific quality of life scales to characterize health status in allergic rhinitis? Allergy 2001;56(10):957–63.

55. Juniper EF, Guyatt GH. Development and testing of a new measure of health status for clinical trials in rhinoconjunctivitis. Clin Exp Allergy 1991;21(1):77–83.

56. Juniper EF, Thompson AK, Ferrie PJ, et al. Development and validation of the mini Rhinoconjunctivitis Quality of Life Questionnaire. Clin Exp Allergy 2000;30(1):132–40.

57. Juniper EF, Guyatt GH, Dolovich J. Assessment of quality of life in adolescents with allergic rhinoconjunctivitis: development and testing of a questionnaire for clinical trials. J Allergy Clin Immunol 1994;93(2):413–23.

58. Juniper EF, Howland WC, Roberts NB, et al. Measuring quality of life in children with rhinoconjunctivitis. J Allergy Clin Immunol 1998;101(2 Pt 1):163–70.

59. Ciprandi G, Klersy C, Cirillo I, et al. Quality of life in allergic rhinitis: relationship with clinical, immunological, and functional aspects. Clin Exp Allergy 2007;37(10):1528–35.

60. Didier A, Melac M, Montagut A, et al. Agreement of efficacy assessments for five-grass pollen sublingual tablet immunotherapy. Allergy 2009;64(1):166–71.

61. Frolund L, Durham SR, Calderon M, et al. Sustained effect of SQ-standardized grass allergy immunotherapy tablet on rhinoconjunctivitis quality of life. Allergy 2010;65(6):753–7.

62. Durham SR, Yang WH, Pedersen MR, et al. Sublingual immunotherapy with once-daily grass allergen tablets: a randomized controlled trial in seasonal allergic rhinoconjunctivitis. J Allergy Clin Immunol 2006;117(4):802–9.

63. Baiardini I, Pasquali M, Giardini A, et al. Rhinasthma: a new specific QoL questionnaire for patients with rhinitis and asthma. Allergy 2003;58(4):289–94.

64. Mosges R, Schmalz P, Koberlein J, et al. [The RHINASTHMA-Quality of Life Scale German Adapted Version: validation of a new disease specific quality of life scale for patients suffering from allergic rhinitis and bronchial hyperreactivity]. HNO 2007;55(5):357–64 [in German].

65. Worm M. 'Well days' after sublingual immunotherapy with a high-dose 6-grass pollen preparation. Allergy 2009;64(7):1104–5.

66. Akerlund A, Andersson M, Leflein J, et al. Clinical trial design, nasal allergen challenge models, and considerations of relevance to pediatrics, nasal polyposis, and different classes of medication. J Allergy Clin Immunol 2005;115(3 Suppl 1):S460–82.

67. Gosepath J, Amedee RG, Mann WJ. Nasal provocation testing as an international standard for evaluation of allergic and nonallergic rhinitis. Laryngoscope 2005;115(3):512–6.

68. Riechelmann H, Bachert C, Goldschmidt O, et al. [Application of the nasal provocation test on diseases of the upper airways. Position paper of the German Society for Allergology and Clinical Immunology (ENT Section) in cooperation with the working team for clinical immunology]. Laryngorhinootologie 2003; 82(3):183–8 [in German].

69. Creticos PS, Schroeder JT, Hamilton RG, et al. Immunotherapy with a ragweed-toll-like receptor 9 agonist vaccine for allergic rhinitis. N Engl J Med 2006; 355(14):1445–55.

70. Purohit A, Niederberger V, Kronqvist M, et al. Clinical effects of immunotherapy with genetically modified recombinant birch pollen Bet v 1 derivatives. Clin Exp Allergy 2008;38(9):1514–25.

71. Keskin O, Tuncer A, Adalioglu G, et al. The effects of grass pollen allergoid immunotherapy on clinical and immunological parameters in children with allergic rhinitis. Pediatr Allergy Immunol 2006;17(6):396–407.

72. Klimek L, Mewes T, Wolf H, et al. The effects of short-term immunotherapy using molecular standardized grass and rye allergens compared with symptomatic drug treatment on rhinoconjunctivitis symptoms, skin sensitivity, and specific nasal reactivity. Otolaryngol Head Neck Surg 2005;133(4):538–43.

73. Senti G, Prinz Vavricka BM, Erdmann I, et al. Intralymphatic allergen administration renders specific immunotherapy faster and safer: a randomized controlled trial. Proc Natl Acad Sci U S A 2008;105(46):17908–12.

74. Senti G, Graf N, Haug S, et al. Epicutaneous allergen administration as a novel method of allergen-specific immunotherapy. J Allergy Clin Immunol 2009; 124(5):997–1002.

75. Kjellman NI, Andersson B. Terfenadine reduces skin and conjunctival reactivity in grass pollen allergic children. Clin Allergy 1986;16(5):441–9.

76. Lofkvist T, Agrell B, Dreborg S, et al. Effects of immunotherapy with a purified standardized allergen preparation of *Dermatophagoides farinae* in adults with perennial allergic rhinoconjunctivitis. Allergy 1994;49(2):100–7.

77. Friedlaender MH. Objective measurement of allergic reactions in the eye. Curr Opin Allergy Clin Immunol 2004;4(5):447–53.

78. La Rosa M, Ranno C, Andre C, et al. Double-blind placebo-controlled evaluation of sublingual-swallow immunotherapy with standardized *Parietaria judaica* extract in children with allergic rhinoconjunctivitis. J Allergy Clin Immunol 1999; 104(2 Pt 1):425–32.

79. Moller C, Dreborg S, Ferdousi HA, et al. Pollen immunotherapy reduces the development of asthma in children with seasonal rhinoconjunctivitis (the PAT-study). J Allergy Clin Immunol 2002;109(2):251–6.

80. Riechelmann H, Epple B, Gropper G. Comparison of conjunctival and nasal provocation test in allergic rhinitis to house dust mite. Int Arch Allergy Immunol 2003;130(1):51–9.

81. Krug N. Usefulness of pollen chamber in the evaluation of clinical trials with allergen products. Arb Paul Ehrlich Inst Bundesamt Sera Impfstoffe Frankf A M 2006;(95):167–70 [discussion: 170–61].

82. Hohlfeld JM, Holland-Letz T, Larbig M, et al. Diagnostic value of outcome measures following allergen exposure in an environmental challenge chamber compared with natural conditions. Clin Exp Allergy 2010;40(7):998–1006.

83. Day JH, Briscoe M, Widlitz MD. Cetirizine, loratadine, or placebo in subjects with seasonal allergic rhinitis: effects after controlled ragweed pollen challenge in an environmental exposure unit. J Allergy Clin Immunol 1998;101(5): 638–45.

84. Day JH, Briscoe MP, Rafeiro E, et al. Onset of action of intranasal budesonide (*Rhinocort aqua*) in seasonal allergic rhinitis studied in a controlled exposure model. J Allergy Clin Immunol 2000;105(3):489–94.
85. Donovan JP, Buckeridge DL, Briscoe MP, et al. Efficacy of immunotherapy to ragweed antigen tested by controlled antigen exposure. Ann Allergy Asthma Immunol 1996;77(1):74–80.
86. Horak F, Stubner P, Berger UE, et al. Immunotherapy with sublingual birch pollen extract. A short-term double-blind placebo study. J Investig Allergol Clin Immunol 1998;8(3):165–71.
87. Devillier P, Le Gall M, Horak F. The allergen challenge chamber: a valuable tool for optimizing the clinical development of pollen immunotherapy. Allergy 2011; 66(2):163–9.
88. Horak F, Zieglmayer P, Zieglmayer R, et al. Early onset of action of a 5-grass-pollen 300-IR sublingual immunotherapy tablet evaluated in an allergen challenge chamber. J Allergy Clin Immunol 2009;124(3):471–7, 477 e1.
89. Bonifazi F, Jutel M, Bilo BM, et al. Prevention and treatment of hymenoptera venom allergy: guidelines for clinical practice. Allergy 2005;60(12):1459–70.
90. Muller U, Golden DB, Lockey RF, et al. Immunotherapy for hymenoptera venom hypersensitivity. Clin Allergy Immunol 2008;21:377–92.
91. Zenner HP, Baumgarten C, Rasp G, et al. Short-term immunotherapy: a prospective, randomized, double-blind, placebo-controlled multicenter study of molecular standardized grass and rye allergens in patients with grass pollen-induced allergic rhinitis. J Allergy Clin Immunol 1997;100(1):23–9.
92. Dahl R, Kapp A, Colombo G, et al. Sublingual grass allergen tablet immunotherapy provides sustained clinical benefit with progressive immunologic changes over 2 years. J Allergy Clin Immunol 2008;121(2):512 e512–8 e512.
93. Quirino T, Iemoli E, Siciliani E, et al. Sublingual versus injective immunotherapy in grass pollen allergic patients: a double blind (double dummy) study. Clin Exp Allergy 1996;26(11):1253–61.
94. Rolinck-Werninghaus C, Kopp M, Liebke C, et al. Lack of detectable alterations in immune responses during sublingual immunotherapy in children with seasonal allergic rhinoconjunctivitis to grass pollen. Int Arch Allergy Immunol 2005;136(2):134–41.
95. Marogna M, Spadolini I, Massolo A, et al. Clinical, functional, and immunologic effects of sublingual immunotherapy in birch pollinosis: a 3-year randomized controlled study. J Allergy Clin Immunol 2005;115(6):1184–8.
96. Durham SR, Ying S, Varney VA, et al. Grass pollen immunotherapy inhibits allergen-induced infiltration of CD4+ T lymphocytes and eosinophils in the nasal mucosa and increases the number of cells expressing messenger RNA for interferon-gamma. J Allergy Clin Immunol 1996;97(6):1356–65.
97. Klimek L, Wolf H, Mewes T, et al. The effect of short-term immunotherapy with molecular standardized grass and rye allergens on eosinophil cationic protein and tryptase in nasal secretions. J Allergy Clin Immunol 1999;103(1 Pt 1):47–53.
98. Juniper EF, Guyatt GH, Epstein RS, et al. Evaluation of impairment of health related quality of life in asthma: development of a questionnaire for use in clinical trials. Thorax 1992;47(2):76–83.
99. Juniper EF, Guyatt GH, Cox FM, et al. Development and validation of the Mini Asthma Quality of Life Questionnaire. Eur Respir J 1999;14(1):32–8.
100. Barley EA, Quirk FH, Jones PW. Asthma health status measurement in clinical practice: validity of a new short and simple instrument. Respir Med 1998; 92(10):1207–14.

Serum Immunologic Markers for Monitoring Allergen-Specific Immunotherapy

Mohamed H. Shamji, MSc, PhD*, Louisa K. James, PhD,
Stephen R. Durham, MD

KEYWORDS

- Allergen immunotherapy • IgE-mediated allergy
- IgE-facilitated allergen binding • IgG4 • IgE-blocking factor

In the early twentieth century, Noon[1] described his initial observations on the effects of pollen-specific injection immunotherapy resulting in amelioration of allergen-induced symptoms. Allergen immunotherapy (SIT) has since become a current standard of practice, particularly in those subjects who are unresponsive to pharmacotherapy.[2] Immunotherapy, either by conventional or sublingual route of administration, is effective in carefully selected individuals with IgE-mediated allergic diseases.[2–5] The clinical benefit of SIT has been demonstrated using several types of allergens including grass and tree pollen,[6,7] house dust mite,[8] insect venom,[9] and animal dander.[10] In a Cochrane systematic review and meta-analysis, Wilson and colleagues[11] reported that the clinical effect size when compared with placebo of the currently available pharmacotherapy for allergic rhinitis was 18% for corticosteroids, 7% for antihistamine, and 5% for leukotriene modifiers. This is less effective than the approximately 30% reduction of symptoms after grass pollen immunotherapy using an alum-adsorbed vaccine.[6] Furthermore, clinical responsiveness to SIT has been shown to

This work was supported by grants from the Immune Tolerance Network, National Institutes of Health USA, a Biotechnology and Biologic Sciences Research Council UK (BBSRC) studentship case award, and ALK-Abelló, Hørsholm, Denmark.

Disclosure of potential conflict of interest: Stephen R. Durham is a member of the Immune Tolerance Network Steering Committee and has consulting arrangements with ALK-Abelló and has received research support from ALK-Abelló. Mohamed H. Shamji and Louisa K. James have no conflicts of interest to declare.

Allergy and Clinical Immunology Section, National Heart and Lung Institute, Medical Research Council and Asthma UK Centre for Allergic Mechanisms of Asthma, Imperial College London, Dovehouse Street, London, SW3 6LY, UK

* Corresponding author.

E-mail address: m.shamji99@imperial.ac.uk

exceed the duration of treatment by several years, a clear advantage over the use of anti-IgE or antiallergic drugs.[3,5,12]

MECHANISMS OF IMMUNOTHERAPY

SIT is the only immunomodulatory treatment that induces long-term immunologic and clinical tolerance for IgE-mediated allergic diseases.[2,13,14] Recent studies have revealed that immunologic mechanisms of conventional and sublingual immuno-therapy are comparable.[14–16] Reduced recruitment and activation of allergy effector cells, in particular eosinophils, basophils, and mast cells, have been shown at the nasal mucosal surfaces.[17–20]

Long-term peripheral tolerance after immunotherapy is associated with a shift in the ratio of Th2 (interleukin [IL]-4 and IL-5) and Th1 (interferon-γ) cytokines. Induction and function of allergen-specific IL-10/transforming growth factor-β producing $CD4^+CD25^+Foxp3^+$ regulatory T after SIT have been reported in several studies.[21–24] The effect of IL-10 on B cells includes class switching to IgG antibody isotypes, in particular IgG_4. These antibodies have antiinflammatory properties and have been shown to inhibit basophil histamine release and prevent IgE-facilitated allergen presentation from B cells reducing subsequent allergen-specific Th2 cell activation.[25]

IL-10 has been measured in allergen-stimulated peripheral blood mononuclear cell cultures harvested before and during immunotherapy.[16,22,23] Studies during 12-month conventional grass pollen immunotherapy using an alum-adsorbed vaccine revealed time-dependent increases in IL-10 as detected by enzyme-linked immunoabsorbent assay.[7] Remarkably, these increases in IL-10 were significant as early as 2 to 4 weeks during the up-dosing immunotherapy protocol and paralleled the early suppression of the grass pollen–induced late cutaneous response.

Several studies have identified IL-10 production by regulatory $CD4^+CD25^+$ T cells after immunotherapy.[21–24] One study showed that these inducible IL-10$^+$ T-regulatory cells suppress antigen-driven proliferative $CD4^+CD25^-$ T-cell responses and Th2 cytokine release in an IL-10–dependent manner.[21] Increased frequency of antigen-specific IL-10$^+$ cells has also been demonstrated.[26]

Recent studies have demonstrated elevated numbers of IL-10$^+CD4^+$, Foxp3$^+CD4^+$, and Foxp3$^+CD25^+$ phenotypic regulatory T cells within the nasal mucosa.[27,28] IL-10 plays a potential dual role during immunotherapy in that it has the potential to both suppress $CD4^+$ Th2 responses and also to induce antibody isotype class switch, in favor of IgG_4. The observed decrease in IgE/IgG_4 ratio during SIT may reflect induction of peripheral tolerance with increased regulatory $CD4^+CD25^+$ T cell activity and damp-ened aberrant Th2 response.

POTENTIAL SURROGATE OR PREDICTIVE BIOMARKER OF SIT

It is tempting to focus on such aberrant changes in T cell responses or B cell responses in the periphery or target organs as putative markers of successful immu-notherapy, to predict responders from nonresponders, or for consideration whether to stop or reinstigate treatment. Unfortunately, such assays are complex and difficult to standardize between laboratories for the purpose of multicenter trials. Similarly, it is tempting to look at measurements of inflammation in target organs by use of lavage fluid or collection of bronchial lavage, or conjunctival tear fluid or nasal secretions on filter paper strips,[29] although the same considerations apply. For these reasons, this article focuses on serum markers that are stable on storage, potentially standar-dizable between laboratories, and accessible for use in multicenter clinical trials.

IMMUNOGLOBULIN E

Increased levels of allergen-specific IgE in the periphery and in local target organs have been reported after exposure to the relevant sensitized allergens in atopic individuals. A natural time-course of IgE in hay fever patients during the season revealed an early transient increase in rye grass pollen (Lol p 1, 2, 3, and 5)–specific IgE followed by a gradual decrease over time.[30] Paradoxically, clinical trials of immunotherapy have revealed transient early increases in allergen-specific IgE that are followed by subsequent blunting of seasonal increases in IgE.[21,31,32] Furthermore, low levels of IgE antibodies to previously unrecognized proteins have been identified in a proportion of patients who received birch pollen injection immunotherapy, suggesting a change of epitope specificity to the sensitizing major allergens.[33]

It is possible that allergen injection immunotherapy may induce initially high IgE antibody levels that are noninflammatory (ie, IgE that may not have the potential effectively to sensitize mast cells for allergen-induced activation). This could occur as a consequence of antibodies that either have low affinity for key grass pollen epitopes or alternatively IgE with a narrow range of grass pollen epitope specificity, both of which might result in poor cross-linking ability of IgE with no implication for worsening of IgE-mediated disease associated with early immunotherapy. In contrast, the usual seasonal elevation observed during the pollen season in hay fever sufferers is likely to be produced by long-lived memory B cells that have been exposed to repeated seasons of pollen exposure, with somatic hypermutation resulting in affinity maturation and a broader range of epitope specificities of IgE, resulting in more effective allergen binding and cross-linking of IgE on the cell surface.

This may explain the apparent paradox of early increases in presumably nonfunctional IgE after immunotherapy, whereas parallel blunting of the superimposed seasonal elevation of functional IgE by immunotherapy could result in clinical protection during the pollen season.

RATIO OF SPECIFIC IGE/TOTAL IGE

The ratio of serum-specific-IgE/total IgE has been recently evaluated in a clinical study of timothy grass pollen immunotherapy as a potential predictive marker.[34] An in vitro analysis of 279 monosensitized patients who received 4 years of conventional (76 patients) or sublingual (203 patients) immunotherapy was performed. Serum t-IgE and s-IgE levels, blood eosinophil counts, and serum s-IgE/t-IgE ratios were determined and assessed for correlation with clinical response as measured by visual analog scores. Receiver-operating characteristic analysis for each in vitro biomarker revealed a superior diagnostic and predictive value in favor of baseline serum s-IgE/t-IgE ratios. A diagnostic and predictive cut-off value of 16.2% to predict successful SIT outcome in both treatment regimes was established and revealed clinical sensitivity and clinical specificity of 97.2% and 88.1%, respectively.[34] However, this was not reproduced in a randomized, controlled, open-labeled, three-parallel group study of house dust mite with 48 monosensitized asthmatic and rhinitis children sensitized to house dust mite who received sublingual immunotherapy (SLIT), subcutaneous immunotherapy (SCIT), or pharmacotherapy. In this study, there was not a significant correlation between combined symptoms and medication scores or visual analog scores and the ratio of serum-specific-IgE/total IgE, which may possibly have been caused by the small sample size in each treated group. Evaluation of serum s-IgE/t-IgE ratios in large randomized double-blind placebo-controlled studies are required to confirm the use or otherwise of s-IgE/t-IgE as a biomarker for effective immunotherapy. Use of recombinant allergens for both accurate in vitro analysis of individual major and minor allergens and the targeted use of a known recombinant or mixture of recombinant allergens for therapy is likely to provide clarification.

IMMUNOREACTIVE IGG ANTIBODIES DURING IMMUNOTHERAPY

Specific IgG subclass measurements in immunotherapy-treated subjects have revealed increases in allergen-specific IgG1 and IgG$_4$ antibody concentrations in serum and in local target organs.[21,35,36] Changes in IgG2 and IgG3 levels were not significant.[37] Despite these increases in levels of allergen-specific antibodies, many studies have failed to show a correlation between allergen-specific IgG1 or IgG$_4$ antibodies and clinical efficacy. Several studies have demonstrated that SIT is associated with elevated concentrations of allergen-specific IgG, in particular IgG$_4$ antibodies, which have inhibitory activity. IgG antibodies have the potential to compete with allergen-specific IgE, inhibit basophil activation, and prevent IgE-facilitated allergen presentation by B cells to T-cell clones.[25,38,39]

IGE-FACILITATED ALLERGEN PRESENTATION

On the surface of B cells, bound immunoglobulin captures and internalizes antigen.[40,41] This process is highly efficient and supports subsequent antigen processing and presentation, and antigen-specific activation of T cells at lower antigen concentrations than those achievable by simple pinocytosis alone. Both FcεRI and CD23 receptors are capable, via interactions with IgE, of facilitating allergen binding and subsequent processing and presentation of allergen-derived peptides.

The trimeric form of CD23 is expressed on antigen-presenting cells, in particular allergen-activated B cells, which can bind allergen-IgE complexes in the periphery or at the mucosal surface and facilitate allergen presentation. Allergen-IgE-CD23 complexes formed are internalized and transported to endosomes. This process is followed by loading of allergen-derived peptides onto major histocompatibility class II molecules (HLA-DR) and presentation to T cells, by way of T-cell receptors, at the cell surface.[42]

In 1989, Kehry and Yamashita[43] were the first to describe CD23-mediated facilitated allergen presentation. These findings were subsequently confirmed for human B cells.[40,41] Four years later, van der Heijden and colleagues[44] demonstrated CD23-mediated IgE-facilitated allergen presentation in allergic patients. Der p II (a major house dust mite allergen) was preincubated in sera from house dust mite–sensitized patients, containing Der p II–specific IgE. The Der p II–IgE complexes were preincubated with CD23-enriched EBV-B cells. When these cells were used as antigen-presenting cells, a Der p II–specific T-cell clone proliferated at 100- to 1000-fold lower allergen concentrations than when using uncomplexed allergen. Follow-up studies revealed that facilitated allergen presentation was dependent on the concentrations of IgE, allergen, and the expression of CD23 on B cells.[25]

Wachholz and colleagues[39] demonstrated that in the grass pollen system the proliferative responses of *Phleum pratense*–specific T-cell clones were proportional to the amount of binding of *P pratense*–specific IgE complexes to B cells. These findings were further reproduced using Bet v 1 antigens in patients treated with birch pollen SIT.[45] These complexes can be detected by a flow cytometric assay, the IgE-facilitated allergen binding (IgE-FAB) assay. These studies clearly demonstrate that allergen complexed to specific IgE can bind to CD23 and can facilitate the presentation of allergens to T cells, resulting in extremely efficient T-cell activation (**Fig. 1**).

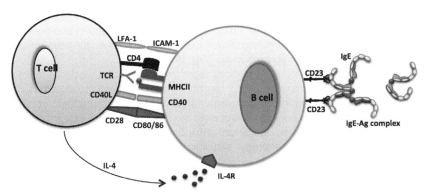

Fig. 1. CD23 receptor-mediated antigen capture and presentation. Cooperative binding of allergen-IgE complexes to CD23 is followed by internalization and presentation of linear epitopes by MHC class II molecules to TCRs. This cognate interaction between Th2 cells and B cells is followed by up-regulation of CD40 on T cells that binds to CD40L on B cells, followed by increased expression and interaction of costimulatory molecules (CD28 by Th2 cells and CD80, CD86 by B cells), and IL-4 receptor resulting in activation of Th2 effector T cells in the presence of 100 to 1000 lower concentration of aeroallergen and IL-4 synthesis and production. Activated B cells undergo affinity maturation, IgE class switching. ICAM, intercellular adhesion molecule; LFA, lymphocyte function associated 1 molecule; MHC, major histocompatibility complex; TCR, T cell receptor.

INHIBITION OF IGE-FACILITATED ALLERGEN PRESENTATION

The inhibitory activity of serum antibodies induced during immunotherapy was first described by Cooke and colleagues in 1935.[46] Later, Lichtenstein and colleagues[47] demonstrated that these inhibitory antibodies could be confined to the IgG fraction in serum. These inhibitory antibodies or 'blocking antibodies' are thought to compete with IgE for allergen binding. IgA antibodies have also been shown to have inhibitory properties.[48]

van Neerven and colleagues[25] demonstrated that serum obtained from subjects after birch pollen immunotherapy was able to inhibit IgE-facilitated allergen presentation by B cells to an allergen-specific T-cell clone, resulting in decreased T-cell proliferation and reduced cytokine production by birch pollen–specific T cells. Wachholz and colleagues[39] showed that serum obtained from subjects who received grass pollen immunotherapy can inhibit IgE-facilitated allergen presentation to a grass-specific T-cell clone.

Elevations in IgG_4 are a consistent feature of allergen immunotherapy. Increases in allergen-specific IgG_4 antibodies are associated with increases in serum IgG-associated inhibitory activity. These antibodies block the interaction of allergen-IgE binding to low-affinity IgE receptors, which prevents IgE-facilitated allergen presentation and subsequent activation of effector Th2 cells. Other studies have demonstrated the functional role of these IgG_4 antibodies in inhibiting FcεRI-mediated basophil histamine release.[7,38] IgG_4 is the least abundant subclass in plasma comprising less than 5% of total IgG with a reference range in adults of 0 to 0.5 g/L.

Elevated levels of IgG_4 are observed after prolonged allergen exposure. IgG_1 and IgG_4 responses to bee venom immunotherapy showed a predominant phospholipase 2–specific IgG_1 response in the first 6 months. Continuation of therapy did not result in further increase of IgG_1 antibodies. Interestingly, a steady increase of phospholipase 2–specific IgG_4 antibodies was reported.[49,50] IgG_4 has low affinity for C1q, Fcγ receptors, and inhibits IgG_1-mediated complement activation.[49,51] IgG_4 antibodies may be distinctively more effective in inhibiting antigen-IgE interaction and preventing complex formation by other immunoglobulin isotypes and thus might have an antiin-flammatory role in immunologic responses (**Fig. 2**).

The IgE-facilitated allergen binding assay represents an in vitro model of facilitated allergen presentation and may be useful for monitoring IgG-associated serum inhibitory activity during allergen immunotherapy. Nouri-Aria and colleagues[52] confirmed increases in allergen-specific IgG_4 antibodies in patients treated with grass pollen immunotherapy. Furthermore, inhibition of IgE-facilitated allergen binding was demonstrated in postimmunotherapy serum and copurified with IgG_4 containing fractions.[14]

In a single center study that involved a randomized double-blind controlled withdrawal of grass pollen subcutaneous immunotherapy, 2 years of treatment resulted in a significant reduction in symptom and medication scores. Symptom and medication scores remained reduced for a further 2 years regardless of whether patients received continued active or placebo injections.[14] A significant increase in serologic blocking activity for grass pollen IgE-FAB was detected in samples obtained after 2 years of allergen immunotherapy compared with samples obtained at baseline. Similarly, IgE-FAB remained strongly inhibited after 2 years in both immunotherapy-continued and immunotherapy-withdrawn groups. Continued immunotherapy treatment was associated with a persistent increase in IgG_4 antibodies for the total 4 years of active therapy. In contrast to results obtained for IgE-FAB inhibition, in those patients who had undergone placebo-controlled withdrawal, IgG_4 antibody levels markedly declined toward baseline levels (**Fig. 3**). Comparable changes in IgG_1 antibody responses were also observed. The relationship between blocking activity and

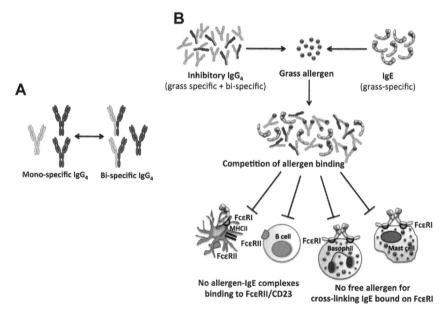

Fig. 2. Serum allergen-specific IgG_4-associated inhibitory antibodies (proposed mechanisms). (*A*) Induction of grass pollen-specific IgG_4 antibodies in the peripheral blood and nasal mucosa after SIT. (*B*) Mono- and bi-specific grass pollen-specific IgG_4 antibodies with inhibitory activity to compete with specific IgE for the allergen binding to FcεRII on B cell and FcεRI on mast cell, basophil, and dendritic cells. MHC, major histocompatibility complex.

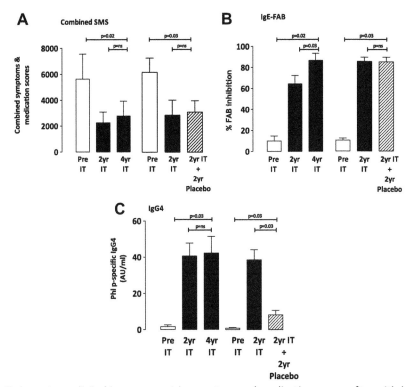

Fig. 3. Long-term clinical improvement in symptom and medication scores after withdrawal of immunotherapy is associated with persistent elevation of serum IgG-associated IgE-FAB inhibitory, whereas immunoreactive allergen-specific IgG$_4$ antibodies return almost to baseline. (A) Combined symptom and medication scores (SMS) were assessed for 13 subjects randomized to receive either 4 years immunotherapy (N = 7) or 2 years of active treatment followed by 2 years of placebo injections (N = 6). IgG$_4$-asssociated blocking activity for allergen-IgE binding was maintained for at least 2 years after discontinuing treatment (B), despite a significant decline of immunotherapy-induced allergen-specific IgG$_4$ antibody (C) concentrations. Data are shown as mean ± SEM. Statistical significance was assessed by using the Wilcoxon matched-pairs comparison.

the clinical response to treatment was examined. IgE-FAB inhibition at 4 years was observed to correlate with combined symptom and medication scores (Spearman correlation coefficient; $r = -0.65$; $P = .02$) (**Fig. 4**). In contrast to serum inhibitory activity for IgE-FAB, specific IgG$_4$ antibodies did not correlate with symptom and medication scores ($r = 0.04$; $P = .5$), nor did specific IgG$_4$ correlate with the blocking antibody response ($r = 0.05$; $P = .9$).[14]

The FAB assay has been demonstrated to be reproducible with within-assay and between-assay reproducibility of 4% and 12%, respectively.[53] In a large multicenter randomized double-blind placebo-controlled study, participants with severe treatment-resistant seasonal allergic rhinitis received grass pollen extract (100,000 SQ-U or 10,000 SQ-U *Phleum pratense*; Alutard) or placebo injections. Serum IgG$_4$-associated inhibitory activity and IgG$_4$ levels were measured before and at intervals after treatment. Subjects had increased levels of serum inhibitory activity and allergen-specific IgG$_4$ after the up-dosing/dose escalation period (8 weeks); at the peak of the grass pollen season (22 weeks); and at the end of treatment (32 weeks).

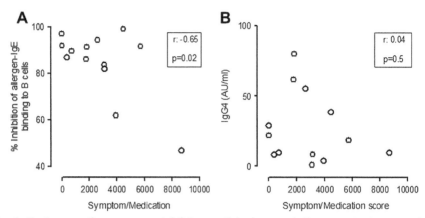

Fig. 4. Postimmunotherapy serum inhibitory activity but not IgG$_4$ concentrations correlate with combined symptom-rescue medication scores. Correlation of combined daily symptom and medication scores with inhibition of (*A*) facilitated allergen binding and (*B*) *Phleum pratense*–specific IgG$_4$. Correlations were obtained using Spearman rank method.

At 32 weeks the increases in IgE-FAB in patients treated with 100,000 and 10,000 SQ-U were 52% (*P*<.001) and 9% (*P*<.001), respectively, and for IgG$_4$ were 29-fold (*P*<.001) and 8-fold (*P*<.001) compared with baseline. A modest but significant inverse correlation was observed between serum inhibitory activity at 8 weeks and combined symptom and rescue medication scores during the pollen season (*r* = −0.25; *P*<.001), whereas no significant correlation was found for serum IgG$_4$ (*r* = −0.09; *P*>.05).[54]

A limitation of these studies to date has been the lack of data from a baseline pollen season that would otherwise permit classification of individual participants as "responders" or "nonresponders." In the absence of a baseline season it is not possible to calculate individual clinical effect sizes before and after treatment for comparison with parallel changes in IgE-FAB inhibition (and IgG$_4$ levels). Such paired measurements would also control for between-participant variability and increase the power to detect an association if one exists.[54] Although further studies are required, these findings support the view that functional IgG-associated blocking antibodies, in particular IgG$_4$ blocking antibodies, may represent a potential marker of successful immunotherapy.

IGE BLOCKING FACTOR

IgE-blocking factor is the amount of IgE actually hindered from binding to allergen.[45,55,56] A functional solid-phase assay has been developed that measures serum blocking antibodies. In a recent study of grass pollen sublingual immunotherapy in North American subjects with seasonal allergic rhinitis, increases in Phl p5–specific IgG$_4$ and IgE blocking factor were observed in the actively treated group compared with those who received placebo tablets.[56] Wurtzen and colleagues[45] evaluated the relationship of IgE-blocking factor with inhibition of facilitated allergen presentation and binding, basophil histamine release. A significant reduction of IgE-FAB, basophil histamine release and an increase in IgE blocking factor was observed after 1 year of treatment and the effect was maintained during the second year of treatment. There was a clear correlation between the CD23-mediated IgE-facilitated allergen binding as a measure of T-cell activation and serum IgE blocking factor and basophil histamine release. IgE-blocking factor accounts for all serum blocking antibodies that compete with IgE for the allergen on a solid-phase matrix. In contrast, IgE-FAB represent a more physiologic readout of functional IgG1 and IgG$_4$ antibodies that seem to correlate more closely with combined symptom and rescue medication scores.[14]

SERUM ALLERGEN-SPECIFIC IGA

Immunoglobulin A, like IgG$_4$, is a noninflammatory isotype that is unable to fix complement or participate in immune complex formation.[57] Elevated levels of allergen-specific IgA$_2$ antibodies and polymeric IgA$_2$ have been reported after grass pollen–specific injection immunotherapy. Passive sensitization of monocytes in vitro using purified polymeric IgA$_2$ from IgA-containing serum obtained after immunotherapy followed by cross-linking in vitro of IgA on monocytes by antigen or anti-IgA resulted in IL-10 production.[28] This indirect production of IL-10 from accessory cells may in turn favor isotype class-switch in favor of IgG$_4$ antibody production. These findings implicate a possible role for IgA antibodies in the induction of tolerance after SIT. Further studies are required to determine whether these increases in allergen-specific IgA correlate with the clinical response to treatment.

SUMMARY

Several in vitro biomarkers have been evaluated to assess clinical efficacy of allergen immunotherapy. To date, identifying individual patient responders and nonresponders remains a major challenge. It would be surprising if a single biologic variable were to correlate closely with the clinical response in terms of reduction in symptoms or other markers of improvement, such as quality of life questionnaires. Various intervening steps include the degree of allergen exposure, the dose and the timing of exposure in relation to symptoms, and the use of rescue medication, all of which might confound the relationship between IgE-FAB and clinical symptoms and response to immunotherapy. There is also the cytokine milieu in which T cells are presented with allergen and the presence or absence of priming, as in exposure to grass pollen, or indeed to other allergens in polysensitized patients, all of which may not be reflected in changes in the IgE-FAB assay during immunotherapy. There is also wide variability in mast cell and basophil reactivity in target organs in response to IgE triggering in humans. The level of bronchial smooth muscle hyperactivity in the lungs or the state of neurogenic control of mucus glands in the nose also vary among patients. For these reasons it is unlikely that a single event in the chain of suppression of antigen presentation would correlate precisely with symptoms after immunotherapy. Nonetheless, what is interesting is that serum inhibitory activity for IgE-FAB correlates more closely than IgG$_4$ levels, a fundamental observation that suggests that it is the functional activity of antibodies rather than immunoreactive IgG per se that is important in determining efficacy.

REFERENCES

1. Noon L. Prophylactic inoculation against hay fever. Lancet 1911;i:1572–3.
2. Bousquet J, Lockey R, Malling HJ. Allergen immunotherapy: therapeutic vaccines for allergic diseases. A WHO position paper. J Allergy Clin Immunol 1998;102(4 Pt 1):558–62.
3. Durham SR, Walker SM, Varga EM, et al. Long-term clinical efficacy of grass-pollen immunotherapy. N Engl J Med 1999;341(7):468–75.

4. Bonifazi F, Jutel M, Bilo BM, et al. Prevention and treatment of hymenoptera venom allergy: guidelines for clinical practice. Allergy 2005;60(12):1459.

5. Durham SR, Emminger W, Kapp A, et al. Long-term clinical efficacy in grass pollen-induced rhinoconjunctivitis after treatment with SQ-standardized grass allergy immunotherapy tablet. J Allergy Clin Immunol 2010;125(1):131–8.

6. Frew AJ, Powell RJ, Corrigan CJ, et al. Efficacy and safety of specific immunotherapy with SQ allergen extract in treatment-resistant seasonal allergic rhinoconjunctivitis. J Allergy Clin Immunol 2006;117(2):319–25.

7. Francis JN, James LK, Paraskevopoulos G, et al. Grass pollen immunotherapy: IL-10 induction and suppression of late responses precedes IgG4 inhibitory antibody activity. J Allergy Clin Immunol 2008;121(5):1120–5.

8. Haugaard L, Dahl R, Jacobsen L. A controlled dose-response study of immunotherapy with standardized, partially purified extract of house dust mite: clinical efficacy and side effects. J Allergy Clin Immunol 1993;91(3):709–22.

9. Hunt KJ, Valentine MD, Sobotka AK, et al. A controlled trial of immunotherapy in insect hypersensitivity. N Engl J Med 1978;299(4):157–61.

10. Varney VA, Edwards J, Tabbah K, et al. Clinical efficacy of specific immunotherapy to cat dander: a double-blind placebo-controlled trial. Clin Exp Allergy 1997;27(8):860–7.

11. Wilson AM, Sims EJ, Orr LC, et al. An evaluation of short-term corticosteroid response in perennial allergic rhinitis using histamine and adenosine monophosphate nasal challenge. Br J Clin Pharmacol 2003;55(4):354–9.

12. Golden DB, Kagey-Sobotka A, Norman PS, et al. Outcomes of allergy to insect stings in children, with and without venom immunotherapy. N Engl J Med 2004; 351(7):668–74.

13. Lockey RF. ARIA: global guidelines and new forms of allergen immunotherapy. J Allergy Clin Immunol 2001;108(4):497–9.

14. James LK, Shamji MH, Walker SM, et al. Long-term tolerance after allergen immunotherapy is accompanied by selective persistence of blocking antibodies. J Allergy Clin Immunol 2011;127(2):509–16.

15. Scadding GW, Shamji MH, Jacobson MR, et al. Sublingual grass pollen immunotherapy is associated with increases in sublingual Foxp3-expressing cells and elevated allergen-specific immunoglobulin G4, immunoglobulin A and serum inhibitory activity for immunoglobulin E-facilitated allergen binding to B cells. Clin Exp Allergy 2010;40(4):598–606.

16. O'Hehir RE, Gardner LM, de Leon MP, et al. House dust mite sublingual immunotherapy: the role for transforming growth factor-beta and functional regulatory T cells. Am J Respir Crit Care Med 2009;180(10):936–47.

17. Passalacqua G, Albano M, Riccio A, et al. Clinical and immunologic effects of a rush sublingual immunotherapy to Parietaria species: a double-blind, placebo-controlled trial. J Allergy Clin Immunol 1999;104(5):964–8.

18. Till SJ, Francis JN, Nouri-Aria K, et al. Mechanisms of immunotherapy. J Allergy Clin Immunol 2004;113(6):1025–34 [quiz: 1035].

19. Ippoliti F, De Santis W, Volterrani A, et al. Immunomodulation during sublingual therapy in allergic children. Pediatr Allergy Immunol 2003;14(3):216–21.

20. Bahceciler NN, Arikan C, Taylor A, et al. Impact of sublingual immunotherapy on specific antibody levels in asthmatic children allergic to house dust mites. Int Arch Allergy Immunol 2005;136(3):287–94.

21. Jutel M, Akdis M, Budak F, et al. IL-10 and TGF-beta cooperate in the regulatory T cell response to mucosal allergens in normal immunity and specific immunotherapy. Eur J Immunol 2003;33(5):1205–14.

22. Francis JN, Till SJ, Durham SR. Induction of IL-10+CD4+CD25+ T cells by grass pollen immunotherapy. J Allergy Clin Immunol 2003;111(6):1255–61.
23. Akdis CA, Blesken T, Akdis M, et al. Role of interleukin 10 in specific immunotherapy. J Clin Invest 1998;102(1):98–106.
24. Ling EM, Smith T, Nguyen XD, et al. Relation of CD4+CD25+ regulatory T-cell suppression of allergen-driven T-cell activation to atopic status and expression of allergic disease. Lancet 2004;363(9409):608–15.
25. van Neerven RJ, Wikborg T, Lund G, et al. Blocking antibodies induced by specific allergy vaccination prevent the activation of CD4+ T cells by inhibiting serum-IgE-facilitated allergen presentation. J Immunol 1999;163(5):2944–52.
26. Mobs C, Slotosch C, Loffler H, et al. Birch pollen immunotherapy leads to differential induction of regulatory T cells and delayed helper T cell immune deviation. J Immunol 2010;184(4):2194–203.
27. Radulovic S, Jacobson MR, Durham SR, et al. Grass pollen immunotherapy induces Foxp3-expressing CD4+ CD25+ cells in the nasal mucosa. J Allergy Clin Immunol 2008;121(6):1467–72.
28. Pilette C, Nouri-Aria KT, Jacobson MR, et al. Grass pollen immunotherapy induces an allergen-specific IgA2 antibody response associated with mucosal TGF-beta expression. J Immunol 2007;178(7):4658–66.
29. Chawes BL, Edwards MJ, Shamji B, et al. A novel method for assessing unchallenged levels of mediators in nasal epithelial lining fluid. J Allergy Clin Immunol 2010;125(6):1387–9.
30. Grindebacke H, Larsson P, Wing K, et al. Specific immunotherapy to birch allergen does not enhance suppression of Th2 cells by CD4(+)CD25(+) regulatory T cells during pollen season. J Clin Immunol 2009;29(6):752–60.
31. Lichtenstein LM, Ishizaka K, Norman PS, et al. IgE antibody measurements in ragweed hay fever. Relationship to clinical severity and the results of immunotherapy. J Clin Invest 1973;52(2):472–82.
32. Gleich GJ, Zimmermann EM, Henderson LL, et al. Effect of immunotherapy on immunoglobulin E and immunoglobulin G antibodies to ragweed antigens: a six-year prospective study. J Allergy Clin Immunol 1982;70(4):261–71.
33. Moverare R, Elfman L, Vesterinen E, et al. Development of new IgE specificities to allergenic components in birch pollen extract during specific immunotherapy studied with immunoblotting and Pharmacia CAP System. Allergy 2002;57(5):423–30.
34. Di Lorenzo G, Mansueto P, Pacor ML, et al. Evaluation of serum s-IgE/total IgE ratio in predicting clinical response to allergen-specific immunotherapy. J Allergy Clin Immunol 2009;123(5):1103–10.
35. Gehlar K, Schlaak M, Becker W-M, et al. Monitoring allergen Im- munotherapy of pollen-allergic patients: the ration of allergen-specificIgG4 to IgG1 correlates with clinical outcome. Clin Exp Allergy 1999;29:497–506.
36. Moverare R, Vesterinen E, Metso T, et al. Pollen-specific rush immunotherapy: clinical efficacy and effects on antibody concentrations. Ann Allergy Asthma Immunol 2001;86(3):337–42.
37. Devey ME, Wilson DV, Wheeler AW. The IgG subclasses of antibodies to grass pollen allergens produced in hay fever patients during hyposensitization. Clin Allergy 1976;6(3):227–36.
38. Garcia BE, Sanz ML, Dieguez I, et al. Modifications in IgG subclasses in the course of immunotherapy with grass pollen. J Investig Allergol Clin Immunol 1993;3(1):19–25.

39. Wachholz PA, Soni NK, Till SJ, et al. Inhibition of allergen-IgE binding to B cells by IgG antibodies after grass pollen immunotherapy. J Allergy Clin Immunol 2003; 112(5):915–22.

40. Pirron U, Schlunck T, Prinz JC, et al. IgE-dependent antigen focusing by human B lymphocytes is mediated by the low-affinity receptor for IgE. Eur J Immunol 1990; 20(7):1547–51.

41. Santamaria LF, Bheekha R, van Reijsen FC, et al. Antigen focusing by specific monomeric immunoglobulin E bound to CD23 on Epstein-Barr virus-transformed B cells. Hum Immunol 1993;37(1):23–30.

42. Karagiannis SN, Warrack JK, Jennings KH, et al. Endocytosis and recycling of the complex between CD23 and HLA-DR in human B cells. Immunology 2001; 103(3):319–31.

43. Kehry MR, Yamashita LC. Low-affinity IgE receptor (CD23) function on mouse B cells: role in IgE-dependent antigen focusing. Proc Natl Acad Sci U S A 1989; 86(19):7556–60.

44. van der Heijden FL, Joost van Neerven RJ, van Katwijk M, et al. Serum-IgE-facilitated allergen presentation in atopic disease. J Immunol 1993;150(8 Pt 1):3643–50.

45. Wurtzen PA, Lund G, Lund K, et al. A double-blind placebo-controlled birch allergy vaccination study II: correlation between inhibition of IgE binding, histamine release and facilitated allergen presentation. Clin Exp Allergy 2008;38(8): 1290–301.

46. Cooke RA, Bernhard JH, Hebald S, et al. Serological evidence of immunity with coexisting sensitization in hay fever type of human allergy. J Exp Med 1935;62: 733–51.

47. Lichtenstein LM, Norman PS, Winkenwerder WL. Antibody response following immunotherapy in ragweed hay fever: Allpyral vs. whole ragweed extract. J Allergy 1968;41(1):49–57.

48. Platts-Mills TA, von Maur RK, Ishizaka K, et al. IgA and IgG anti-ragweed anti-bodies in nasal secretions. Quantitative measurements of antibodies and correlation with inhibition of histamine release. J Clin Invest 1976;57(4):1041–50.

49. Aalberse RC, van der Gaag R, van Leeuwen J. Serologic aspects of IgG4 anti-bodies. I. Prolonged immunization results in an IgG4-restricted response. J Immunol 1983;130(2):722–6.

50. van der Zee JS, van Swieten P, Aalberse RC. Serologic aspects of IgG4 anti-bodies. II. IgG4 antibodies form small, nonprecipitating immune complexes due to functional monovalency. J Immunol 1986;137(11):3566–71.

51. Aalberse RC, Schuurman J. IgG4 breaking the rules. Immunology 2002; 105(1):9–19.

52. Nouri-Aria KT, Wachholz PA, Francis JN, et al. Grass pollen immunotherapy induces mucosal and peripheral IL-10 responses and blocking IgG activity. J Immunol 2004;172(5):3252–9.

53. Shamji MH, Wilcock LK, Wachholz PA, et al. The IgE-facilitated allergen binding (FAB) assay: validation of a novel flow-cytometric based method for the detection of inhibitory antibody responses. J Immunol Methods 2006; 317(1–2):71–9.

54. Shamji M, Ljørring C, Francis JN, et al. Blocking antibodies: relationship between IgG4-associated inhibitory activity and clinical response to grass-pollen immunotherapy. J Allergy Clin Immunol 2010;125(2 Suppl 1):AB131.

55. Petersen AB, Gudmann P, Milvang-Gronager P, et al. Performance evaluation of a specific IgE assay developed for the ADVIA centaur immunoassay system. Clin Biochem 2004;37(10):882–92.

56. Nelson HS, Nolte H, Creticos P, et al. Efficacy and safety of timothy grass allergy immunotherapy tablet treatment in North American adults. J Allergy Clin Immunol 2011;127(1):72–80.
57. Russell MW, Mansa B. Complement-fixing properties of human IgA antibodies. Alternative pathway complement activation by plastic-bound, but not specific antigen-bound, IgA. Scand J Immunol 1989;30(2):175–83.

The Health Economics of Allergen Immunotherapy

Cheryl S. Hankin, PhD[a],*, Linda Cox, MD[b], Amy Bronstone, PhD[a]

KEYWORDS

- Health economics • Allergen immunotherapy • Allergic rhinitis
- Asthma

More than 50 million people in the United States are affected by allergic diseases, making allergies the sixth leading cause of chronic disease among Americans.[1] Allergic rhinitis (AR), the most common allergic disease, is characterized by congestion, rhinorrhea, sneezing, and itching.[2] AR affects up to 30% of adults and 40% of children,[1] and ranks as the third-leading US chronic disease of individuals younger than 45.[3] AR prevalence is increasing globally, particularly in developed countries.[4]

Although sometimes mistakenly viewed as a trivial disease,[2] AR is associated with substantial clinical burden.[5] Typically a lifelong condition,[6] AR causes year-around symptoms in more than half of sufferers.[7] Symptoms of the illness can significantly reduce quality of life by causing physical discomfort and negative mood; disrupted sleep leading to daytime somnolence and reduced alertness; impaired cognitive functioning and learning; and lost time from work, school, and leisure activities.[8]

Health care expenditures for AR were estimated at $11.2 billion in 2004 ($13.5 billion in 2010).[9] Outpatient visits account for approximately one-third (36%) of AR-related direct costs and prescription medications account for nearly the entire remainder (59%).[9] Because costs for over-the-counter (OTC) medications, which were not included in the estimated expenditures shown in the first sentence of this paragraph, are reportedly equivalent to costs for prescription medications, health care expenditures attributable to AR may be substantially underestimated. AR often precedes the development of other chronic related diseases, including chronic sinusitis, otitis media with effusion, recurrent nasal polyps, and asthma.[8] The presence of AR with asthma significantly increases health services use in general,[10,11] and childhood hospitalizations in particular.[11]

In contrast to symptomatic drug treatment (SDT), which only temporarily relieves allergy symptoms,[12] allergen-specific immunotherapy (SIT) has the potential to alter

a BioMedEcon, LLC, Moss Beach, PO Box, 129 Moss Beach, CA 94038, USA
b 5333 North Dixie Highway, Suite 210, Fort Lauderdale, FL 33334, USA
* Corresponding author.
E-mail address: CHankin@biomedecon.com

Immunol Allergy Clin N Am 31 (2011) 325–341
doi:10.1016/j.iac.2011.03.007
0889-8561/11/$ – see front matter © 2011 Elsevier Inc. All rights reserved.
immunology.theclinics.com

the course of allergic disease, thereby reducing the need for long-term treatment, the progression of allergic rhinitis to asthma[13,14] and the development of new allergies.[10,11] The clinical benefits of SIT have been shown to persist for an additional 3 to 12 years after discontinuation of a 2.5- to 5.0-year treatment.[15] It therefore stands to reason that the clinical benefits of SIT also extend to economic benefits.

METHODOLOGIC APPROACHES TO ECONOMIC ANALYSES

Given the substantial economic burden associated with allergic disease, it is important to understand how different treatment strategies may mitigate allergy-related outcomes and costs of care (**Table 1**).[16] Cost-effectiveness analysis (CEA) is a method used to evaluate the tradeoffs involved in choosing among interventions.[16] Data regarding resource use may be captured from a variety of sources, including prospective clinical trials, patient or physician reports, or retrospective administrative claims data. Costs may be derived from standardized costs (eg, Medicare reimbursement rates for procedures or wholesale acquisition costs for drugs) or actual charges. Analytic approaches may include decision-tree modeling, Markov modeling, or between-group comparisons of actual mean or median costs. Results may be expressed through the use of a "cost-effectiveness ratio," in which all health effects of an intervention relative to a stated alternative are captured in the denominator, and changes in resource use relative to the alternative are captured in the numerator and valued in monetary terms.[16] Or, results may be expressed in terms of the health care cost differences between groups (eg, those who receive a specified treatment vs those who do not).

ECONOMIC ANALYSES OF ALLERGIC RHINITIS TREATMENTS

Treatment of AR may include allergen avoidance, pharmacologic treatments, and SIT.[17] Unfortunately, there have been no economic analyses of allergen avoidance measures and only 5 economic studies of pharmacologic treatments for AR to date.[18,19] The few existing economic analyses of pharmacotherapies for AR have been plagued by methodological flaws, such as small sample sizes, extrapolation of costs from short-term outcomes, limited information on the clinical benefits of comparators, and lack of standardized effectiveness measures, which significantly detract from the value of their findings.[18,19]

In contrast, a growing number of studies have evaluated the economic benefits of SIT in patients with AR and/or asthma.[20–34] We critically examine each of these studies from their first published appearance in 1995, to present. Costs reported in foreign currencies were translated to US dollars using specified exchange rates[35] and were updated to 2010 values using the Consumer Price Index for Health Care.[36]

1995
Donahue

The earliest study was a retrospective analysis of administrative claims for 294,000 US health plan enrollees who filed a claim during the period 1988 to 1992.[33] Investigators identified 603 adults and children with AR and/or asthma who had received at least 1 SIT injection and who had continuous membership during the year before and 2 years after their initial SIT administration. Costs related to SIT included all encounters with an SIT code, an allergen skin test, or a code for allergic reaction to SIT. Costs of care for asthma and rhinitis not related to SIT were defined as all encounters or claims with codes for asthma, rhinitis, sinusitis, nasal polyps, and a variety of tests, procedures, and dispensing for certain prescription drugs. No other costs were considered in this analysis.

The mean annual cost per patient following SIT initiation was $438 for all patients, $212 for those with asthma only, $416 for those with AR only, and $496 for those with both AR and asthma. The cost of SIT was significantly lower for patients age 10 to 20 years ($P<.03$). Only 33% of patients who initiated SIT completed the desired 3.5 years of treatment. The average annual costs for SIT per patient who completed 3.5 years of treatment were $698 compared with $247 for patients who prematurely terminated SIT. Patients who completed SIT also had 20% greater nonimmunotherapy costs than patients who received SIT of shorter duration (mean of $508 vs $421 per person-year), primarily attributable to higher prescription costs in the former group.

Several possible explanations have been proposed for the finding of higher costs in patients who completed SIT of longer duration. First, SIT completers may have had a greater disease burden than noncompleters, because the costs for asthma and AR treatment for this group were 30% higher during the year before starting SIT. Second, the follow-up period after completion of SIT (mean of 7 months) may have been too brief to begin to see a cost reduction among SIT completers. Third, the different SIT completion rates in the 2 groups may reflect an underlying tendency toward better adherence among SIT completers, who may have had higher medication costs because they were more likely to follow medical advice.

Buchner

In the same year, a German article described a theoretical cost-benefit analysis of SIT for the treatment of AR and allergic asthma based upon published literature.[27] Two models were created: one for patients with AR, and another for patients with allergic asthma. Among those with AR who received SDT alone, 57% were assumed to continue to experience AR symptoms over 10 years, and 43% were assumed to progress to allergic asthma. For those with AR who initiated SIT, a 90% therapeutic success rate was assumed over a 3-year treatment course (ie, use of SDT would decreased to 30% in the first year, 20% in the second year, and to 10% in the third year of treatment); for the 10% with AR who did not achieve treatment success with SIT, 57% would continue to experience AR symptoms (requiring SDT), and 43% would progress to allergic asthma after 8 years. In the second model, among patients with extant allergic asthma who initiated SIT, a 90% success rate again was assumed, in which the need for SDT would diminish in a parallel manner. Cost components included direct costs of treatment (drugs, physician and hospital services and SIT if appropriate) and indirect costs (days lost from work, disability, and premature death). According to these models, the cost advantage shifted in favor of SIT during the sixth year of treatment for AR. The 10-year total cost per AR patient treated with SDT was 11,054 in 1990 DM ($16,311 in 2010 USD) compared with 6083 in 1990 DM ($8976 in 2010 USD) for treatment with SIT. The cost advantage shifted to SIT during the fourth year of treatment for allergic asthma. The 10-year total cost per asthma patient treated with SDT was 16,430 in 1990 DM ($24,243 in 2010 USD) compared with 6849 in 1990 DM ($10,106 in 2010 USD) for SIT.

This relatively simplistic model, based on the assumption that 10% of patients receiving SIT would not achieve therapeutic success, had several limitations. First, the investigators provide no justification for their determinations of specific indirect and direct costs. Second, no sensitivity analyses were conducted to test the robustness of the model. Finally, the model examined patients with AR and asthma separately and did not account for that fact that many patients would be diagnosed with both disorders at the onset of treatment.

Table 1
Summary of SIT economic analyses

Pub Date	Author	Country	Source of Cost Data	Subject Characteristics	Comparisons	Results
1995	Donahue[33]	USA	RACD	603 adults & children with AR ± asthma	Patients completing 3.5 y SIT vs patients not completing 3.5 y SIT	Mean direct costs per patient-year: 3.5 y SIT: $698 (1988–2992) <3.5 y SIT: $247 (1988–1992)
1995	Buchner[27]	Germany	Cost-of-illness study	400,000 adults & children with AR; 400,000 adults & children with asthma	10 y SIT vs SDT	Mean direct costs per AR patient over 10 y: SIT: $8976 (2010) SDT: $16,311 (2010) Mean direct costs per asthma patient over 10 y: SIT: $10,106 (2010) SDT: $24,243 (2010)
1997	Le Pen[32]	France	Physician survey	851 adults & children with AR ± asthma (6% other dx)	Various duration of SIT	Mean cost allergy medications per patient-year: <1 y SIT: $37 (2010) ≥1 y SIT: $23 (2010)
1999	Bernstein[34]	USA	Published literature	Patients with AR at 3 medical facilities	5 y SIT + SDT vs SDT	Mean direct costs per patient over 5 y: SIT: $5000 SDT: $10,200
2000	Schadlich[24]	Germany	Published literature, cost-of-illness studies	Hypothetical cohort of 2000 patients with AR ± asthma	10 y SIT vs SDT	Difference (SIT-SDT) in direct costs per patient with AR (pollen) over 10 y: −$960 (2010) Difference (SIT-SDT) in direct costs per patient with AR (mite) over 10 y: −$1190 (2010)
2005	Berto[21]	Italy	Medical records	135 children with AR ± asthma	1 y before SLIT vs 3 y during SLIT	Mean direct costs per patient-year: Before SLIT: $651 (2010) During SLIT: $288 (2010)

Year	Author	Country	Design	Population	Comparison	Outcome
2005	Petersen[23]	Denmark	Medical records & patient survey	253 patients aged 16–60 with AR ± asthma	4 y SIT vs SDT	Mean direct costs per patient over 4 y: SIT: $2802 (2010) SDT: $1335 (2010)
2006	Ariano[20]	Italy	Randomized controlled trial	30 adults with AR ± asthma	3 y SIT vs SDT; 3 y FU	Difference (SIT-SDT) in direct costs per patient in the 6th year: −$932
2006	Berto[22]	Italy	Physician survey	Hypothetical cohort of 1000 patients aged 16–45 with AR ± asthma	3 y SLIT + SDT vs SDT; 3 y FU	Difference (SIT-SDT) in direct costs per patient over 6 y: −$759
2007	Bachert[25]	Northern Europe	Randomized controlled trial	634 adults with AR ± asthma	3 y SLIT + SDT vs SDT; 6 y FU	$19,345 to $27,324 (2010) cost per QALY gained (payer perspective)
2007	Keiding[26]	UK	Randomized controlled trial	306 adults with AR	3 y SLIT + SDT vs SDT; 6 y FU	$14,536 to $38,695 (2010) cost per QALY gained (payer perspective)
2007	Omnes[28]	France	Delphi panel	Hypothetical cohort of 1000 adults & children with AR ± asthma	3–4 y SIT; 3 y FU	ICER per additional improved patient: SCIT vs SDT: $517 to $1069 (2010) SLIT vs SDT: $933 to $3509 (2010) ICER per additional asthma case avoided: SCIT vs SDT: $582 to $1964 (2010) SLIT vs SDT: $1120 to $5829 (2010)
2008	Hankin[29]	USA	RACD	354 children with AR ± asthma	6 months before SIT vs 6 months after SIT	Difference (postSIT-preSIT) in direct costs (excluding cost of SIT) per patient over 6 months: $401
2010	Hankin[30]	USA	RACD	13,781 children with AR ± asthma	18 months SIT vs SDT	Difference (SIT-SDT) in direct costs per patient over 18 months: −$1625 over 18 months
2011	Hankin[31]	USA	RACD	6443 adults with AR ± asthma	18 months SIT vs SDT	Difference (SIT-SDT) in direct costs per patient over 18 months: −$7286 over 18 months

Abbreviations: AR, allergic rhinitis; dx, diagnosis; FU, follow-up; QALY, quality-adjusted life year; RACD, retrospective administrative claims database; SDT, symptomatic drug treatment; SIT, allergen-specific immunotherapy; SLIT, sublingual allergen immunotherapy; ±, with or without.
Note: For cost differences, negative numbers indicate a cost savings conferred by SIT.

1997
Le Pen

In a French study, investigators used physician survey data of patients receiving SIT to test the hypothesis that greater duration of SIT is directly related to the magnitude of decrease in the use of SDT.[32] Among 1000 patients who had received SIT for a variety of allergies, 851 (85%) had completed surveys regarding aspects of their SIT treatment (duration and reasons for desensitization), and past 15-day allergy symptoms, other allergy treatments received, physician visits, allergy-related hospitalizations, and work missed. Among respondents, 333 (29%) had received SIT for less than 1 year. For all respondents regardless of SIT duration, past 15-day self-reported physician visits accounted for 150 F (1996 value, $49.98 in 2010 USD), SDT 55 F (1996 value, $18.30 in 2010 USD), SIT 14.5 F (1996 value, $4.82 in 2010 USD), hospitalizations 1.6 F (1996 value, $0.53 in 2010 USD), and missed work 28.9 F (1996 value, $9.62 in 2010 USD). Costs for SDT were significantly lower (P-value not provided) for patients who received 1 to 2 years of SIT versus those who received less than 1 year. This benefit plateaued after 1 to 2 years; in other words, there were no significant additional cost benefits for SIT duration of more than 2 years.

This short-term retrospective study was limited by some key weaknesses. First, data were derived from a physician survey rather than from an administrative database. Thus, self-selection (149 refused participation) and/or biases associated with self-reported data may have affected the results. Second, SDT costs were estimated over a very short period of time (15 days). Third, as the investigators acknowledge, only a small proportion (undisclosed) of patients completed more than 2 years of SIT. Fourth, the absolute between-group differences in SDT costs and P-values were not provided. Finally, the authors did not compare total medical costs among patients with different durations of SIT. Although the cost of SDT appeared to be reduced among patients with longer duration of SIT, the meaning of this finding is questionable unless SIT also reduced the total costs of care.

1999
Bernstein

A 1999 US study used data from a 1996 American College of Allergy, Asthma and Immunology report to compare the estimated the 5-year average cost of SIT plus SDT versus SDT alone among patients with AR.[34] Data from 3 allergy treatment centers in different geographic regions in the United States provided the basis for estimating costs. Costs for SIT were based on the assumption that patients with AR would require daily use of an antihistamine/decongestant and intranasal corticosteroid spray. The authors estimated 5-year SIT costs to be $5000 ($8511 in 2010 USD) versus SDT $10,200 ($17,362 in 2010 USD) for SDT, and concluded that SIT was more "cost-effective" than SDT. This casual analysis is limited by rough estimates of costs that were not further substantiated or validated, assumptions that patients who received SIT do not concomitantly use symptomatic drug treatment, and the exclusion of other costs of care associated with SIT, or undertreated AR.

2000
Schadlich

In 2000, a study used retrospective data from clinical trials, observational studies, and epidemiologic sources to model health outcomes associated with 3 years of SIT versus SDT in patients with AR over 10 years of follow-up.[24] Direct costs included outpatient medical services, outpatient drug treatment, inpatient medical services, allergy-related diagnostic tests, treatment for adverse events, SIT allergen extract, and allergy medications. Resource use (physician visits, diagnostic tests) for patients receiving SIT was estimated based on results of a provider survey and the quantity of allergen extract used each year was estimated based on expert interviews. The frequency of systemic adverse events was based on clinical trial and observational study results.

A decision-tree model was constructed using change in the proportion of patients with asthma as the measure of effectiveness. Clinical trials data suggested that the proportion of patients with asthma would decrease from 30% at the start of treatment to 19% after 10 years in the SIT-treated group and would increase from 30% to 35% in patients treated with SDT. The costs incurred by patients treated with SIT were modeled and compared with the annual costs for patients with AR and/or asthma based on cost-of-illness studies.

The total direct costs associated with SIT were higher for the first 6 years, after which SIT became cost saving relative to SDT. The average, 10-year, per-patient net savings with SIT, as evaluated from the payer perspective, ranged from 580 DM (1997 value, $960 in 2010 USD) for mite allergy to 670 DM (1997 value, $1109 in 2010 USD) for pollen allergy. Although this study used a sophisticated model, estimation of cost savings was based strictly on the potential of SIT to reduce the development of asthma, and therefore likely underestimated the true savings that are possible with SIT. In addition, the model assumed that patients were 100% adherent to SIT, which is unrealistic and contradictory to SIT adherence data reported in various studies.[33,37–40]

2005
Berto

In another study, investigators analyzed the medical records of children receiving care for allergic disease at a single allergy center in Italy.[21] Subjects who had 1 year of data before receiving sublingual immunotherapy (SLIT) and at least 3 years of data while on SLIT were selected. Of the 135 identified children, 34% had seasonal allergies and 66% had perennial allergy (house dust mites). About 61% had AR and asthma, 38% had asthma, and fewer than 1% had AR only. Outcome measures used to calculate direct costs included the number of physician and specialist office visits, pharmacologic treatment, and use of SLIT. Data on hospitalizations were not available from the patient medical records. The number of school absences served as a proxy for the number of lost work days by parents, which was used to estimate indirect costs.

Clinical effectiveness, indicated by the number of asthma and rhinitis exacerbations, improved after SLIT: the mean number of exacerbations was 5 times lower during the 3 years on SLIT compared with the year before SLIT. The number of medical visits decreased threefold during an average year under SLIT compared with the year before SLIT. The mean cost per patient was €506 ($651 in 2010 USD) during the year before SLIT and €224 ($288 in 2010 USD) per year during the 3 years of SLIT. When indirect costs were included, the total cost per patient decreased from €2672 ($3436 in 2010 USD) in the year before SLIT to €629 ($809 in 2010 USD) per year during SLIT.

Investigators also conducted a case-control analysis involving a subgroup of SLIT-treated patients with allergic asthma who were matched with a group of similar patients who had not received SLIT and were not from the same data source as those who received SLIT. This analysis revealed comparable direct costs between SLIT-treated patients (€1182 in 2002; $1520 in 2010 USD) and controls (€1100 in 2002; $1414 in 2010 USD) over 4 years of follow-up.

Although the results of this study suggest that SLIT reduces the use of health care resources and can alleviate the economic burden of allergic illness, several limitations should be noted. First, the investigators apparently did not conduct significance testing, and so it is impossible to conclude that SLIT significantly reduced direct or total costs. Second, because the economic analyses did not include hospitalizations, the true effect of SLIT on costs may have been underestimated. Third, the involvement of allergic children from a single allergy center limits the generalizability of study findings. In addition, the case-control analysis was limited by the selection of matched controls from a different database than the one used to select SLIT-treated patients, and by the lack of matching based on demographic or illness characteristics.

Petersen

A 6-year retrospective analysis involving 253 adults who received SIT for grass pollen and/or dust mite allergy at a hospital or allergy specialist office in Denmark from 1996 to 2002 was one of the few studies that failed to find a reduction in direct costs related to SIT.[23] Patients were surveyed regarding the number of emergency visits and hospital admissions they had during the year before starting SIT, 4 years of SIT, and the year following SIT. Information on outpatient visits was obtained from local county records for the period 1997 to 2002. Outpatient visit data were not available for 26 patients who initiated SIT in 1996. Because medical records contained only medication use data for the latest 16 months, information on pre-SIT medication use was obtained from a different cohort of 53 patients who started SIT in 2002. Post-SIT medication use was based on data from a minority of patients who had completed SIT; because only 7 months of medication use data were available for these patients, data were extrapolated to estimate 1-year post-SIT medication use. Indirect costs were estimated using the number of lost work and leisure days.

Costs for medications (2002 values) averaged Danish krone (DKK) 1309 ($226 in 2010 USD) per patient in the year before SIT, increased to DKK 2776 ($479 in 2010 USD) during the first year of SIT, and fell to DKK 1629 ($281 in 2010 USD) during years 2 to 4 of SIT and to DKK 338 ($58 in 2010 USD) in the year following SIT completion. Use of medical doctors increased after the initiation of SIT and continued to be higher after SIT was completed. Outpatient costs increased from DKK 609 ($105 in 2010 USD) before SIT to between DKK 1041 ($180 in 2010 USD) and DKK 3247 ($560 in 2010 USD) during SIT and DKK 825 ($142) in the year after SIT. Finally, costs for hospitalizations and emergency visits fell from DKK 46 ($8 in 2010 USD) before SIT to DKK 13 ($2 in 2010 USD) after SIT after increasing to DKK 127 ($22 in 2010 USD) per year during SIT.

Although the total mean direct cost per patient decreased from DKK 1964 ($445 in 2010 USD) in the year before SIT to DKK 1176 ($203 in 2010 USD) in the year after SIT, the average cost for 4 years of SIT (DKK 16,248 or $2802 in 2010 USD) exceeded that for 4 years of SDT (DKK 7856 or $1355 in 2010 USD). Based on these calculations, breakeven with SIT would not occur until the 10th year following a 4-year course of SIT (Year 15).

This study had several methodological flaws that should be noted. First, hospital and emergency department use over 6 years were obtained by self-report, and it is likely that patient recall was imprecise over this period of time. Second, indirect costs were also obtained by patient self-report, which was subject to bias. Specifically, patients were asked whether SIT had improved the quality of their well-being over the previous 1 to 7 years, and they were asked to provide the number of work and leisure days lost due to allergy and asthma prior, during and following SIT. Third, investigators collected data on pre-SIT medication use from a different sample, and extrapolated 7 months of post-SIT medication use to 12 months to calculate pre- versus post-SIT changes in medication costs. Furthermore, because the 7-month period post-SIT medication use information included the grass pollen season, when allergy medication use peaks, medication use during the 12-month post-SIT period may have been overestimated. Finally, patients were followed for only 1 year after SIT was completed, and potential long-term reductions in costs could not be detected.

2006
Ariano

An economic analysis of SIT was performed using data from a prospective, single-site study in which 30 Italian adults with *Parietaria* pollen-induced rhinitis and asthma were randomly assigned to 3 years of SIT plus SDT (n = 20) or SDT alone (n = 10) and then followed for 3 years after completion of SIT.[20] During the 4-month pollen season, patients recorded symptom scores, allergy drug use, and adverse drug reactions on a daily diary card; each month during the study, they recorded the number of general practitioner or specialist office visits attended, SIT injections received, and boxes of allergy medications used. At 6-month intervals, patients completed study visits and turned in their daily diary and health care use cards.

Patients in the SIT plus SDT group began to show a significant reduction in allergy symptoms and medication use compared with the SDT-alone group beginning in the first year of treatment. The superior effectiveness in the SIT plus SDT group continued throughout the 6-year study, even during the 3 years after discontinuation of SIT.

The mean annual cost for patients in the SIT plus SDT group was similar to that of patients in the SDT-only group for the first 2 years of treatment. In the third year, the SIT plus SDT group showed a 48% reduction in costs (*P*<.0001) compared with the SDT-only group. This cost reduction progressively increased over time, such that, in year 6 of the study, annual costs were 80% lower (€623 in 2005, $932 in 2010 USD) in the SIT plus SDT group.

The main strength of this study was its use of data from a prospective, randomized, long-term study. Investigators were able to show that, even though significant clinical benefits were evident during the first year of treatment with SIT, cost benefits were not seen until the third year. Further, maximum cost benefits did not occur until 3 years after discontinuation of SIT, indicating that a long-term perspective is critical when evaluating the economic impact of SIT.

A disadvantage of this study was its reliance on patient self-report to assess health care use. Although patients were to record doctor visits, SIT injections, and allergy medication use every month, the only monitoring of this activity occurred at the 6-month study visits. In addition, because this economic analysis did not take into account hospital admissions or emergency room visits (except for drug reactions), the results may have underestimated the true cost savings associated with SIT. Finally, the ability to generalize from these study findings is limited by the nature of the sample (adults with seasonal AR and asthma), the small number of patients involved, recruitment of patients from a single allergy center.

Berto

The Sublingual Immunotherapy Pollen Allergy Italy (SPAI) study compared costs, clinical outcomes, and cost-effectiveness ratios for 2 AR and asthma management strategies: SLIT with SDT and SDT alone.[22] A decision-tree model was populated using retrospective data from the clinical records of 100 young adults (age 16–45) with pollen-induced AR with or without asthma who were treated by a panel of 27 physicians from 25 allergy centers in Italy. Retrospective data included allergy treatments received, use of health care resources (office visits, diagnostic procedures, and hospital admissions), physician ratings of improvement, and patient diagnoses;

however, it was unclear as to whether the source(s) of health care resource data were patient self-report, medical records, or administrative claims. Direct costs included physician office visits, diagnostic procedures, hospitalizations, SLIT, and antiallergy drugs; indirect costs included lost workdays. The cost of SLIT and antiallergy medications was based on recommended dosing schedules as opposed to actual use. The number of follow-up visits per year by disease severity and number of hospital admissions was obtained from analysis of data provided by the physician panel; the same rate of hospitalizations was applied to both treatment groups.

A cost analysis was performed to determine, from the payer perspective, the mean direct cost per patient during a 6-year period for patients receiving 3 years of SLIT plus SDT (€1901 or $2844 in 2010 USD) or SDT alone (€2408 or $3603 in 2010 USD; net savings = $759 in 2010 USD). The break-even point occurred 4 years after the initiation of SLIT, even though reduction in costs began in the first year of treatment. From the societal perspective, which included direct costs paid by the patient and indirect costs, the break-even point was reached in year 2, and the net savings in 6-year total costs was €2113 ($3161 in 2010 USD) for patients receiving SLIT.

A decision-tree model was constructed to determine the cost per improved patient and per asthma case avoided for SLIT versus no SLIT. For a hypothetical cohort of 1000 patients, physicians estimated that SLIT would have improved symptoms of 631 patients versus 232 patients in the no SLIT arm and that SLIT would have prevented asthma in 518 patients versus 289 in the no SLIT arm. From the payer perspective, the cost per additional improved patient was €4313 ($6453 in 2010 USD) for SLIT plus SDT and €6426 ($9614 in 2010 USD) for SDT alone and the cost per additional asthma case avoided was €1901 ($2844 in 2010 USD) for SLIT plus SDT and €2408 ($3603 in 2010 USD) for SDT alone. SLIT was less costly for both endpoints from the societal perspective as well.

It is unfortunate that the cost analysis was based on health care use data of questionable validity. Although these data were supposedly derived from patient "clinical records," investigators failed to specify the precise methods used to estimate these outcomes. For example, it is unclear why investigators assumed that hospital admission rates were equal in the 2 treatment groups if objective data were available to determine these rates. Patient use of allergy medications and SLIT were estimated based on the prescribed regimens rather than on actual patient use. It is possible, for example, that patients who were experiencing symptom relief may have used less medication than was prescribed. Finally, outcomes were determined by unblinded physician ratings, which may have been influenced by physicians' knowledge of the treatments patients had received.

2007
Bachert

A cost-utility analysis was conducted using data from a large, international (8 countries), randomized, double-blind, placebo-controlled trial in which 316 patients were randomized to a grass allergen tablet arm and 318 to a placebo (SDT) arm.[25] During the clinical trial, patients received preseasonal SLIT for 16 to 35 weeks. To estimate the long-term effectiveness of SLIT, it was assumed that 3 years of treatment with the grass allergen tablet would result in sustained clinical benefits for another 6 years.

All study patients were permitted the use of allergy medications according to need. Patient use of health care resources (physician visits, use of allergy medication, hospitalizations, and time missed from work because of AR) and quality of life data were collected prospectively. Medication use was assessed by daily patient diaries and physician visits and missed work assessed by weekly patient diaries. In addition to the physician visit data collected during the weekly diaries during the pollen season, the annual number of physician visits for patients receiving SLIT was estimated using data from a European survey.

Patients who received SLIT experienced a 30% reduction in allergy symptoms and a 38% reduction in medication score ($P<.0001$) compared with placebo during the allergy season of the first treatment year. SLIT-treated patients gained 0.0287 additional quality-adjusted life years (QALYs) per season (0.222 QALYs gained over 9 years) compared with patients receiving only SDT ($P<.001$). No patients were hospitalized and there were no significant differences between groups in the number of physician visits during the pollen season. The mean use of symptomatic medication and hours of lost work because of AR were significantly higher in the placebo group. From a payer perspective, assuming an annual cost of SLIT of €1500 ($2244 in 2010 USD), the cost per QALY gained ranged from €12,930 ($19,345 in 2010 USD) in the Netherlands to €18,263 ($27,324 in 2010 USD) in Germany.

Although this study incorporated data from a well-controlled and large clinical trial, the trial was relatively short in duration and long-term outcomes were based on assumptions that may have resulted in the overestimation or underestimation of cost effectiveness. For example, patient-reported health care resource use over the first pollen season after treatment was extrapolated to a 9-year period, yet there is no reason to assume that health care use remained constant throughout this long period. In addition, the assumption that 3 years of SLIT would result in sustained clinical benefits for all patients is doubtful; it is likely that some long-term users of SLIT would have experienced a relapse of symptoms after discontinuation of treatment.

Keiding and Jørgensen

Similar to the study just described, Keiding and Jørgensen conducted a 9-year cost-effectiveness analysis of SIT based on results of a 1-year clinical trial.[26] The UK Immunotherapy Study Group (UKIS) trial was a 1-year, multicenter, randomized, double-blind, parallel-group study comparing SIT (Alutard SQ; ALK-Abelló, Hoersholm, Denmark) and placebo (SDT) in patients with seasonal grass pollen–induced rhinoconjunctivitis whose symptoms were uncontrolled using SDT.[41] Patients received 15 injections over the first 7 to 8 weeks (induction period) followed by maintenance injections every 6 weeks. Acrivastine, fluticasone propionate nasal spray, and sodium cromoglycate eye drops were freely available throughout the study for both groups. Where necessary, rescue medication was given according to written protocols. Clinical outcomes, including symptom and medication scores and quality of life, were assessed before and after a 15-week pollen season.

The direct costs of treatment were estimated by combining the resource use found in the UKIS study (cost of SIT, follow-up visits to specialists/general practitioners, and use of pharmacologic treatments) with national price data from 6 European countries. Although use of pharmacologic medications was documented by patients, and visits to health care professionals for SIT administration were documented by investigators, other use of health care resources during the study does not appear to have been captured. The cost of maintenance SIT was included for an additional 2 years (assuming a 3-year SIT treatment period); differences between groups in the use of emergency medications observed during the clinical trial were assumed to continue through the remaining 8 years. Indirect costs were estimated using the number of workdays lost (0.6 for SIT and 2.7 for SDT) in a previous study of rhinoconjunctivitis. A 3% discount rate was applied. Treatment effects were measured as the percentage of symptom-free days (31.2% for SIT and 23.6% for SDT) and well days (36.6% for SIT and 28.2% for SDT) during the pollen season in the UKIS.

The incremental cost-effectiveness ratio (ICER), calculated as the cost difference between SIT and SDT divided by the difference in effect, for direct cost per symptom-free day and well day ranged from €26 ($39 in 2010 USD) in Austria to €68 ($102 in 2010 USD) in the Netherlands and from €24 ($36 in 2010 USD) in Austria to €61 ($91 in 2010 USD) in the Netherlands, respectively. When indirect costs were included, SIT dominated SDT (ie, reduced costs and increased effects) in 4 of the 6 countries for both variables. When only direct costs were considered, the cost-effectiveness ratio ranged from €9716 ($14,536 in 2010 USD) to €25,863 ($38,695 in 2010 USD) per QALY, below the $40,000 to $60,000 threshold for cost-effective therapies established by the National Institute for Clinical Excellence.[42] When indirect costs were included, SIT was dominant over SDT in all countries except the Netherlands and Sweden. Sensitivity analyses conducted on the number of up-dosing visits, cost of IT visit, cost of general practitioner and/or specialist visit, cost of emergency medicine, and effectiveness of SIT showed that only very considerable changes in the base values turned the cost-effectiveness ratios into unfavorable ones that exceeded the threshold of $60,000.

As with the Bachert and colleagues study,[25] the main weakness of this analysis is the extrapolation of short-term costs and effects to 9 years. This may have resulted in an underestimation of cost savings associated with SIT, as it failed to account for the potential reduction in the use of health care resources over time (due to lower rates of asthma and other comorbid disorders) among those receiving SIT. Further, documentation of health care resource use during the clinical trial appears to be incomplete in that non–allergy-related outpatient visits, inpatient care, and emergency services use were not assessed.

Omnes

A cost-effectiveness analysis conducted from a French health insurance perspective compared SCIT, SLIT, and SDT in pollen or dust mite allergic patients with AR or asthma.[28] Unlike the previous 2 economic modeling studies, which used data from a clinical trial to estimate key variables, this study used a Delphi expert panel to populate a decision-tree model with both efficacy (number of improved patients and asthma cases avoided) and resource use variables (clinic visits, diagnosis and follow-up tests, drugs, and SIT); hospitalization costs were not included.

The model time horizon was 6 years for adults and 7 for children. Patients were assumed to receive SIT for 3 (adults) or 4 (children) years. After 1 year of SIT, patients were (1) asymptomatic and assumed to stop use of rescue medications, (2) improved and assumed to reduce rescue medication use, or (3) unchanged or worse, resulting in treatment discontinuation and initiation of SDT. Treatment was discontinued after 3 or 4 years of SIT and patients were assumed to be either stabilized or worse at the end of the 6- to 7-year study. Patients receiving SDT were assumed to continue therapy throughout the study and symptoms were either improved, stabilized, or worsened.

SIT was found to be more effective both in terms of the number of patients with improved symptoms and asthma cases avoided. SDT was the least expensive treatment regardless of group (adult vs child) or indication (pollen vs dust mite allergy). SCIT was more cost effective than SLIT. Comparing SCIT to SDT, the ICER per additional improved patient ranged from €349/$517 in 2010 USD (children-dust mite allergy) to €722/$1069 in 2010 USD (adults-pollen allergy) and ICER per additional case of asthma avoided ranged from €393/$582 in 2010 USD (adults-dust mite allergy) to €1327/$1964 in 2010 USD (adults-pollen allergy). Comparing SLIT to

SDT, the ICER per additional improved patient ranged from €630/$933 in 2010 USD (children-pollen allergy) to €2371/$3509 in 2010 USD (children-dust mite allergy) and ICER per additional case of asthma avoided ranged from €824/$1220 in 2010 USD (children-pollen allergy) to €3938/$5829 in 2010 USD (children-dust mite allergy).

The main limitation of this study was its use of an expert panel to estimate both efficacy and health care resource variables. Although decision models commonly use expert opinion to develop and populate models, groups of experts often disagree and the notion of expert "consensus" may be an illusion.[43] The investigators claimed to have "cross-validated" the medical outcomes of the model with those of published clinical trials, but it is not clear whether these clinical trials were selected to develop the model efficacy parameters (and whether other trial data were rejected) or whether these parameters were estimated using other sources. In addition, the expert panel's assumptions regarding health care resource use were faulty in at least one respect. Although the expert panel had determined that hospitalization was a rare event in patients with AR and asthma, and thus did not include inpatient use in the model, subsequent examination of French retrospective data indicated that hospitalization of asthmatic children and adults occurred each year. The investigators acknowledged that the failure to include hospitalization costs likely underestimated the cost effectiveness of SIT relative to SDT.

2008
Hankin

A 7-year (1997–2004) retrospective analysis of Florida Medicaid claims data evaluated treatment outcomes and costs of children who were newly diagnosed with allergic rhinitis and naïve to SIT.[29] Patients were selected who were newly diagnosed with AR, had at least 1 year of data preceding and 4 years of data following their first AR diagnosis, had received SIT following their first AR diagnosis, and had at least 6 months of data following termination of SIT. Among these 354 patients, medical costs accrued during the 6 months before SIT initiation were compared with costs accrued during the 6 months following termination of SIT. Although only 16% of patients completed at least 3 years of SIT, and more than half of patients received 1 year or less of SIT, pharmacy, outpatient, and inpatient costs were significantly reduced in the 6 months post-SIT compared with the 6 months before SIT initiation. The mean weighted 6-month cost reduction was $401 per patient, which offset the mean cost of SIT ($424 per patient). The main limitations of this study were its short-term follow-up and the specialized nature of the sample.

2010
Hankin

A 10-year (1997–2007), retrospective claims, matched cohort study compared the median, 18-month, per-patient direct costs (pharmacy, outpatient visits, inpatient admissions) of Florida Medicaid-enrolled children (age <18 years) newly diagnosed with AR who subsequently received versus did not receive SIT.[30] Those with AR who received at least 2 administrations of SIT were matched by age at AR diagnosis, sex, race/ethnicity, comorbid illness burden, and the presence of asthma, conjunctivitis, or dermatitis to children newly diagnosed with AR who did not subsequently receive SIT.

Compared with matched controls who did not receive SIT, children who received SIT had significantly lower 18-month, median, per-patient, total health care costs ($3247 vs $4872), outpatient costs exclusive of SIT ($1107 vs $2626) or inclusive of SIT ($1829 vs $2594), and pharmacy costs ($1108 vs $1316; $P<.001$ for all).

Significant differences in total median health care costs were evident as early as 3 months after SIT initiation and increased throughout the 18-month analysis. At 3, 6, 12, and 18 months, median, per-patient, total health care cost savings in favor of SIT were $248, $527, $1061, and $1625, respectively, (P<.001 at all time points). As previously noted, limitations include the short-term follow-up and the specialized nature of the sample.

2011
Hankin

In an 11-year (1997–2008), matched cohort, retrospective claims analysis of Florida Medicaid adult enrollees newly-diagnosed with AR, investigators reported even more compelling findings than those reported for children.[31] At 18 months, total mean health care costs for inpatient ($10,352 vs $14,796, P = .003), outpatient excluding ($2466 vs $4181, P<.0001) or including ($2668 vs $4101, P<.0001) SIT, pharmacy ($5636 vs $6321, P<.0001) and total health care services ($10,626 vs $17,912, P<.0001) were significantly lower for patients who received versus did not receive SIT. Significant total health care savings were realized within 3 months of SIT initiation ($1932 vs $3189, P<.0001), and exceeded the mean 18-month outlay for SIT ($337). Per-patient, 18-month total cost savings with SIT were 41%. Again, limitations include the short-term follow-up and the specialized nature of the sample.

SUMMARY

We identified 15 studies from 1995 to 2011 that have examined the health economics of SIT. All focus on AR with or without asthma. Five studies specifically pertain to treatment of US patients[29–31,33,34] and the remainder examine the economics of SIT among patients in Europe. Routes of SIT administration include subcutaneous injection,[20,23,24,27–34] and sublingual immunotherapy.[21,22,25,26] There is wide variation in primary sources for health services use and costs: retrospective administrative claims data were the basis for 4 studies,[29–31,33] randomized, controlled trials for 3 studies[20,25,26] published literature for 3 studies,[24,27,34] physician surveys for 2 studies,[22,32] and medical records,[21] medical records and patient survey,[23] and Delphi panel expert opinion,[28] for 1 study each. Duration of evaluated outcomes ranges from 6 months pre- versus post-SIT[29] to 6-year follow-up after a 3-year course of SIT.[25,26]

Despite the wide variation in AR comorbidity, geographic location of analysis, route of administration, sources from which economic evaluations are based, and duration of treatment outcomes, the resounding message is that SIT provides cost benefit that ranges from $96[24] to $5465[31] per year. Of the 2 studies that reported a cost disadvantage for SIT, one failed to adjust for group differences in baseline illness severity[33] and the other[23] predicated much of its findings upon potentially biased patient self-report and extrapolations from unrelated populations.

There are unique limitations associated with each type of economic analysis included in this review. Whereas analyses based upon prospective, randomized trials offer the greatest control of clinical and economic variables, particularly with regard to the quality and quantity of treatment received, clinical trials may be limited by their lack of generalizability due to potentially contrived study design, recruitment of patients who are unrepresentative of those who actually receive treatment, unrealistically intensive patient attention and monitoring, and short time horizons.[44] In contrast, although retrospective analysis of administrative claims data does not allow for the selection of variables beyond those already provided within the database, this type of analysis offers objective information about medical resource utilization of patients receiving treatment in the "real world." Finally, while economic analyses based upon pharmacoeconomic models have consistently found SIT to confer cost advantages relative to SDT over an 8- to 10-year period,[22,24–28] the underlying assumptions upon which these analyses are based often remain opaque to the reader, have not been well validated, and are not routinely tested for sensitivities.

Compared to SDT, which provides temporary symptomatic relief, SIT is the only potentially disease-modifying treatment currently available.[15] Unfortunately, SIT is initiated by only a minority (2–6%) of potentially appropriate patients in the US[29,33,45] and patient adherence to the generally recommended 3-year minimum course of treatment[46] is rare.[29] Underserved populations are generally the least likely to initiate SIT, and are the most likely to prematurely discontinue treatment.[47]

The magnitude of cost savings associated with SIT varies across studies cited in this review. Savings of as much as 80% have been reported among Italian adults with AR and asthma 3 years after completion of a 3-year course of SIT.[20] In the US, total health care cost savings of 33% and 41% have been reported for US children[29] and adults[30] with AR (with or without asthma), respectively, within 18 months of SIT initiation. Given the suboptimal duration of SIT reported for US patients[30,33] estimated US cost savings conferred by SIT are likely to be greater among patients who adhere to the suggested 3-year minimum course of treatment.

Although SIT lacks the glamor and allure of more sophisticated (and more expensive) SDTs, SIT remains the current, albeit underutilized, standard of care for the treatment of allergic disease. As new SDTs proliferate and health care costs continue to spiral, the comparative clinical and cost effectiveness conferred by these new market entries over SIT must be carefully and thoughtfully examined.

REFERENCES

1. The American Academy of Allergy, Asthma and Immunology (AAAAI). The Allergy Report. Milwaukee (WI): AAAAI; 2000.
2. Wallace D, Dykewicz M, Bernstein D, et al. The diagnosis and management of rhinitis: an updated practice parameter. J Allergy Clin Immunol 2008;122(2): S1–84.
3. Chronic conditions - a challenge for the 21st century. Washington, DC: National Academy on an Aging Society; 1999.
4. Schoenwetter WF. Allergic rhinitis: epidemiology and natural history. Allergy Asthma Proc 2000;21(1):1–6.
5. Meltzer EO, Blaiss MS, Derebery MJ, et al. Burden of allergic rhinitis: results from the Pediatric Allergies in America survey. J Allergy Clin Immunol 2009;124(Suppl 3):S43–70.
6. Schoenwetter WF, Dupclay L Jr, Appajosyula S, et al. Economic impact and quality-of-life burden of allergic rhinitis. Curr Med Res Opin 2004;20(3):305–17.
7. Allergies in America. A landmark survey of nasal allergy sufferers. Allergies in America: executive summary 2006. [January 9, 2007]; Available at: http://www.myallergiesinamerica.com/healthcare/overview.aspx. Accessed August 16, 2010.
8. Meltzer EO. Quality of life in adults and children with allergic rhinitis. J Allergy Clin Immunol 2001;108(1):S45–53.
9. Soni A. Allergic rhinitis: trends in use and expenditures, 2000 and 2005; Statistical brief #204. Bethesda (MD): Agency for Healthcare Research and Quality; 2008.
10. Halpern MT, Schmier JK, Richner R, et al. Allergic rhinitis: a potential cause of increased asthma medication use, costs, and morbidity. J Asthma 2004;41(1): 117–26.

11. Thomas M, Kocevar VS, Zhang Q, et al. Asthma-related health care resource use among asthmatic children with and without concomitant allergic rhinitis. Pediatrics 2005;115(1):129–34.

12. Guilbert TW, Morgan WJ, Zeiger RS, et al. Long-term inhaled corticosteroids in preschool children at high risk for asthma. N Engl J Med 2006;354(19):1985–97.

13. Leger D, Annesi-Maesano I, Carat F, et al. Allergic rhinitis and its consequences on quality of sleep: an unexplored area. Arch Intern Med 2006;166(16):1744–8.

14. Stewart MG. Identification and management of undiagnosed and undertreated allergic rhinitis in adults and children. Clin Exp Allergy 2008;38(5):751–60.

15. Cox L, Atwater S. Allergen immunotherapy for allergic rhinitis and asthma. Drug Benefit Trends 2008;20:1–6.

16. Gold MR, Siegel JE, Russell LB, et al. Cost-Effectiveness in Health and Medicine. New York (NY): Oxford University Press; 1996.

17. Cox L, Nelson H, Lockey R, et al. Allergen immunotherapy: a practice parameter third update. J Allergy Clin Immunol 2011;127(Suppl 1):S1–55.

18. Sullivan SD, Weiss KB. Health economics of asthma and rhinitis. II. Assessing the value of interventions. J Allergy Clin Immunol 2001;107(2):203–10.

19. Reed SD, Lee TA, McCrory DC. The economic burden of allergic rhinitis: a critical evaluation of the literature. Pharmacoeconomics 2004;22(6):345–61.

20. Ariano R, Berto P, Tracci D, et al. Pharmacoeconomics of allergen immunotherapy compared with symptomatic drug treatment in patients with allergic rhinitis and asthma. Allergy Asthma Proc 2006;27(2):159–63.

21. Berto P, Bassi M, Incorvaia C, et al. Cost effectiveness of sublingual immunotherapy in children with allergic rhinitis and asthma. Eur Ann Allergy Clin Immunol 2005;37(8):303–8.

22. Berto P, Passalacqua G, Crimi N, et al. Economic evaluation of sublingual immunotherapy vs symptomatic treatment in adults with pollen-induced respiratory allergy: the Sublingual Immunotherapy Pollen Allergy Italy (SPAI) study. Ann Allergy Asthma Immunol 2006;97(5):615–21.

23. Petersen KD, Gyrd-Hansen D, Dahl R. Health-economic analyses of subcutaneous specific immunotherapy for grass pollen and mite allergy. Allergol Immunopathol (Madr) 2005;33(6):296–302.

24. Schadlich PK, Brecht JG. Economic evaluation of specific immunotherapy versus symptomatic treatment of allergic rhinitis in Germany. Pharmacoeconomics 2000;17(1):37–52.

25. Bachert C, Vestenbaek U, Christensen J, et al. Cost-effectiveness of grass allergen tablet (GRAZAX(R)) for the prevention of seasonal grass pollen induced rhinoconjunctivitis—a Northern European perspective. Clin Exp Allergy 2007;37(5):772–9.

26. Keiding H, Jorgensen KP. A cost-effectiveness analysis of immunotherapy with SQ allergen extract for patients with seasonal allergic rhinoconjunctivitis in selected European countries. Curr Med Res Opin 2007;23(5):1113–20.

27. Buchner K, Siepe M. Nutzen der Hyposensibilierung unter wirtschaftlichen Aspekten. Allergo J 1995;4:156–63 [in German].

28. Omnes LF, Bousquet J, Scheinmann P, et al. Pharmacoeconomic assessment of specific immunotherapy versus current symptomatic treatment for allergic rhinitis and asthma in France. Eur Ann Allergy Clin Immunol 2007;39(5):148–56.

29. Hankin CS, Cox L, Lang D, et al. Allergy immunotherapy among Medicaid-enrolled children with allergic rhinitis: patterns of care, resource use, and costs. J Allergy Clin Immunol 2008;121(1):227–32.

30. Hankin CS, Cox L, Lang D, et al. Allergen immunotherapy and health care cost benefits for children with allergic rhinitis: a large-scale, retrospective, matched cohort study. Ann Allergy Asthma Immunol 2010;104:79–85.

31. Hankin CS, Cox L, Wang Z, et al. Does allergen-specific immunotherapy provide cost benefits for children and adults with allergic rhinitis? Results from large-scale retrospective analyses jointly funded by AAAAI and ACAAI. Oral presentation to be presented at the 2011 Annual Conference of the American Academy of Allergy, Asthma and Immunology. San Francisco (CA), March 18–22, 2011.

32. Le Pen C, Rumeau-Pichen C, Lillin H. L'impact de l'immunothérapie specifique sur le couts directs de la maladie allergique: une etude pragmatique. Rev Franc Allergol Immunol Clin 1997;37:11–4 [in French].

33. Donahue JG, Greineder DK, Connor-Lacke L, et al. Utilization and cost of immunotherapy for allergic asthma and rhinitis. Ann Allergy Asthma Immunol 1999; 82(4):339–47.

34. Bernstein JA. Pharmacoeconomic considerations for allergen immunotherapy. In: Lockey RF, Bukantz SC, editors. Allergens and allergen immunotherapy. New York: Marcel Dekker, Inc; 1999. p. 445–53.

35. Available at: http://www.measuringworth.com/index.php. Accessed February 15, 2011.

36. Bureau of Labor Statistics. Consumer Price Index. Available at: http://data.bls. gov/cgi-bin/surveymost?cu. Accessed February 15, 2011.

37. Lower T, Henry J, Mandik L, et al. Compliance with allergen immunotherapy. Ann Allergy 1993;70(6):480–2.

38. Cohn JR, Pizzi A. Determinants of patient compliance with allergen immunotherapy. J Allergy Clin Immunol 1993;91(3):734–7.

39. Tinkelman D, Smith F, Cole WQ 3rd, et al. Compliance with an allergen immunotherapy regime. Ann Allergy Asthma Immunol 1995;74(3):241–6.

40. More DR, Hagan LL. Factors affecting compliance with allergen immunotherapy at a military medical center. Ann Allergy Asthma Immunol 2002;88(4):391–4.

41. Frew AJ, Powell RJ, Corrigan CJ, et al. Efficacy and safety of specific immunotherapy with SQ allergen extract in treatment-resistant seasonal allergic rhinoconjunctivitis. J Allergy Clin Immunol 2006;117(2):319–25.

42. National Institute for Clinical Excellence. Guide to the methods of technology appraisal. London: NICE; 2004.

43. Sheldon TA. Problems of using modelling in the econonomic evaluation of health care. Health Econ 1996;5:1–11.

44. Sculpher MJ, Claxton K, Drummond M, et al. Whither trial-based economic evaluation for health care decision making? Health Econ 2006;15(7):677–87.

45. Law AW, Reed SD, Sundy JS, et al. Direct costs of allergic rhinitis in the United States: estimates from the 1996 Medical Expenditure Panel Survey. J Allergy Clin Immunol 2003;111(2):296–300.

46. Cox L, Cohn JR. Duration of allergen immunotherapy in respiratory allergy: when is enough, enough? Ann Allergy Asthma Immunol 2007;98:416–26.

47. Hankin CS, Lockey RF. Patient characteristics associated with allergen immunotherapy initiation and adherence. J Allergy Clin Immunol 2011;127:46–8.

Future Forms of Immunotherapy and Immunomodulators in Allergic Disease

Tran-Hoai T. Nguyen, MD, Jeffrey R. Stokes, MD,
Thomas B. Casale, MD*

KEYWORDS

- Immunotherapy • Immunomodulator • Cytokine
- Allergic rhinitis • Asthma

Novel agents for treating allergic diseases are being developed based on our expanding knowledge of innate and adaptive responses of the immune system at the molecular level. Immunomodulators are agents that cause a decrease in the pathologic immune response, rather than necessarily a return to an immunologically naive, or unresponsive state. Allergen-specific subcutaneous immunotherapy (IT) is the only form of immunomodulator that has been shown to induce immune tolerance, that is, long-lasting therapeutic effects that persist after discontinuation of therapy. It may also prevent further progression to multiple aeroallergen sensitization. However, with the benefits of IT come rare but real risks of severe adverse reactions, including anaphylaxis and death. Several immunomodulators are being developed that may improve the immunogenicity of IT without increasing its allergenicity, thereby improving its risk/benefit profile and it is to be hoped improving quality of life (QOL) and reducing the burden of disease (**Fig. 1**).

This review discusses future forms of IT, specifically toll-like receptor (TLR) agonists as adjuvants, but also other immunomodulators of allergic disease, including cytokine blockers (oral, parenteral, subcutaneous, and inhaled), transcription factor inhibitors, synthesis inhibitors, anti-IgE monoclonal antibodies (mAbs), receptor antagonists, and

Disclosures of potential conflicts of interest: T.T. Nguyen has nothing to disclose; J.R. Stokes has received speaker's honoraria from the Advancing Respiratory Care Network subset of the Respiratory Allergic Disease Foundation and has received research support from Novartis, Genentech, Stallergenes, and Schering-Plough; T.B. Casale is on the Stallergenes advisory board, has received research support from Novartis, Genentech, Stallergenes, and Schering-Plough, and is Executive Vice President of the American Academy of Allergy, Asthma & Immunology.
Department of Medicine, Division of Allergy and Immunology, Creighton University School of Medicine, 601 North 30th Street, Suite 3M100, Omaha, NE 68131, USA
* Corresponding author.
E-mail address: thomascasale@creighton.edu

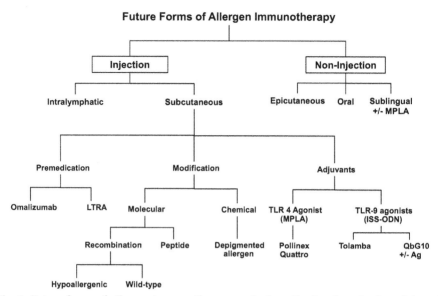

Fig. 1. Future forms of allergen immunotherapy under investigation in animal models and/ or clinical trials. Toll-like receptor (TLR) agonists, particularly TLR-4 and TLR-9, are discussed in this article, whereas the other forms are addressed elsewhere in this issue. MPLA, mono-phosphoryl lipid A; QbG10, Q β protein G10; LTRA, leukotriene receptor antagonist.

other receptor modulators (**Fig. 2**). Rationale and preclinical in vitro and animal study data are reviewed for each agent but the focus is on presenting human clinical trial results on safety, tolerability, and efficacy that determine the risk/benefit profiles and likelihood of further development and usefulness in human allergic diseases.

Other promising forms of IT, including sublingual, peptide, recombinant, epicutaneous, and intralymphatic IT, and use of adjuvants other than TLRs are discussed in other sections with these respective themes (see **Fig. 1**).

TLRS

TLRs are cell surface or intracellular receptors that recognize pathogen-associated molecular patterns commonly conserved in bacteria, viruses, and some fungi. Binding of these TLRs activates antigen-presenting cells (APCs), such as macrophages and dendritic cells, to commence both innate and adaptive immune responses. Agents directed against TLRs may skew the cytokine balance from Th2 toward Th1, thereby affecting allergic diseases. Eleven TLRs have been identified in humans, and agonists for 4 TLRs (TLR-1, TLR-4, TLR-8, and TLR-9) have been studied in clinical trials for allergic diseases. Of these, ligands for TLR-4 and TLR-9 have been most studied and are the focus of the following discussion.

TLR-9 Agonists (Immunostimulatory Oligodeoxynucleotides)

TLR-9 (CD289) recognizes unmethylated CpG DNA motifs from bacteria that are engulfed by endosomes that are either exposed after proteolytic degradation or produced de novo if these pathogens persist intracellularly. In vertebrates, CpG sequences are often silenced by methylation. In humans, plasmacytoid dendritic cells (pDCs) and B cells express the highest concentrations of TLR-9. On TLR-9 activation,

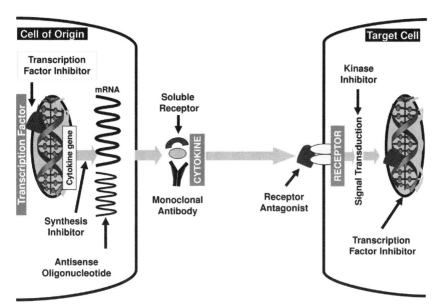

Fig. 2. Strategies to inhibit inflammatory pathways. Overview of different targets and mechanisms of action studied in inhibition of inflammatory pathways using drugs covered in this article. (*Adapted from* Casale TB, Stokes J. Immunomodulation for allergic respiratory disorders. J Allergy Clin Immunol 2008;121(2):294; with permission.)

pDCs produce interferon α (IFN-α), leading to secondary activation of neutrophils, monocytes, and natural killer T cells, whereas B cells produce interleukin 6 (IL-6) and IL-10 and induce B-cell differentiation into plasma cells and trigger IgG isotype switching and antibody production.[1] TLR-9 agonists act by these mechanisms to activate both innate and adaptive immune responses.

There are 3 known classes of immunostimulatory CpG oligodeoxynucleotides (ISS-ODNs): A, B, and C, which differ in length, motif, and which immune responses each elicits; A and B have been studied as adjuvants in allergen IT, and B and C in infectious diseases and malignancy.

Tolamba (Dynavax Technologies, Berkeley, CA, USA) is a B-type ISS-ODN, ISS-1018, covalently linked to the major ragweed allergen, *Amb a 1*. A phase 2 clinical trial was conducted in 25 adult patients with seasonal ragweed allergic rhinitis who were treated with 6 weekly subcutaneous injections of Tolamba or placebo before the ragweed season and then monitored for 2 ragweed seasons. Patients receiving Tolamba reported better QOL and rhinitis symptoms than the placebo group and had suppression of seasonal increases in *Amb a 1*-specific IgE, which persisted over both ragweed seasons.[2] A subsequent study reported reduction in IL-4 and IFN-γ mRNA-positive cells and also eosinophils from nasal biopsies in Tolamba-treated patients, but did not reproduce significant reductions in nasal symptoms.[3] Questions about efficacy continued after the interim analysis of a large, multicenter phase 2 clinical trial, the Dynavax Allergic Rhinitis Tolamba Trial (DARTT), failed to meet its primary end point (difference in total nasal symptom score), possibly because symptom scores were too low in both study groups even during the ragweed season to detect a treatment effect.[4] Further development of Tolamba has been placed on hold.

An inhaled form of ISS-1018 has been studied in atopic asthmatic patients.[5] Although treatment significantly increased IFN-γ and IFN-γ-inducing genes, it did not attenuate early-phase or late-phase asthmatic responses to allergen challenge nor were there significant reductions in sputum eosinophils or Th2-related gene expression.

A-type ISS-ODNs, with and without conjugation to allergen, have also been studied in allergen IT. A-type ISS-ODNs are more potent inducers of IFN-γ than B-type ISS-ODNs but their unstable phosphodiester backbones made them less clinically useful until they were stabilized by association to viruslike particles such as the bacteriophage Qβ coat protein. A single-center, open-label phase 1/2a study of 20 patients with perennial rhinitis with house dust mite (HDM) allergy reported that subcutaneous allergen IT of HDM extract conjugated to an A-type ISS-ODN (G10) and contained in Qβ protein (Qb) over a 10-week period was well tolerated and still reduced symptoms and skin test responses at least 38 weeks after treatment completion.[6] In a more recent phase 2 study, CYT003-QbG10 (Cytos Biotechnology, Zurich, Switzerland) was used without allergen in 80 patients with mild to moderate perennial allergic rhinoconjunctivitis to HDM and/or cat allergens. Patients received 6 weekly subcutaneous injections of CYT003-QbG10 or placebo; after 8 weeks the treatment group had significantly improved total rhinoconjunctivitis symptom scores, and median allergen tolerance on nasal allergen provocation improved 100-fold.[7]

In another phase 2 trial, 63 persistent allergic asthmatic patients on inhaled corticosteroids (ICS) received either 7 weekly subcutaneous injections of CYT003-QbG10 or placebo, and were monitored over a 12-week period. During the run-in period, all patients were stabilized on an ICS, beclomethasone, and then 4 weeks into the study, the ICS was reduced by 50%, and if possible, reduced to zero in another 4 weeks. From weeks 6 to 12, the treatment group had significantly better combined symptom and medication scores than placebo, and at 12 weeks, had stable forced expiratory volume after 1 second (FEV_1) compared with placebo. A subgroup analysis of patients who were able to come off ICS after week 8 suggests that CYT003-QbG10 may be as effective as an ICS in asthma.[8]

TLR-4 Agonists

TLR-4 (CD284) is expressed on the cell surface and, with the adaptor molecule CD14, binds lipopolysaccharide (LPS) found on gram-negative bacteria leading to proinflammatory Th1 responses. Monophosphoryl lipid A (MPLA) is derived from the active component of LPS of *Salmonella minnesota* R595. It has been used as an adjuvant in the anthrax vaccine used by the US Armed Forces and has been investigated in allergen rhinitis and allergen IT.

CRX-675, an intranasal formulation of MPLA, was administered in patients with ragweed allergic rhinitis at varying doses (2, 20, 100, and 200 μg) 24 hours before ragweed intranasal challenge. It was tolerated well, but there was no inhibition of nasal allergen challenge responses compared with placebo; however, improvement in nasal symptom scores was observed at the 100-μg dose.[9]

Pollinex Quattro (Allergy Therapeutics, West Sussex, UK) is an allergy vaccine that contains pollen extract (available with grass, tree, parietaria, or ragweed) that is chemically modified by glutaraldehyde and adsorbed onto an L-tyrosine depot with an MPLA adjuvant. It has been used in Europe and Canada as a preseasonal ultrashort-course IT consisting of 4 weekly subcutaneous injections. A large multicenter phase 3 study of G301 (Pollinex Quattro-Grass) that enrolled 1028 patients to receive ultrashort-course IT or placebo for 4 weeks reported significant improvement in symptom plus medication scores during the peak (12%) and entire pollen season (13%) and improved QOL scores over placebo. Active treatment was well tolerated. A prospective study of 34 patients with seasonal grass pollen allergic rhinitis was conducted with Pollinex Quattro-G given over 2 seasons.[10] Specific grass IgG and IgG4 levels increased slightly the first season but only significantly after the second season along with an increase in FoxP3+ regulatory T cells, suggesting that at least 2 seasonal IT courses are needed to establish tolerance. A controlled field study of 29 *Parietaria* seasonal allergic patients who underwent MPLA-adjuvanted IT compared with 28 who refused, showed persistent improvement in rhinoconjunctivitis and asthma symptoms, although no effect on lung function, after 3 years of IT and 5 years after discontinuation in the treated group.[11] Although Pollinex Quattro appeared to be well tolerated and effective in adults and children,[12] clinical trials in the United States were halted because of a reported serious adverse event of transverse myelitis in 1 patient. A recent study has reported the potential of using MPLA to augment the clinical and biologic responses to sublingual IT (SLIT) in grass allergic patients.[13]

CYTOKINE BLOCKERS

Th2 cytokines, particularly IL-4, IL-5, and IL-13, play essential roles in allergic diseases and have been targeted by immunomodulators such as mAbs directed against the cytokines themselves or their receptors. Other unique blocking strategies have been studied in phase 1 and 2 clinical trials. Therapies directed against other cytokines including IL-2, IL-9, and tumor necrosis factor α (TNF-α) have also been investigated for their roles in treating allergic diseases. Cytokine-blocking therapies must be evaluated carefully, because redundancy of effector mechanisms may render single cytokine-directed therapy ineffective, yet inhibition of pleotropic cytokines may lead to undesired or unexpected side effects and risks that outweigh benefits in patients.

ORAL SYNTHESIS INHIBITORS

Two oral inhibitors of cytokine synthesis have undergone human clinical trials. Suplatast tosilate (IPD-1151T, Taiho Pharmaceutical, Tokyo, Japan) is an oral dimethylsulfonium compound that selectively inhibits Th2 type cytokine production and is taken 3 times daily but is available only in Japan. In murine models of asthma, suplatast reduced levels of IL-4, IL-5, IL-13, eotaxin-1, and transforming growth factor β (TGF-β) in bronchoalveolar lavage fluid and inhibited airway remodeling.[14] Pretreatment with suplatast in rats and mice significantly suppressed allergen-induced nasal symptoms, mucus secretion, and nasal eosinophilia and blunted the increase in mRNA expression of histamine H_1 receptors and IL-4.[15,16]

In human asthmatic patients, suplatast inhibited monocyte-derived dendritic cells in vitro from stimulating CD4+ T cells to produce IL-5 and IFN-γ.[17] Suplatast administered during the first 6 months of IT in adults with perennial allergic rhinitis to HDM significantly decreased serum IL-4 and specific IgE compared with placebo and perhaps may improve efficacy and or tolerability to IT.[18] Moderate to severe asthmatic patients who received suplatast reported significantly better FEV_1, peak expiratory flow, and asthma symptom scores than placebo when their stable dose of ICS was reduced by half. Suplatast may be effective in mild asthmatic patients who do not respond to leukotriene receptor antagonist monotherapy.[19,20] Suplatast has also been shown to improve lung eosinophilia and airway hyperresponsiveness (AHR).[21–23] Topical suplatast formulations inhibited expression of IL-4 and IL-5 in skin of a mouse model of atopic dermatitis, and may be effective as an adjunctive, sparing agent to topical calcineurin inhibitors in humans.[24,25]

A phase 1 clinical trial with AVP-13,358, a novel, orally available 2-(substituted phenyl)benzimidazole derivative (Avanir Pharmaceuticals, Aliso Viejo, CA, USA) reported safety and tolerability at all tested doses in 54 healthy volunteers and was able to suppress antigen-stimulated IL-4 and IL-5 responses, but is not in development.

SOLUBLE RECEPTOR/MAB THERAPIES
Chemokine Receptor CCR3 and Common β Chain Antagonist

CCR3 is the chemokine receptor for eotaxin-3 and is involved in eosinophil trafficking. GM-CSF, IL-3, and IL-5 are critical to eosinophil development in the bone marrow. TPI-ASM8 (Pharmaxis, Frenchs Forest, Australia) is a nebulized drug containing 2 modified phosphorothioate antisense oligonucleotides: one targeting CCR3, the other targeting the common β chain of the receptors for GM-CSF, IL-3, and IL-5. In mild asthmatic patients, TPI-ASM8 attenuated allergen-induced increases in mRNA of the common β chain and CCR3 and also significantly reduced the early asthmatic response and sputum eosinophilia.[26] A subsequent study reported dose-response relationships for these effects, significant attenuation of the late asthmatic response, and tolerability at all tested doses.[27] In an asthmatic rat model, TPI-ASM8 added to nebulized budesonide showed a synergistic, dose-dependent reduction of eosinophil recruitment induced by allergen challenge and decreased bronchoalveolar lavage fluid levels of monocyte chemoattractant protein 1 and IL-13, suggesting that TPI-ASM8 may be an effective adjunctive treatment in asthma.[28] A phase 2 3-way crossover study of TPI-ASM8 in mild asthmatic patients started in late 2010.[29]

Anti-IL-5 mAb

IL-5 is critical to the differentiation and maturation of eosinophils in the bone marrow and their subsequent egress to the circulation, and may be important in the pathogenesis of several allergic disorders, including certain asthma phenotypes, eosinophilic esophagitis, and hypereosinophilic syndrome. There are currently 2 anti-IL-5 mAbs in active development for allergic diseases: mepolizumab and reslizumab. Initial data from animal models had been promising, but clinical trials thus far have only been able to show decreases in eosinophilia with significant concurrent improvements in clinical outcomes only in subsets of patients.

Mepolizumab

Mepolizumab (Bosatria, GlaxoSmithKline, Vienna, Austria) is a recombinant humanized anti-IL-5 mAb that has been studied in asthma, atopic dermatitis, and eosinophilic esophagitis. Two single intravenous infusions of mepolizumab 750 mg given 1 week apart were studied in patients with moderate to severe atopic dermatitis and resulted in significant decreases in peripheral blood eosinophilia but not clinically significant changes in symptoms.[30] In eosinophilic esophagitis, mepolizumab showed improved mean esophageal eosinophilia histologically and decreased TGF-β1 expression, but resulted in limited improvement in clinical symptoms.[31] In asthma, several initial clinical trials failed to show clinical outcome improvement despite reduction in sputum and blood eosinophilia. However, a recent clinical trial of 1 year's duration reported effectiveness of mepolizumab in reducing blood and sputum eosinophilia in patients with refractory eosinophilic asthma, and also in clinical parameters, namely exacerbations and asthma QOL scores.[32] Another trial also reported improved FEV_1, asthma control, and reductions in sputum and serum eosinophils in asthmatic patients with persistent sputum eosinophilia despite prednisone treatment, over a 5-month treatment period and up to 8 weeks after the last infusion.[33]

Reslizumab

Reslizumab (Cinquil [SCH55700] Ception Therapeutics Inc, Frazer, PA, USA) is a humanized IgG2 anti-IL-5 mAb that has been shown to block pulmonary eosinophilia induced by antigen challenge in monkeys and AHR and pulmonary eosinophilia in allergic guinea pigs.[34] A phase 2 clinical trial of patients with eosinophilic asthma receiving monthly intravenous reslizumab for 4 months was recently completed, but no results have been reported yet. Reslizumab has been granted orphan drug status by the US Food and Drug Administration (FDA) for treatment of pediatric eosinophilic esophagitis, and a phase 2/3 clinical trial was completed in early 2010.[35]

Anti-IL-5Rα mAb

Benralizumab (MEDI-563, Medimmune LLC, Gaithersburg, MD, USA) is a humanized anti-IL-5 receptor α (anti-IL-5Rα) IgG1 mAb that induces apoptosis of eosinophils and basophils by antibody-dependent cell-mediated cytotoxicity.[36] A phase 1 trial of intravenous benralizumab reported acceptable safety and tolerability, and phase 2 trials in asthma are under way.[36,37]

Anti-IL-9 mAb

IL-9 is implicated in asthma because it increases numbers of mast cells and Th2 lymphocytes in the lung, and leads to increased airway inflammation, AHR, and mucus production. Expression of IL-9 and its receptor are also higher in asthmatic airways, and the chromosomal region 5q31–33, where the IL-9 gene is located, has been linked to asthma in gene association studies. Murine models of asthma also show that IL-9 induces airway eosinophilia and IgE production.[38,39] MEDI-528 (Medimmune LLC) is a humanized IgG1 anti-IL-9 mAb currently undergoing a phase 2b clinical study in uncontrolled adult asthmatic patients receiving either subcutaneous MEDI-528 or placebo biweekly for 24 weeks.[40] A recent pilot study reported that MEDI-528 may improve exercise-induced bronchospasm by reducing the maximum mean decrease in FEV_1 after exercise.[41]

IL-4 Antagonists

IL-4 induces immunoglobulin isotype switching to IgE and promotes differentiation of naive T lymphocytes to the Th2 lineage, leading to subsequent production of IL-4, IL-5, and IL-13. Altrakincept is a nebulized, soluble recombinant human IL-4 receptor (Amgen, Thousand Oaks, CA, USA) that binds IL-4 without mediating cellular activation because it only is the extracellular component. Although an initial study showed some promise, a subsequent study was not so favorable and this molecule is no longer under development for asthma.[42]

Clinical trials of pascolizumab (SB 240,683), a fully humanized anti-IL-4 mAb, and a similar mAb made by PDL, had disappointing results and neither is being developed further. Targeting IL-4 alone may be ineffective because of redundant mechanisms shared with other cytokines, particularly IL-13.

Anti-IL-13 mAbs

Blockade of IL-13 may be an important strategy in treatment of allergic diseases, particularly asthma, because of the effects of IL-13 on IgE production, AHR, mucus production, and airway remodeling in animal and in vitro models. IL-13 blockade reduced lung inflammation in monkey and mouse studies.[43,44] Several anti-IL-13 mAbs are undergoing or have completed phase 2 human clinical trials.

QAX576 (Novartis, Basel, Switzerland) is an intravenous anti-IL-13 mAb being developed for several allergic diseases. QAX576 failed to attenuate nasal symptoms and eosinophilia in patients undergoing nasal antigen challenge with Timothy grass pollen, though nasal IL-13 was inhibited.[45] A phase 2 study of QAX576 in moderate to severe atopic asthmatic patients was withdrawn because of complexity of the design and lack of enrollment.[46] An ongoing phase 2 trial is evaluating its effectiveness in eosinophilic esophagitis.[47]

Anrukinzumab (IMA-638, Pfizer, New York, NY, USA) is a humanized anti-IL-13 mAb administered subcutaneously. Although an initial phase 2 trial in mild atopic asthmatic patients reported attenuation of postallergen early and late asthmatic responses, a subsequent trial of persistent asthmatic patients did not meet its end point in clinical efficacy and its development was halted in May 2009. However, Pfizer is developing another anti-IL-13 mAb, IMA-026, which completed a phase 2 asthma study in 2009.[48–50]

Tralokinumab (CAT-354, MedImmune, Gaithersburg, MD, USA) is a humanized IgG4 anti-IL-13 mAb in development for asthma. Intraperitoneal injection of CAT-354 attenuated intratracheal human IL-13-induced AHR as well as airway and esophageal eosinophilia in a murine model of asthma.[44] Tolerability and safety have been reported in phase 1 studies.[51] A phase 2 trial has been completed, but the results have not yet been published.[52]

Lebrikizumab (Genentech, South San Francisco, CA, USA) is a humanized anti-IL-13 mAb undergoing phase 2 studies in asthmatic patients inadequately controlled on only ICS.[53]

Anti-IL-4Rα Antagonists

IL-4 has 2 receptors that are heterodimers consisting of 1 IL-4Rα subunit and either the common γ chain (type I) or the IL-13Rα1 subunit (type II). Binding of the type II IL-4 receptor by either IL-4 or IL-13 results in common pleotropic effects, mediated via the JAK/STAT pathway, to promote Th2 cytokine production, eosinophil transmigration into tissue, and immunoglobulin class switching to IgE. Several therapies targeting IL-4Rα in allergic diseases have been evaluated in clinical trials.

AMG 317 (Amgen, Thousand Oaks, CA, USA) is a fully human IgG2 anti-IL-4Rα mAb being developed for allergic asthma. A phase 2 clinical trial of weekly subcutaneous AMG 317 in asthmatic patients did not significantly improve asthma control questionnaire scores, its primary end point, but did decrease frequency of and time to exacerbations in patients in the higher-dose groups. Patients with more asthma symptoms at baseline were more likely to respond to AMG 317, which was also well tolerated.[54]

AIR 645 (Altair Therapeutics, San Diego, CA, USA) is a 2'-O-methoxyethyl 2-MOE Gapmer antisense oligonucleotide that targets the mRNA encoding IL-4Rα. A phase 1 trial of nebulized AIR 645 in healthy volunteers reported low systemic absorption and no severe adverse events.[55] A phase 2a trial in mild allergic asthmatic patients was recently completed although no results have been reported yet.[56]

Pitrakinra (Aerovant [also AER 001 or BAY 16-9996], Aerovance, Berkeley, CA, USA) is a recombinant IL-4 mutein that interferes with binding to IL-4-Rα and is being developed for use in allergic asthma. Two phase 2a studies were conducted in atopic asthmatic patients receiving pitrakinra, either as daily subcutaneous injection or twice-daily nebulization versus placebo.[57] Late-phase asthmatic response after allergen challenge, measured by maximum percentage decrease in FEV_1, was decreased in both treatment groups, although statistically significant only in the nebulized pitrakinra group. There were significantly fewer adverse events related to asthma in the subcutaneous pitrakinra group compared with placebo. A phase 2b trial of an inhaled dry powder formulation is under way. Aerovance is also developing Aeroderm

(AER 003), a PEGylated mutein of pitrakinra, as a weekly or every-2-weeks subcutaneous injection for severe eczema. A phase 2a study of patients with moderate to severe eczema receiving subcutaneous Aeroderm twice daily reported significant reductions in eczema symptom score at 28 days and also fewer exacerbations compared with placebo.[58]

Anti-IL-2R mAb

IL-2 is critical to the proliferation of T and B cells and natural killer cells, and also enhances cytokine synthesis in T cells. Daclizumab (Hoffman-Roche, Basel, Switzerland) is a humanized IgG1 mAb directed against CD25, the α subunit of the high-affinity receptor for IL-2. Although currently approved for prophylaxis of renal allograft rejection, a phase 2 study of intravenous administration in moderate to severe persistent asthmatic patients demonstrated significantly improved lung function, reduced daytime symptoms and rescue inhaler use, and prolonged time to exacerbation.[59] Daclizumab was well tolerated, but caution must be taken in pursuing therapies against a pleotropic cytokine such as IL-2.

TNF-α Inhibitors

TNF-α is a pleotropic proinflammatory cytokine with biologic effects that may be important in refractory asthma, such as increased AHR and expression of chemokines and adhesion molecules that promote neutrophil recruitment. Small clinical trials reported promising results with TNF-α receptor antagonists, such as etanercept, which reduced AHR and improved asthma-related QOL scores.[60] However, larger trials have been disappointing. Golimumab (CNTO 148 or Simponi, Centocor, Horsham, PA, USA), a human anti-TNF-α mAb, was investigated in a phase 2 clinical trial of 309 subjects with severe persistent asthma; however, the study was terminated at its interim 24-week analysis because of an unfavorable risk/benefit profile, in which the treatment group failed to achieve significant improvement in FEV_1 or incidence of severe asthma exacerbations but had significantly more respiratory infections and an increase in malignancy.[61] There are no further efforts to pursue this strategy in allergic disease, although it is approved for several rheumatologic conditions.

TRANSCRIPTION FACTOR INHIBITION

Transcription factors are proteins that bind to promoter regions of genes to stimulate or inhibit transcription, and regulate gene expression for proinflammatory cytokines and mediators; thus, they are attractive targets for immunomodulation of allergic disease.

Spleen Tyrosine Kinase Inhibitors

Spleen tyrosine kinase (Syk) is an intracellular enzyme that is activated after allergen cross-links IgE bound to the high-affinity IgE receptor (FcεRI) on mast cells and transduces signals leading to degranulation of preformed mediators such as histamine, production of proinflammatory cytokines such as TNF-α, and synthesis of lipid mediators including leukotriene C4. R112 (Rigel Pharmaceuticals, South San Francisco, CA, USA) is a potent, rapid-onset, reversible Syk inhibitor discovered by a human mast cell culture screen to inhibit all mast cell reactions mediated by FcεRI cross-linking.[62] A phase 2 study compared an intranasal formulation of R112 administered twice daily with placebo in patients with seasonal allergic rhinitis in a park setting over a 2-day period, reported significant symptomatic improvement with onset of action within 30 to 90 minutes, and was well tolerated.[63] However, in a subsequent phase 2 trial comparing intranasal R112 and beclomethasone with placebo over a 7-day period in patients with allergic rhinitis, R112 did not significantly improve symptoms over placebo, although beclomethasone did.[64] Although the company has halted development of R112, it has brought R343, a dry powder inhaler formulation of R112, to phase 1 clinical trials for asthma.

Peroxisome Proliferator-activated Receptor-γ Agonists

GATA-3 is a key transcription factor of Th2 cytokines IL-4, IL-5, and IL-13, which are all involved in allergic diseases. Downregulation of GATA-3 using a dominant negative mutation in a murine model of asthma attenuated Th2-driven inflammatory responses including mucus production, airway eosinophilia, and cytokine and IgE synthesis.[65] Peroxisome proliferator-activated receptors (PPARs), particularly the α and γ subtypes, can also downregulate GATA-3 with similar effects but also inhibit in vitro chemotaxis of eosinophils and antibody-dependent cellular cytotoxicity.[66] Agonists of PPAR-γ include the thiazolidinediones rosiglitazone and pioglitazone, which are oral hypoglycemic agents used in noninsulin-dependent diabetes mellitus. PPAR-γ agonists can bind to and inhibit other transcription factors such as activated protein (AP)-1, signal transducer and activator of transcription 1(STAT-1), nuclear factor κB (NF-κB), and nuclear factor of activated T cells, and attenuate production of reactive oxygen and nitrogen metabolites and cyclooxygenase 2 expression.[67,68]

Bronchodilatory effects of rosiglitazone were studied in 46 mild to moderate asthmatic patients who were current smokers, and were randomized to either rosiglitazone 8 mg daily or inhaled beclomethasone dipropionate 200 μg daily for 4 weeks. At 28 days, patients on rosiglitazone had significantly improved FEV_1, FEV_{25-75}, and forced vital capacity than those on beclomethasone, but no significant improvement in asthma symptoms.[69] Results of an open-label pilot study were recently reported in 14 steroid-naive asthmatic patients given rosiglitazone 4 mg daily for 8 weeks then 8 mg daily for 4 additional weeks. Trends favored improvement in AHR and FEV_1 in a dose-dependent and time-dependent manner; however, incomplete data likely precluded statistically significant results.[70]

Further studies of rosiglitazone in asthma are unlikely to take place because the modest potential for benefit is largely outweighed by association of increased adverse cardiovascular events in patients already taking this drug, which has prompted its withdrawal in Europe and severe restrictions in the United States for use only in diabetes not controlled on other medications. However, pioglitazone does not have such known associations and is being investigated in 2 phase 2 clinical trials for asthma.[71,72]

NF-κB Inhibition

NF-κB is a key transcription factor that enhances expression of many genes involved in allergic diseases. Corticosteroids can suppress NF-κB activity as part of their anti-inflammatory effects, but long-term use is associated with an undesirable side effect profile. One nonsteroidal strategy involves decoy oligonucleotides that mimic consensus binding sequences of the promoter region normally bound by NF-κB to effectively silence transcription factor activity without altering its expression. Another strategy involves inhibiting the inhibitor of κB kinase (IKK2/IKKβ) to prevent release and activation of NF-κB and its translocation to the cell nucleus.[73] No human trial data have been reported with either strategy in allergic diseases.

STAT-6 Inhibition

The biologic effects of IL-4 and IL-13 are mediated, in part, through STAT-6, leading to upregulation of proinflammatory genes, and thus STAT-6 may be an important target in allergic disease. AS1517499 is a STAT-6 inhibitor found to inhibit allergen-induced bronchial hyperresponsiveness in mice and also blunts upregulation of RhoA, a protein involved in airway smooth-muscle contraction.[74] This may be a novel strategy in treating allergic diseases, especially asthma.

RGS2

G-protein coupled receptor (GPCR) signaling pathways are involved in airway contraction, and GPCR agonists and antagonists are used in treatment of asthma. Some regulators of G-protein signaling (RGS) proteins inhibit GPCRs and may be important in asthma pathophysiology. Nguyen and colleagues found that RGS2 knockout mice have increased AHR, equivalent to allergen sensitization (Nguyen TT and colleagues, unpublished data, 2011).[75] Nguyen and colleagues recently completed a pilot study examining whether RGS2 expression is lower in human asthmatic patients and if the degree of AHR was related to RGS2 expression using isolated monocytes as a model. Fifteen nonatopic, nonasthmatic patients and 15 treatment-naive atopic mild to moderate asthmatic patients underwent methacholine challenge to determine the degree of AHR, measured by PD20. Peripheral blood mononuclear cells (PBMCs) from these patients were analyzed for RGS2 mRNA and protein expression. RGS2 mRNA expression and protein levels were lower in asthmatic patients than normal patients, and amongst asthmatic patients, there is a statistically significant correlation between lower AHR and higher RGS2 mRNA expression.[75] Future studies aimed at elucidating the exact role of RGS2 in asthma could lead to new therapeutic opportunities.

ENDOTHELIAL ADHESION RECEPTOR ANTAGONISTS

Extravasation of leukocytes plays a central role in chronic inflammation seen in asthma. Animal models have shown that P-selectins, E-selectins, and L-selectins, are involved in rolling, adhesion, and transmigration, respectively, of leukocytes from bloodstream into peribronchial tissue. Preventing entry of these cells by blocking key adhesion molecules may inhibit inflammation.

Panselectin Antagonists

Panselectin antagonists including bimosiamose (TBC1269, Revotar Biopharmaceuticals AG, Germany) target all 3 selectins. An inhaled formulation of bimosiamose administered twice daily in 12 mild atopic asthmatic patients showed significant attenuation of late asthmatic reactions after allergen challenge although it had no significant effect on early asthmatic response, AHR, or exhaled nitric oxide.[76] Bimosiamose has also undergone phase 2 studies for chronic obstructive pulmonary disease (COPD) and for psoriasis and atopic dermatitis, as a topical microemulsion cream.[77–79]

Very Late Antigen 4 Antagonists

Very late antigen 4 (VLA-4, $\alpha4\beta1$) is upregulated by IL-4 and IL-13 and binds to vascular cell adhesion molecule 1, which halts rolling of eosinophils and mononuclear cells and promotes their extravasation and accumulation, which may contribute to airway inflammation in asthma. IVL745 (Sanofi-Aventis, Bridgeport, NJ, USA) is a VLA-4 antagonist that was administered via dry powder inhaler to mild to moderate asthmatic patients and resulted in modest reduction in sputum eosinophils but after allergen challenge failed to show a significant difference in early or late asthmatic response, AHR, or peak expiratory flow.[80]

Vascular Adhesion Protein 1 Antagonists

Vascular adhesion protein 1 (VAP-1), also known as human semicarbazide-sensitive amine oxidase, is an inflammation-inducible endothelial cell adhesion molecule that mediates interaction between leukocytes and activated endothelial cells. LJP 1207 (La Jolla Pharmaceuticals, La Jolla, CA, USA) is an oral VAP-1 inhibitor that reduced mortality in murine models of ulcerative colitis and levels of TNF-α and IL-6 in LPS-challenged mice.[81] LJP 1207 also reduced adhesion and infiltration of leukocytes in cerebral vessels in animal models of stroke.[82] VAP-1 is expressed at higher levels in the serum and skin of patients with atopic dermatitis compared with healthy controls, and decreases after treatment of eczema.[83] Although there are no known plans to develop LJP 1207 for allergic diseases, another VAP-1 inhibitor, PXS4159 (Pharmaxis, Frenchs Forest, Australia), is undergoing review for phase 1 trials for asthma treatment.

ANTI-IGE MABS
Omalizumab

Omalizumab (Xolair, Genentech, South San Francisco, CA, USA) is a 95% humanized mAb that forms soluble immune complexes with free IgE at the same site, which normally binds the high-affinity IgE receptor, FcεRI, thus preventing cross-linking of FcεRI and subsequent basophil and mast cell activation. Omalizumab can reduce serum free IgE levels by 99% within 2 hours of administration, and within 2 weeks of therapy initiation can reduce nasal allergen challenge responses.[84] Omalizumab also induces downregulation of FcεRI on basophils, dendritic cells, and monocytes within 7 days.[84,85] In patients with allergic rhinitis, omalizumab reduced serum eosinophils. In asthmatic patients, omalizumab reduced serum, tissue, and sputum eosinophilia and cells positive for FcεRI and CD4+ lymphocytes.[86]

Several studies have established the safety and efficacy of omalizumab, including 3 phase 3 clinical trials conducted on a total of 1405 patients with moderate to severe persistent allergic asthma.[87–89] All 3 studies reported that omalizumab, compared with placebo, reduced asthma exacerbations and had a corticosteroid-sparing effect. Significantly more omalizumab-treated patients were able to reduce their ICS dose by 50% and also to discontinue ICS, compared with placebo (39.1% vs 19.1%, $P<.01$).[87] Omalizumab was also associated with decreased rescue medication use, fewer asthma symptoms, and improved QOL scores. Small but significant improvements in peak expiratory flow and FEV_1 were observed in adolescent and adult patients on omalizumab.[89] Omalizumab-treated patients have also sought significantly fewer unscheduled outpatient visits and emergency department visits, and required fewer hospitalizations.[90]

In light of the supporting evidence for omalizumab, the FDA has approved it for the treatment of moderate to severe persistent allergic asthma in patients 12 years of age and older. Recent expert panel guidelines recommend consideration of omalizumab as adjunctive therapy in perennial allergic asthmatic patients who fail to achieve adequate control on medium-dose ICS in conjunction with a long-acting β agonist. Patients with greater disease severity seem to benefit more from therapeutic addition of omalizumab, although cost-benefit analysis is not favorable for all severe asthmatic patients.[91] Omalizumab is administered subcutaneously every 2 to 4 weeks, with initial dosing determined by 2 factors: pretreatment serum total IgE, up to 700 IU/mL, and patient weight, up to 150 kg.

Patients with seasonal allergic rhinitis also show improvement on omalizumab, including improved rhinitis QOL scores, reduced nasal symptom scores, and antihistamine use, compared with placebo.[92] Omalizumab was effective in attenuating responses to nasal allergen challenge in patients with allergic rhinitis and has been shown to be effective in treating perennial allergic rhinitis in adults and adolescents.[93,94] Several phase 2 trials are under way investigating the effects of omalizumab on chronic rhinosinusitis.[95,96]

Omalizumab as adjunctive therapy to subcutaneous IT in children allergic to birch tree and grass was shown to reduce seasonal allergic rhinitis symptoms, rescue medication use, and symptom load.[97] Omalizumab has also been shown to reduce systemic reactions from and improve tolerability to traditional and accelerated schedules of subcutaneous IT.[98,99] This use of omalizumab as premedication for IT is discussed elsewhere in this issue.

Omalizumab is also being investigated as a novel immunomodulator in several other allergic disorders in which IgE may play a key role in pathophysiology, including eosinophilic esophagitis, allergic bronchopulmonary aspergillosis, hyper-IgE syndrome, idiopathic anaphylaxis, and peanut allergy.[100–105] There have been few case reports of omalizumab used with varying success in atopic dermatitis and chronic urticaria, which also has an ongoing phase 2 trial.[106–108]

Omalizumab is generally well tolerated, with the most common adverse events noted as local reactions at the injection site. There was a higher rate of malignancy in omalizumab-treated patients reported during initial clinical trials compared with controls, but causal association is unclear and is being closely monitored during post-marketing surveillance, including the phase 4 prospective observational cohort study, Xolair to Evaluate Effectiveness and Long-Term Safety in Patients With Moderate to Severe Asthma (EXCELS). The EXCELS study has also identified the potential association between omalizumab and cardiovascular events, but final conclusions await adjudication of events in relationship to patient characteristics. In 2007, the FDA ordered a black-box warning to be placed on omalizumab because of possible association with increased risk of anaphylaxis. A review of data from approximately 57,000 patients treated with omalizumab has indicated that anaphylaxis can occur at any dose and there can be delayed onset of symptoms beyond 2 hours and also a protracted course, with signs and symptoms lasting many hours.[109] Mechanisms of omalizumab-associated anaphylaxis and predisposing risk factors have yet to be elucidated. Current recommendations are to observe patients for 2 hours after each of their first 3 injections, and then for 30 minutes after each subsequent injection, which would have captured 75% of anaphylactic reactions that were reviewed by the Joint Task Force of the American Academy of Allergy, Asthma & Immunology and American College of Allergy, Asthma and Immunology.[110] There may also be an association with Churg-Strauss syndrome and omalizumab, although causation is questionable because this effect may result from reduction of oral steroids that unmasks the underlying disease.[111]

Genentech, which manufactures and markets omalizumab under the trade name Xolair, is also developing a phase 1 trial in asthma for anti-M1 prime, a humanized mAb that binds to the M1 prime segment of membrane IgE and targets B lymphocytes before they produce IgE, rather than neutralizing existing IgE.

CD23

CD23 is the low-affinity receptor for IgE (FcεRII) and its expression on monocytes, alveolar macrophages, and B lymphocytes is increased in allergic patients. In vitro studies have shown that cross-linking CD23 downregulates IgE synthesis. Lumiliximab (IDEC-152, Biogen Idec Pharmaceuticals, Westin, MA, USA) is a primatized, IgG1, anti-CD23 mAb that was studied in PBMCs of atopic patients and shown to reduce allergen-induced PBMC proliferation and levels of proinflammatory cytokines such as IL-1β, IL-5, and TNF-α.[112] Anti-CD23 mAb has not been shown to be effective for allergic rhinitis or asthma despite a significant effect on IgE levels, albeit much less than omalizumab.[113,114] No additional clinical trials have been planned for lumiliximab in allergic diseases, but it has been investigated for chronic lymphocytic leukemia.

OTHER IMMUNOMODULATORS
OX40L mAbs

OX40L is expressed on APCs such as macrophages, dendritic cells, and endothelial cells, and also B and T lymphocytes. In the absence of IL-12, dendritic cells activated by thymic stromal lymphopoietin upregulate OX40L, which binds to OX40, and leads to Th2 cell differentiation and expansion of Th2 memory cells.[115] OX40L-deficient transgenic mice had attenuated asthmatic responses to allergen challenge compared with wild-type, and administration of an OX40L antibody to wild-type mice during sensitization also prevented asthmatic responses.[116] R0498991 (Hoffman-Roche Pharmaceuticals, Basel, Switzerland) is a humanized anti-OX40L mAb. Phase 2 trials of RO4989991 are under way to assess safety of a subcutaneous formulation in patients with allergic rhinitis and efficacy of an intravenous formulation to attenuate allergen-induced responses in asthmatic patients.[117,118]

Chemoattractant Receptor-homologous Molecule Expressed on Th2 Lymphocytes Antagonists

Prostaglandin D_2 (PGD$_2$) is a potent prostanoid released on mast cell activation linking early-phase and late-phase allergen responses. Chemoattractant receptor-homologous molecule expressed on Th2 lymphocytes (CRTh2) is the biologically relevant GPCR for PGD$_2$ and its metabolites, as is the D prostanoid receptor, DP1.[119] Several CRTh2 antagonists are in active development and have completed or are undergoing clinical trials.

OC000459 (Oxagen Ltd, Oxfordshire, UK), an oral CRTH2 antagonist, was evaluated in 132 moderate to persistent asthmatic patients randomized to receive OC000459 twice daily or placebo for 28 days. The treatment group had significant improvement in FEV$_1$ (7.4%) compared with placebo, which continued to improve even at the study end point. QOL significantly improved on OC000459 and there was a significant reduction in total serum IgE and trend toward reduced sputum eosinophilia.[120] OC000459 has now completed phase 2 studies in both asthma and allergic rhinitis with enrollment of more than 600 patients and has been well tolerated. In addition, a phase 2 proof-of-concept clinical trial for use in eosinophilic esophagitis is under way.[121] AMG 853 (Amgen Pharmaceuticals, Thousand Oaks, CA, USA) is an oral CRTH2 and DP1 antagonist that was tolerated well in a phase 1 study and is currently being evaluated in a phase 2 study in patients with inadequately controlled asthma.[122] ACT-129,968 (Actelion Pharmaceuticals, South San Francisco, CA, USA) is another oral CRTH2 antagonist scheduled to undergo phase 2 clinical trials in both asthma and allergic rhinitis. In a recently completed 28-day phase 2 study in patients with mild to moderate asthma ACT-129,968 improved AHR by 1 to 1.5 doubling doses, FEV$_1$ by 10% to 14%, and asthma QOF questionnaire scores by 0.7 and decreased in sputum eosinophils and IgE.

ARRY-005 (Array BioPharma, Boulder, CO, USA) is an oral CRTh2 antagonist shown to dose-dependently inhibit early-phase and late-phase responses in a murine model of allergic rhinitis and improve clinical scores and inhibit scratching behavior in a murine model of atopic dermatitis. ARRY-006, another candidate CRTh2 antagonist developed by Array BioPharma, inhibited airway hyperreactivity and cellular infiltration in bronchoal-veolar lavage fluid after allergen challenge in ovalbumin-sensitized BALB/c mice.[123]

Phosphodiesterase 4 Inhibitors

Phosphodiesterase (PDE) is a major cyclic adenosine monophosphate metabolizing enzyme, and 1 type, PDE-4, is upregulated in inflammatory cells in asthma and COPD. Theophylline, a nonselective PDE inhibitor, has been used to treat asthma or COPD; however, selective PDE inhibitors may provide better benefit-to-risk ratios. PDE4 inhibitors have shown antiinflammatory activity in murine models of asthma and COPD.

Roflumilast (Daxas, Forest Laboratories, New York, NY, USA) is an oral once-daily PDE4 inhibitor currently approved in Europe for COPD, but has been evaluated for both asthma and allergic rhinitis. A phase 2/3 clinical trial of roflumilast was conducted in asthmatic patients over a 12-week period and showed significant improvement in FEV_1 amongst all tested doses.[124] Roflumilast, given for 9 days in atopic patients, improved nasal airflow and subjective obstruction scores compared with placebo on intranasal allergen provocation.[125] In mild atopic asthmatic patients, roflumilast atten-uated both early and late asthmatic reactions to allergen challenge.[126] Roflumilast, compared with inhaled beclomethasone dipropionate, was similar in improving FEV_1 and asthma symptoms and in reducing medication use in a study of 499 asthmatic patients over a 12-week period.[127] Promising results of phase 3 trials in which roflumi-last was added to patients with COPD already treated with salmeterol or tiotropium included significant mean improvement in baseline FEV_1, (0.49 L, 0.8 L, respectively) and health-related QOL scores over a 24-week period.[128] However, this same study reported increased incidence of suicide and suicide attempts and malignancy in the

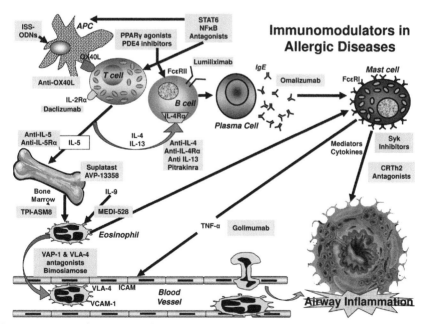

Fig. 3. Summary of immunomodulators in allergic diseases discussed in this article and their sites of action. (*Adapted from* Casale TB, Stokes J. Immunomodulation for allergic respiratory disorders. J Allergy Clin Immunol 2008;121(2):290; with permission.)

treatment group, prompting an FDA panel to vote against its use for COPD in the United States, and likely precluding use in asthma and other allergic diseases.

An inhaled PDE4 inhibitor, GSK256066 (GlaxoSmithKline, Vienna, Austria) given over a 7-day period to 24 steroid-naive atopic asthmatic patients was shown to attenuate early-phase and late-phase allergic responses to allergen challenge compared with placebo.[129] An intranasal formulation of GSK256066 has been evaluated in 2 crossover clinical trials, comparing it with fluticasone propionate and also with azelastine hydrochloride in patients with seasonal allergic rhinitis over an 8-day period, although results have not yet been released.[130,131]

SUMMARY

Many immunomodulators are on the horizon for treatment of allergic diseases, especially TLRs as potent adjuvants for allergen IT or perhaps as allergen-free IT themselves. (**Fig. 3**) Many therapies began with promising outlooks after initial in vitro or animal studies only to fail to translate into successful human clinical trials. Despite these disappointments, many important lessons have been learned about the pleotropic effects of cytokines and the redundancies of their effector mechanisms, and also of the heterogeneity of allergic disease phenotypes. Several immunomodulators that have failed or been abandoned for development in allergic diseases live on in active clinical trials or have been approved for diseases common to other disciplines, including pulmonology, rheumatology, oncology, dermatology, and infectious diseases. Clinical studies with immunomodulators have helped define asthma pathogenesis. The goals for new immunomodulator therapies are to provide better therapeutic options by decreasing symptoms and improving QOL, preventing and favorably altering disease course, and having a good risk/benefit ratio with a cost-effective profile.

REFERENCES

1. Krieg AM. Therapeutic potential of toll-like receptor 9 activation. Nat Rev Drug Discov 2006;5(6):471–84.
2. Creticos PS, Schroeder JT, Hamilton RG, et al. Immunotherapy with a ragweed-toll-like receptor 9 agonist vaccine for allergic rhinitis. N Engl J Med 2006; 355(14):1445–55.
3. Tulic MK, Fiset PO, Christodoulopoulos P, et al. Amb a 1-immunostimulatory oligodeoxynucleotide conjugate immunotherapy decreases the nasal inflammatory response. J Allergy Clin Immunol 2004;113(2):235–41.
4. Bernstein D, Segall N, Nayak A, et al. Safety and efficacy of the novel vaccine Tolamba in ragweed allergic adults, a dose finding study. J Allergy Clin Immunol 2007;119(Suppl):S78–9.
5. Gauvreau GM, Hessel EM, Boulet L, et al. Immunostimulatory sequences regulate interferon-inducible genes but not allergic airway responses. Am J Respir Crit Care Med 2006;174(1):15–20.
6. Senti G, Johansen P, Haug S, et al. Use of A-type CpG oligodeoxynucleotides as an adjuvant in allergen-specific immunotherapy in humans: a phase I/IIa clinical trial. Clin Exp Allergy 2009;39(4):562–70.
7. Blaziene A, Leisyte P, Sitkauskine B, et al. CYT003-QbG10, a novel allergen-independent immunotherapy, shown to be safe and efficacious in placebo-controlled phase II study. Ann Allergy Asthma Immunol 2009;102:A19.
8. Placebo-controlled phase II study shows CYT003-QbG10 is safe and efficacious for the treatment of allergic asthma. 2010. Available at: http://www.cytos.com/userfiles/file/Cytos_Press_E_100521.pdf. Accessed May 10, 2010.

9. Casale TB, Kessler J, Romero FA. Safety of the intranasal toll-like receptor 4 agonist CRX-675 in allergic rhinitis. Ann Allergy Asthma Immunol 2006;97(4): 454–6.

10. Rosewich M, Schulze J, Eickmeier O, et al. Tolerance induction after specific immunotherapy with pollen allergoids adjuvanted by monophosphoryl lipid A in children. Clin Exp Immunol 2010;160(3):403–10.

11. Musarra A, Bignardi D, Troise C, et al. Long-lasting effect of a monophosphoryl lipid-adjuvanted immunotherapy to parietaria. A controlled field study. Eur Ann Allergy Clin Immunol 2010;42(3):115–9.

12. Rosewich M. Ultra-short course immunotherapy in children and adolescents during a 3-yrs post-marketing surveillance study. Pediatr Allergy Immunol 2010;21(1 Pt 2):e185–9.

13. Pfaar O, Barth C, Jaschke C, et al. Sublingual allergen-specific immunotherapy adjuvanted with monophosphoryl lipid A: a phase I/IIa study. Int Arch Allergy Immunol 2010;154(4):336–44.

14. Tanaka A, Watanabe Y, Ohta S, et al. Suplatast tosilate, a potent anti-allergic agent, inhibits a remodeling in a mouse model of bronchial asthma. Am J Respir Crit Care Med 2010;181:A5678 1_MeetingAbstracts.

15. Shimizu S, Hattori R, Majima Y, et al. Th2 cytokine inhibitor suplatast tosilate inhibits antigen-induced mucus hypersecretion in the nasal epithelium of sensitized rats. Ann Otol Rhinol Laryngol 2009;118(1):67–72.

16. Shahriar M, Mizuguchi H, Maeyama K, et al. Suplatast tosilate inhibits histamine signaling by direct and indirect down-regulation of histamine H1 receptor gene expression through suppression of histidine decarboxylase and IL-4 gene transcriptions. J Immunol 2009;183(3):2133–41.

17. Tanaka A, Minoguchi K, Samson KT, et al. Inhibitory effects of suplatast tosilate on the differentiation and function of monocyte-derived dendritic cells from patients with asthma. Clin Exp Allergy 2007;37(7):1083–9.

18. Washio Y, Ohashi Y, Tanaka A, et al. Suplatast tosilate affects the initial increase in specific IgE and interleukin-4 during immunotherapy for perennial allergic rhinitis. Acta Otolaryngol Suppl 1998;538:126–32.

19. Tamaoki J, Kondo M, Sakai N, et al. Effect of suplatast tosilate, a Th2 cytokine inhibitor, on steroid-dependent asthma: a double-blind randomised study. Lancet 2000;356(9226):273–8.

20. Wada M, Nagata S, Kudo T, et al. Effect of suplatast tosilate on antileukotriene non-responders with mild-to-moderate persistent asthma. Allergol Int 2009; 58(3):389–93.

21. Hoshino M, Fujita Y, Saji J, et al. Effect of suplatast tosilate on goblet cell metaplasia in patients with asthma. Allergy 2005;60(11):1394–400.

22. Sano Y, Suzuki N, Yamada H, et al. Effects of suplatast tosilate on allergic eosinophilic airway inflammation in patients with mild asthma. J Allergy Clin Immunol 2003;111(5):958–66.

23. Yoshida M, Aizawa H, Inoue H, et al. Effect of suplatast tosilate on airway hyperresponsiveness and inflammation in asthma patients. J Asthma 2002;39(6): 545–52.

24. Miyachi Y, Katayama I, Furue M. Suplatast/tacrolimus combination therapy for refractory facial erythema in adult patients with atopic dermatitis: a meta-analysis study. Allergol Int 2007;56(3):269–75.

25. Murakami T, Yamanaka K, Tokime K, et al. Topical suplatast tosilate (IPD) ameliorates Th2 cytokine-mediated dermatitis in caspase-1 transgenic mice by down-regulating interleukin-4 and interleukin-5. Br J Dermatol 2006;155(1):27–32.

26. Gauvreau GM, Boulet LP, Cockcroft DW, et al. Antisense therapy against CCR3 and the common beta chain attenuates allergen-induced eosinophilic responses. Am J Respir Crit Care Med 2008;177(9):952–8.

27. Gauvreau G, Pageau R, Seguin R, et al. Efficacy of increasing doses of TPI ASM8 on allergen inhalation challenges in asthmatics. Am J Respir Crit Care Med 2010;181:A5669.

28. Fortin M, Moktefi K, Court M, et al. TPI ASM8, an inhaled antisense oligonucleotide drug candidate targeting CCR3 and the common beta chain of IL-3, IL-5 and GM-CSF receptors, potentiates the anti-inflammatory activity of an inhaled corticosteroid in a rat model of asthma. Am J Respir Crit Care Med 2010;181:A5694.

29. Efficacy of TPI ASM8 during a 14-day allergen challenge. 2010. Available at: clinicaltrials.gov/ct2/show/NCT01158898. Accessed July 6, 2010.

30. Oldhoff JM, Darsow U, Werfel T, et al. Anti-IL-5 recombinant humanized monoclonal antibody (mepolizumab) for the treatment of atopic dermatitis. Allergy 2005;60(5):693–6.

31. Straumann A, Conus S, Grzonka P, et al. Anti-interleukin-5 antibody treatment (mepolizumab) in active eosinophilic oesophagitis: a randomised, placebo-controlled, double-blind trial. Gut 2010;59(01):21–30.

32. Haldar P, Brightling CE, Hargadon B, et al. Mepolizumab and exacerbations of refractory eosinophilic asthma. N Engl J Med 2009;360(10):973–84.

33. Nair P, Pizzichini MM, Kjarsgaard M, et al. Mepolizumab for prednisone-dependent asthma with sputum eosinophilia. N Engl J Med 2009;360(10):985–93.

34. Walsh GM. Reslizumab, a humanized anti-IL-5 mAb for the treatment of eosinophil-mediated inflammatory conditions. Curr Opin Mol Ther 2009;11(3):329–36.

35. Open-label extension study of reslizumab in pediatric subjects with eosinophilic esophagitis. 2010. Available at: http://clinicaltrials.gov/show/NCT00635089. Accessed May 24, 2010.

36. Kolbeck R, Kozhich A, Koike M, et al. MEDI-563, a humanized anti-IL-5 receptor alpha mAb with enhanced antibody-dependent cell-mediated cytotoxicity function. J Allergy Clin Immunol 2010;125(6):1344–53 e2.

37. Busse WW, Katial R, Gossage D, et al. Safety profile, pharmacokinetics, and biologic activity of MEDI-563, an anti-IL-5 receptor alpha antibody, in a phase I study of subjects with mild asthma. J Allergy Clin Immunol 2010;125(6):1237–44 e2.

38. Temann UA, Ray P, Flavell RA. Pulmonary overexpression of IL-9 induces Th2 cytokine expression, leading to immune pathology. J Clin Invest 2002;109(1):29–39.

39. Levitt RC, McLane MP, MacDonald D, et al. IL-9 pathway in asthma: new therapeutic targets for allergic inflammatory disorders. J Allergy Clin Immunol 1999;103(5 Pt 2):S485–91.

40. A study to evaluate the effectiveness and safety of MEDI-528 in adults. 2010. Available at: clinicaltrials.gov/ct2/show/NCT00968669. Accessed June 24, 2010.

41. Parker J, Brazinsky S, Miller DS, et al. Randomized, double-blind, placebo-controlled, multicenter phase 2A study to evaluate the effect of a humanized interleukin-9 monoclonal antibody (MEDI-528) on exercise-induced bronchospasm. Am J Respir Crit Care Med 2010;181:A5394.

42. Borish LC, Nelson HS, Corren J, et al. Efficacy of soluble IL-4 receptor for the treatment of adults with asthma. J Allergy Clin Immunol 2001;107(6):963–70.

43. Bree A, Schlerman FJ, Wadanoli M, et al. IL-13 blockade reduces lung inflammation after Ascaris suum challenge in cynomolgus monkeys. J Allergy Clin Immunol 2007;119(5):1251–7.

44. Blanchard C, Mishra A, Saito-Akei H, et al. Inhibition of human interleukin-13-induced respiratory and oesophageal inflammation by anti-human-interleukin-13 antibody (CAT-354). Clin Exp Allergy 2005;35(8):1096–103.

45. Kariyawasam HH, Nicholson GC, Tan AJ, et al. Effects of anti–IL–13 (Novartis QAX576) on inflammatory responses following nasal allergen challenge (NAC). Am J Respir Crit Care Med 2009;179:A3642.

46. Efficacy of QAX576 in asthma; 2010. Available at: Clinicaltrials.gov; http://clinicaltrials.gov/ct2/show/NCT01130064?term=QAX576&rank=5. Accessed June 10, 2010.

47. Efficacy and safety of QAX576 in patients with eosinophilic esophagitis. 2010. Available at: http://clinicaltrials.gov/ct2/show/NCT01022970?term=QAX576&rank=4. Accessed September 8, 2010.

48. Study evaluating the effect of IMA-026 on allergen-induced late asthma response in mild asthma. 2009. Available at: clinicaltrials.gov/ct2/show/NCT00725582. Accessed June 1, 2009.

49. Study evaluating the effect of IMA-638 in subjects with persistent asthma. 2009. Available at: clinicaltrials.gov/ct2/show/NCT00425061. Accessed July 6, 2009.

50. Study evaluating the effects of IMA-638 on allergen-induced airway responses in subjects with mild atopic asthma. 2008. Available at: clinicaltrials.gov/ct2/show/NCT00410280. Accessed June 26, 2008.

51. Oh CK, Faggioni R, Jin F, et al. An open-label, single-dose bioavailability study of the pharmacokinetics of CAT-354 after subcutaneous and intravenous administration in healthy males. Br J Clin Pharmacol 2010;69(6):645–55.

52. Study to evaluate the safety and efficacy of CAT-354.2010. Available at: Clinical trials.gov; http://clinicaltrials.gov/ct2/show/NCT00873860. Accessed April 6, 2010.

53. A study of lebrikizumab (MILR1444A) in adult patients with asthma who are inadequately controlled on inhaled corticosteroids (MILLY). 2010. Available at: http://clinicaltrials.gov/ct2/show/NCT00930163. Accessed June 7, 2010.

54. Corren J, Busse W, Meltzer EO, et al. A randomized, controlled, phase 2 study of AMG 317, an IL-4Ralpha antagonist, in patients with asthma. Am J Respir Crit Care Med 2010;181(8):788–96.

55. Hodges MR, Castelloe E, Chen A, et al. Randomized, double-blind, placebo controlled first in human study of inhaled AIR645, an IL–4Ra oligonucleotide, in healthy volunteers. Am J Respir Crit Care Med 2009;179:A3640.

56. Study evaluating the effects of AIR 645 on allergen-induced airway responses in subjects with mild atopic asthma. 2010. Available at: http://clinicaltrials.gov/ct2/show/NCT00941577. Accessed July 21, 2010.

57. Wenzel S, Wilbraham D, Fuller R, et al. Effect of an interleukin-4 variant on late phase asthmatic response to allergen challenge in asthmatic patients: results of two phase 2a studies. Lancet 2007;370(9596):1422–31.

58. Aeroderm. 2010. Available at: http://www.aerovance.com/pipeline/aeroderm/. Accessed November 2, 2010.

59. Busse WW, Israel E, Nelson HS, et al. Daclizumab improves asthma control in patients with moderate to severe persistent asthma: a randomized, controlled trial. Am J Respir Crit Care Med 2008;178(10):1002–8.

60. Berry MA, Hargadon B, Shelley M, et al. Evidence of a role of tumor necrosis factor alpha in refractory asthma. N Engl J Med 2006;354(7):697–708.

61. Wenzel SE, Barnes PJ, Bleecker ER, et al. A randomized, double-blind, placebo-controlled study of tumor necrosis factor-alpha blockade in severe persistent asthma. Am J Respir Crit Care Med 2009;179(7):549–58.

62. Rossi AB, Herlaar E, Braselmann S, et al. Identification of the syk kinase inhibitor R112 by a human mast cell screen. J Allergy Clin Immunol 2006;118(3):749–55.

63. Meltzer EO, Berkowitz RB, Grossbard EB. An intranasal syk-kinase inhibitor (R112) improves the symptoms of seasonal allergic rhinitis in a park environment. J Allergy Clin Immunol 2005;115(4):791–6.

64. Rigel announces disappointing results from phase II study of R112 for the treatment of allergic rhinitis. 2005. Available at: http://www.rigel.com/rigel/pr_1133385395. Accessed December 1, 2005.

65. Zhang DH, Yang L, Cohn L, et al. Inhibition of allergic inflammation in a murine model of asthma by expression of a dominant-negative mutant of GATA-3. Immunity 1999;11(4):473–82.

66. Woerly G, Honda K, Loyens M, et al. Peroxisome proliferator-activated receptors alpha and gamma down-regulate allergic inflammation and eosinophil activation. J Exp Med 2003;198(3):411–21.

67. Belvisi MG, Hele DJ. Peroxisome proliferator-activated receptors as novel targets in lung disease. Chest 2008;134(1):152–7.

68. Denning GM, Stoll LL. Peroxisome proliferator-activated receptors: potential therapeutic targets in lung disease? Pediatr Pulmonol 2006;41(1):23–34.

69. Spears M, Donnelly I, Jolly L, et al. Bronchodilatory effect of the PPAR-gamma agonist rosiglitazone in smokers with asthma. Clin Pharmacol Ther 2009;86(1):49–53.

70. Sandhu MS, Dimov V, Romero T, et al. Effects of rosiglitazone on airway hyperresponsiveness and obstruction in asthma. J Allergy Clin Immunol 2010;125(2):AB66.

71. Pilot study of pioglitazone for the treatment of moderate to severe asthma in obese asthmatics (GLITZ). 2010. Available at: clinicaltrials.gov/ct2/show/NCT00787644. Accessed July 7, 2010.

72. A randomized, placebo-controlled, double-blind pilot study of pioglitazone hydrochloride in severe, refractory asthma. 2010. Available at: clinicaltrials.gov/ct2/show/NCT00994175. Accessed September 17, 2010.

73. Karin M, Yamamoto Y, Wang QM. The IKK NF-kappa B system: a treasure trove for drug development. Nat Rev Drug Discov 2004;3(1):17–26.

74. Chiba Y, Todoroki M, Nishida Y, et al. A novel STAT6 inhibitor AS1517499 ameliorates antigen-induced bronchial hypercontractility in mice. Am J Respir Cell Mol Biol 2009;41(5):516–24.

75. Nguyen TT, Xie Y, Berro AI, et al. Relationship of airway hyperresponsiveness and RGS2 expression in asthma. J Allergy Clin Immunol 2011;127(2):AB55.

76. Beeh KM, Beier J, Meyer M, et al. Bimosiamose, an inhaled small-molecule pan-selectin antagonist, attenuates late asthmatic reactions following allergen challenge in mild asthmatics: a randomized, double-blind, placebo-controlled clinical cross-over-trial. Pulm Pharmacol Ther 2006;19(4):233–41.

77. Study to evaluate safety and efficacy of inhaled bimosiamose for the treatment of patients with moderate to severe chronic obstructive pulmonary disease (COPD). 2010. Available at: clinicaltrials.gov/ct2/show/NCT01108913. Accessed May 20, 2010.

78. Study to evaluate the effect of bimosiamose on ozone induced sputum neutrophilia. 2010. Available at: clinicaltrials.gov/ct2/show/NCT00962481. Accessed January 5, 2010.

79. Safety and efficacy study of bimosiamose cream to treat psoriasis. 2009. Available at: clinicaltrials.gov/ct2/show/NCT00823693. Accessed August 20, 2009.

80. Norris V, Choong L, Tran D, et al. Effect of IVL745, a VLA-4 antagonist, on allergen-induced bronchoconstriction in patients with asthma. J Allergy Clin Immunol 2005;116(4):761–7.

81. Salter-Cid LM, Wang E, O'Rourke AM, et al. Anti-inflammatory effects of inhibiting the amine oxidase activity of semicarbazide-sensitive amine oxidase. J Pharmacol Exp Ther 2005;315(2):553–62.

82. Xu HL, Salter-Cid L, Linnik MD, et al. Vascular adhesion protein-1 plays an important role in postischemic inflammation and neuropathology in diabetic, estrogen-treated ovariectomized female rats subjected to transient forebrain ischemia. J Pharmacol Exp Ther 2006;317(1):19–29.

83. Madej A, Reich A, Orda A, et al. Expression of vascular adhesion protein-1 in atopic eczema. Int Arch Allergy Immunol 2006;139(2):114–21.

84. Lin H, Boesel KM, Griffith DT, et al. Omalizumab rapidly decreases nasal allergic response and FcepsilonRI on basophils. J Allergy Clin Immunol 2004;113(2): 297–302.

85. Prussin C, Griffith DT, Boesel KM, et al. Omalizumab treatment downregulates dendritic cell FcepsilonRI expression. J Allergy Clin Immunol 2003;112(6): 1147–54.

86. van Rensen EL, Evertse CE, van Schadewijk WA, et al. Eosinophils in bronchial mucosa of asthmatics after allergen challenge: effect of anti-IgE treatment. Allergy 2009;64(1):72–80.

87. Busse W, Corren J, Lanier BQ, et al. Omalizumab, anti-IgE recombinant humanized monoclonal antibody, for the treatment of severe allergic asthma. J Allergy Clin Immunol 2001;108(2):184–90.

88. Milgrom H, Berger W, Nayak A, et al. Treatment of childhood asthma with anti-immunoglobulin E antibody (omalizumab). Pediatrics 2001;108(2):E36.

89. Soler M, Matz J, Townley R, et al. The anti-IgE antibody omalizumab reduces exacerbations and steroid requirement in allergic asthmatics. Eur Respir J 2001;18(2):254–61.

90. Corren J, Casale T, Deniz Y, et al. Omalizumab, a recombinant humanized anti-IgE antibody, reduces asthma-related emergency room visits and hospitalizations in patients with allergic asthma. J Allergy Clin Immunol 2003;111(1):87–90.

91. Wu AC, Paltiel AD, Kuntz KM, et al. Cost-effectiveness of omalizumab in adults with severe asthma: results from the asthma policy model. J Allergy Clin Immunol 2007;120(5):1146–52.

92. Casale TB, Condemi J, LaForce C, et al. Effect of omalizumab on symptoms of seasonal allergic rhinitis: a randomized controlled trial. JAMA 2001;286(23): 2956–67.

93. Hanf G, Noga O, O'Connor A, et al. Omalizumab inhibits allergen challenge-induced nasal response. Eur Respir J 2004;23(3):414–8.

94. Chervinsky P, Casale T, Townley R, et al. Omalizumab, an anti-IgE antibody, in the treatment of adults and adolescents with perennial allergic rhinitis. Ann Allergy Asthma Immunol 2003;91(2):160–7.

95. Subcutaneous omalizumab for treatment of chronic rhinosinusitis with nasal polyposis (Xolair CRS). 2010. Available at: clinicaltrials.gov/ct2/show/ NCT01066104. Accessed February 9, 2010.

96. Xolair in patients with chronic sinusitis. 2008. Available at: clinicaltrials.gov/ct2/ show/NCT00117611. Accessed July 16, 2008.

97. Kuehr J, Brauburger J, Zielen S, et al. Efficacy of combination treatment with anti-IgE plus specific immunotherapy in polysensitized children and adolescents with seasonal allergic rhinitis. J Allergy Clin Immunol 2002;109(2): 274–80.

98. Casale TB, Busse WW, Kline JN, et al. Omalizumab pretreatment decreases acute reactions after rush immunotherapy for ragweed-induced seasonal allergic rhinitis. J Allergy Clin Immunol 2006;117(1):134–40.

99. Massanari M, Nelson H, Casale T, et al. Effect of pretreatment with omalizumab on the tolerability of specific immunotherapy in allergic asthma. J Allergy Clin Immunol 2010;125(2):383–9.

100. A pilot study of the treatment of eosinophilic esophagitis with omalizumab. 2010. Available at: clinicaltrials.gov/ct2/show/NCT0012360. Accessed February 2, 2010.

101. Omalizumab to treat hyper-IgE (job's) syndrome. 2010. Available at: clinicaltrials.gov/ct2/show/NCT00260702. Accessed March 20, 2010.

102. A randomized, double-blind, placebo-controlled study of omalizumab for idiopathic anaphylaxis. 2010. Available at: clinicaltrials.gov/ct2/show/ NCT00890162. Accessed October 1, 2010.

103. Identifying responders to Xolair (omalizumab) using eosinophilic esophagitis as a disease model. 2009. Available at: clinicaltrials.gov/ct2/show/NCT01040598. Accessed December 28, 2009.

104. Omalizumab in the treatment of peanut allergy. 2009. Available at: clinicaltrials. gov/ct2/show/NCT00949078. Accessed July 29, 2009.

105. An exploratory study to assess multiple doses of omalizumab in patients with cystic fibrosis complicated by ABPA. 2010. Available at: clinicaltrials.gov/ct2/ show/NCT00787917. Accessed June 24, 2010.

106. Lane JE, Cheyney JM, Lane TN, et al. Treatment of recalcitrant atopic dermatitis with omalizumab. J Am Acad Dermatol 2006;54(1):68–72.

107. Spector SL, Tan RA. Effect of omalizumab on patients with chronic urticaria. Ann Allergy Asthma Immunol 2007;99(2):190–3.

108. A study of Xolair (omalizumab) in patients with chronic idiopathic urticaria (CIU) who remain symptomatic with antihistamine treatment (H1). 2010. Available at: clinicaltrials.gov/ct2/show/NCT00866788. Accessed January 15, 2010.

109. Limb SL, Starke PR, Lee CE, et al. Delayed onset and protracted progression of anaphylaxis after omalizumab administration in patients with asthma. J Allergy Clin Immunol 2007;120(6):1378–81.

110. Cox L, Platts-Mills TA, Finegold I, et al. American Academy of Allergy, Asthma & Immunology/American College of Allergy, Asthma and Immunology Joint Task Force Report on omalizumab-associated anaphylaxis. J Allergy Clin Immunol 2007;120(6):1373–7.

111. Wechsler ME, Wong DA, Miller MK, et al. Churg-Strauss syndrome in patients treated with omalizumab. Chest 2009;136(2):507–18.

112. Poole JA, Meng J, Reff M, et al. Anti-CD23 monoclonal antibody, lumiliximab, inhibited allergen-induced responses in antigen-presenting cells and T cells from atopic subjects. J Allergy Clin Immunol 2005;116(4):780–8.

113. Casale T, Busse W, Lizambri R. Results of a phase II, multiple-dose, randomized trial of an anti-CD23 monoclonal antibody (IDEC-152) in patients with seasonal allergic rhinitis. J Allergy Clin Immunol 2003;111(2):S75.

114. Rosenwasser LJ, Busse WW, Lizambri RG, et al. Allergic asthma and an anti-CD23 mAb (IDEC-152): results of a phase I, single-dose, dose-escalating clinical trial. J Allergy Clin Immunol 2003;112(3):563–70.

115. Wang YH, Liu YJ. OX40-OX40L interactions: a promising therapeutic target for allergic diseases? J Clin Invest 2007;117(12):3655–7.
116. Hoshino A, Tanaka Y, Akiba H, et al. Critical role for OX40 ligand in the development of pathogenic Th2 cells in a murine model of asthma. Eur J Immunol 2003; 33(4):861–9.
117. A study of RO4989991 in patients with allergic rhinitis. 2010. Available at: clinicaltrials.gov/ct2/show/NCT01152619. Accessed September 23, 2010.
118. A study of huMAb OX40L in the prevention of allergen-induced airway obstruction in adults with mild allergic asthma. 2010. Available at: clinicaltrials.gov/ct2/show/NCT00983658. Accessed May 14, 2010.
119. Pettipher R. The roles of the prostaglandin D(2) receptors DP(1) and CRTH2 in promoting allergic responses. Br J Pharmacol 2008;153(Suppl 1):S191–9.
120. Barnes NB, Pavord IP, Chuchalin AC, et al. A randomised, double-blind, placebo-controlled study of the CRTH2 antagonist OC000459 on moderate persistent asthma [abstract 3267]. European Respiratory Society Annual Meeting. Vienna, Austria, September 15, 2009.
121. Proof of concept study of OC000459 in eosinophilic esophagitis. 2010. Available at: clinicaltrials.gov/ct2/show/NCT01056783. Accessed September 1, 2010.
122. AMG 853 phase 2 study in subjects with inadequately controlled asthma. 2010. Available at: clinicaltrials.gov/ct2/show/NCT01018550. Accessed October 7, 2010.
123. Carter LL, Shiraishi Y, Shin Y, et al. Potent and selective CRTh2 antagonists are efficacious in models of asthma, allergic rhinitis and atopic dermatitis. J Allergy Clin Immunol 2010;5(2):AB490.
124. Bateman ED, Izquierdo JL, Harnest U, et al. Efficacy and safety of roflumilast in the treatment of asthma. Ann Allergy Asthma Immunol 2006;96(5):679–86.
125. Schmidt BM, Kusma M, Feuring M, et al. The phosphodiesterase 4 inhibitor roflumilast is effective in the treatment of allergic rhinitis. J Allergy Clin Immunol 2001;108(4):530–6.
126. van Schalkwyk E, Strydom K, Williams Z, et al. Roflumilast, an oral, once-daily phosphodiesterase 4 inhibitor, attenuates allergen-induced asthmatic reactions. J Allergy Clin Immunol 2005;116(2):292–8.
127. Bousquet J, Aubier M, Sastre J, et al. Comparison of roflumilast, an oral anti-inflammatory, with beclomethasone dipropionate in the treatment of persistent asthma. Allergy 2006;61(1):72–8.
128. Fabbri LM, Calverley PM, Izquierdo-Alonso JL, et al. Roflumilast in moderate-to-severe chronic obstructive pulmonary disease treated with longacting bronchodilators: two randomised clinical trials. Lancet 2009;374(9691):695–703.
129. Singh D, Petavy F, Macdonald AJ, et al. The inhaled phosphodiesterase 4 inhibitor GSK256066 reduces allergen challenge responses in asthma. Respir Res 2010;11:26.
130. A phase II study evaluating intranasal GSK256066 and azelastine hydrochloride in subjects with seasonal allergic rhinitis. 2009. Available at: clinicaltrials.gov/ct2/show/NCT00612118. Accessed July 22, 2009.
131. A phase II study evaluating intranasal GSK256066 and fluticasone propionate in subjects with seasonal allergic rhinitis (SAR). 2008. Available at: clinicaltrials.gov/ct2/show/NCT00612820. Accessed October 9, 2008.

Oral Desensitization for Food Hypersensitivity

Michael H. Land, MD*, Edwin H. Kim, MD, A. Wesley Burks, MD

KEYWORDS

- Food allergy • Oral tolerance • Oral immunotherapy
- Sublingual immunotherapy

Food allergies are adverse reactions to foods that have an immunologic basis, as opposed to food intolerance, which does not involve the immune system.[1] The clinical reactions that occur in food allergy may be immunoglobulin E (IgE)–mediated or non–IgE-mediated. Non–IgE-mediated reactions to foods can involve other components of the immune system and are not discussed in this article. Typical IgE-mediated symptoms of a reaction may include hives, swelling, vomiting, abdominal pain, wheezing, dyspnea, and shock. These symptoms occur within a few minutes and up to 2 hours following ingestion of the food. Food-related anaphylaxis is the leading cause of anaphylaxis that is treated in emergency departments in America and Europe, and is estimated to cause as many as 30,000 anaphylactic reactions, 2000 hospital admissions, and 200 deaths per year in the United States alone.[2] In general, food allergies have been increasing, affecting 6% to 8% of children less than 4 years of age, and approximately 4% of Americans more than 10 years of age.[3,4] The prevalence of food allergy is also increasing with time. The true prevalence of food allergy has been difficult to establish because most prevalence studies have focused on the most common foods and studies differ in design and definition of food allergies. It has been estimated by the Centers for Disease Control and Prevention that, in a 10-year period, the prevalence of childhood food allergy increased by 18%, with approximately 3.9% of children currently being affected.[5] Recent guidelines by a National Institute of Allergy and Infectious Diseases (NIAID) expert panel released

This work was supported in part by a training grant from the National Institutes of Health # 5T32–AI007062–32.

Disclosures: Dr Burks has served as a consultant for ActoGeniX NV, Intelliject, McNeil Nutritionals, Novartis, and Schering-Plough and owns stock/stock options in Allertein Therapeutics and Mast Cell Pharmaceuticals. Dr Land and Dr Kim have nothing to disclose.

Division of Pediatric Allergy and Immunology, Duke University Medical Center, Medical Sciences Research Building I, DUMC Box 2644, Durham, NC 27710, USA

* Corresponding author.

E-mail address: m.land@duke.edu

in December 2010 have focused on a best-practice clinical guideline on the diagnosis and management of food allergies.[6]

The most common food allergens in the United States include milk, egg, peanuts, tree nuts, wheat, soy, fish, and shellfish.[6] Among these foods, allergies to peanuts and tree nuts are considered significant because they may be lifelong and reactions can often be severe. It is estimated that only 21% of children with peanut allergy spontaneously outgrow their allergy.[7] Furthermore, clinical reactions in peanut allergic patients are the most common causes of food-related anaphylaxis.[8] In contrast, milk and egg allergies generally resolve in most children with the allergies compared with those with peanut, tree nut, fish, or shellfish allergy. Despite this trend, recent data have shown that milk and egg allergies are becoming more persistent and children may be outgrowing these allergies by adolescence rather than in the first 5 to 6 years of life, as had been previously believed.[9,10]

Although fatal reactions to foods implicated in food allergy are not common,[11] the burden of disease is significant not only to the patients but to the families, schools, and communities of the patients. In a study on quality of life in children with peanut allergy compared with children with insulin-dependent diabetes mellitus, the patients with peanut allergy reported a poorer quality of life.[12] Fear of a potential reaction, such as severe anaphylaxis, and needing to take preventative measures may affect participation in social activities, eating outside the home, and choosing to homeschool children.[13]

Once a patient is given a diagnosis of food allergies, the current standard of care dictates strict avoidance of the food allergen and ensuring availability of rescue medications in the case of a mild or severe reaction. These medications are typically an antihistamine such as diphenhydramine for milder symptoms, and injectable epinephrine for more severe, life-threatening symptoms. A food allergy action plan is recommended for patients and their families to have available as a guide during a suspected reaction.

Aside from avoidance, active disease-modifying therapy for food allergy has been studied in recent years. Traditional subcutaneous immunotherapy, also known as allergy shots, has been studied more than 10 years ago, and this type of therapy was able to induce desensitization. However, because of the high rate of systemic reactions during immunotherapy,[14,15] this type of treatment is not appropriate. Given the safety issues from subcutaneous immunotherapy, oral immunotherapy and sublingual immunotherapy have been more heavily studied and are the focus of this article.

GASTROINTESTINAL IMMUNITY AND ORAL TOLERANCE

The largest immunologic organ in the body is the gastrointestinal (GI) tract, which has continual exposure to the external environment through the large surface area of its epithelial layer. Through this large surface area, a tremendous amount and variety of food proteins come in contact with our immune cells. Rather than mount an immune response against these proteins, the normal reaction of the immune system is not to react to them. This concept is known as tolerance, which refers to active suppression by the immune system of an immune response. A failure to develop oral tolerance or a loss of oral tolerance is hypothesized to be the primary problem in food allergy.[16]

When a food is ingested in a nonallergic person, the food proteins are broken down and digested by gastric acids and digestive enzymes within the lumen of the GI tract. This process decreases the immunogenicity of the proteins. The normal process of digestion may be disrupted and lead to a breakdown in oral tolerance induction.[17] The lining of the GI tract consists of a single layer of epithelium overlying loose connective tissue containing lymphocytes. Food protein antigens are absorbed by several specialized cells including the dendritic cell, microfold cell (M cell), and epithelial cells themselves. These cells may then process and present the food antigens to gut-associated lymphoid tissues (in the case of GI dendritic cells), subepithelial antigen-presenting cells (in the case of M-cells), or to primed T cells (in the case of epithelial cells).[17]

The development of tolerance relies on several important factors, including the form and dose of the antigen, genetics of the host, normal intestinal flora of the host, and age of the host. As mentioned earlier, gastric acidity in addition to GI proteases are important in normal digestion, and a breakdown in this process leads to a change in the form of the antigen. Antigens in the soluble form are more tolerogenic than antigens in particulate form. The solubility of food proteins may be affected by how the foods are prepared. For example, in peanuts, roasting decreases the solubility and enhances binding of peanut-specific IgE.[18]

The dose of food antigen exposure influences how oral tolerance develops. High doses of antigen favor an anergy-driven pathway to tolerance, whereas low doses of antigen promote a suppressive pathway to tolerance via regulatory T cells (T_{Regs}). T_{Regs} are a subset of T lymphocytes that possess the ability to decrease the proliferative activity of other lymphocytes. The pathway to high-dose tolerance involves T cell receptor ligation in the absence of costimulatory signals such as soluble interleukin (IL)-2, or interactions between CD28 on T cells with either CD80 or CD86 on antigen-presenting cells.[17] Low-dose tolerance can be achieved by the action of T_{Regs} and CD8+ T cells through production of cytokines such as IL-10 and transforming growth factor (TGF)$-\beta$. An important clinical model of food allergy occurs in a condition in which T_{Regs} fail to develop, known as immune dysregulation, polyendocrinopathy, enteropathy, X-linked (IPEX). In patients with IPEX, significant food allergies develop along with eczema, endocrinopathy, enteropathy, and immune dysregulation.[19]

The genetics of the host influence the development of tolerance, but the role of genetic factors has not been as clearly understood. In murine models, strain-dependent susceptibility to food allergy has been shown, whereas, in humans, limited studies examining associations between specific human leukocyte antigens (HLA) with food allergies has shown variable results. There is some evidence that, in peanut allergies, specific HLA class II genotypes may be found in a higher frequency of peanut allergic patients compared with controls.[17] This area continues to be investigated. The normal flora of the host also may affect tolerance induction, suggested by some evidence in studies of germ-free versus conventional murine models.

The age of the host is another factor that may be important in the development of tolerance. Early introduction of allergen may be important to prevent the development of food allergies in young children. In some countries where a peanut-based snack is introduced in the diet of young children (such as Israel), the rates of peanut allergies are low compared with other countries with children who are genetically similar (such as Jewish children in the United Kingdom).[20,21] A study investigating the roles of age and timing in the development of allergy is currently underway in the United Kingdom. This study, the Learning Early About Peanut Allergy (LEAP) study, involves children between 4 and 10 months of age who are randomized to either eat peanuts regularly 3 times a week or to avoid peanuts until the age of 3 years. Study completion is anticipated by 2013 (http://www.leapstudy.co.uk).

These normal mechanisms and factors that influence the development of oral tolerance are lost or insufficient in patients with food allergy. Methods to regain or induce tolerance are now being studied. It is important to understand the difference between desensitization and tolerance when reviewing immunotherapy. Desensitization is a state in which effector cells involved in a specific immune response develop reduced reactivity or become nonreactive on increased introduction of an allergen. In a desensitized state, an individual may be nonreactive while regularly receiving the allergen. However, when the regular administration ends, the previous amount of reactivity returns. This condition is not the goal of immunotherapy, which is to reach a state of tolerance, in which the nonreactive state remains present permanently.

ORAL IMMUNOTHERAPY

Oral immunotherapy (OIT) involves the regular administration of small amounts of allergen by the oral route to first rapidly induce desensitization and then, in time, induce tolerance to the allergen. Some reports have considered immunotherapy that is ingested and immunotherapy that is administered sublingually as 2 forms of oral immunotherapy. For the purposes of this article, OIT refers specifically to ingested immunotherapy and sublingual immunotherapy (SLIT) refers to immunotherapy that is administered under the tongue. Patients undergoing OIT generally ingest a mixture of protein powder in a vehicle food such as apple sauce. Patients undergoing SLIT generally receive a small amount of liquid extract under the tongue. Both treatments are typically initiated in a controlled setting where gradually increasing doses of allergen are given up to a targeted dose. Following this, in standard protocols, most dosing is done at home.

Although there have been scattered reports in the literature on the use of OIT for food allergy in the last 100 years, most research on OIT has occurred in the last 25 years, beginning with work by Patriarca and colleagues,[22] who showed the successful treatment of allergies to cow's milk, egg, fish, and fruits with standardized OIT protocols. Bauer and colleagues,[23] in a 1999 case report of a 12-year-old girl with cow's milk allergy, showed that OIT using a rush protocol could also be effective. Further work by Patriarca and colleagues[24,25] showed that clinical desensitization using OIT was accompanied by changes in allergen-specific IgE and immunoglobulin G4 (IgG4) similar to that seen in subcutaneous aeroallergen immunotherapy. Although skepticism in the scientific community remained, these studies suggested that the defect in oral tolerance causing food allergy could potentially be overcome through OIT. This realization, combined with the increase in public awareness of food allergies, prompted the significant increase in OIT research in the past 5 years (**Table 1**).

To broaden the scope of OIT, the next generation of OIT studies shifted the focus of treatment from adults to children and began to investigate the potential of OIT to induce long-term tolerance. In a pilot study of OIT for egg allergy in children, Buchanan and colleagues[26] showed the safety of a 24-month egg OIT protocol involving a modified rush desensitization phase, buildup phase, and maintenance phase. Successful desensitization by the protocol was shown by double-blind, placebo-controlled food challenges (DBPCFC) but no conclusions could be made regarding long-term tolerance. A randomized study of OIT versus an elimination diet for cow's milk allergy and egg allergy by Staden and colleagues[27] focused on the persistence of induced tolerance as measured by DBPCFC 2 months after the discontinuation of therapy. This larger study of 45 children, 25 receiving OIT and 20 on elimination diets, showed similar rates of allergy resolution in the OIT and elimination diet groups marked by significant reductions in allergen-specific IgE. However, partial responders in the OIT group also showed reduced allergen-specific IgE, but to a lesser degree, whereas nonresponders showed no change in allergen-specific IgE. This result suggested immunologic suppression through OIT but its effectiveness in inducing tolerance remained unclear.

Table 1
Results of recent prospective studies of OIT and SLIT for food allergy (excluding individual case reports)

Year	Author	Food Allergen	Type	Age	Blinded	Total Subjects	Completed Treatment	Completed Food Challenge	Immunoglobulin Changes
1984	Patriarca et al[22]	Milk, egg, other	OIT	—	No	19	15/19	14/15	n/a
2003	Patriarca et al[25]	Milk, egg, other	OIT	3–55	No	59	38/59	n/a	↓IgE, ↑IgG4
2004	Meglio[40]	Milk	OIT	5–10	No	21	15/21	n/a	IgE no change
2007	Buchanan et al[26]	Egg	OIT	1–7	No	7	7/7	4/7	↓IgE, ↑IgG
2007	Staden et al[27]	Milk, egg	OIT	1–13	No	25	16/25	9/16	↓IgE
2008	Longo et al[28]	Milk	OIT	5–17	No	30	27/30	11/27	↓IgE
2008	Skripak et al[29]	Milk	OIT	6–17	Yes	13	12/13	4/12	IgE no change, ↑IgG4
2008	Staden[41]	Milk	OIT	3–14	No	9	6/9	n/a	n/a
2008	Zapatero[42]	Milk	OIT	4–8	No	18	16/18	n/a	IgE no change
2009	Clark et al[30]	Peanut	OIT	9–13	No	4	4/4	3/4	n/a
2009	Jones et al[31]	Peanut	OIT	1–16	No	39	29/39	27/29	↓IgE, ↑IgG4
2010	Blumchen et al[32]	Peanut	OIT	3–14	No	23	14/23	3/14	IgE no change, ↑IgG4
2010	Itoh[43]	Egg	OIT	7–12	No	6	6/6	3/6	↓IgE, ↑IgG4
2005	Enrique et al[36]	Hazelnut	SLIT	19–53	Yes	12	11/12	5/11	IgE no change, ↑IgG4
2011	Kim et al[37]	Peanut	SLIT	1–11	Yes	11	11/11	0	↓IgE, ↑IgG4

Abbreviation: n/a, not applicable.

A common criticism of the early OIT studies was the exclusion of patients with more severe disease. To address this concern, Longo and colleagues[28] conducted a study of OIT on children with severe reactions to cow's milk that typically resulted in exclusion from other OIT studies. In addition, the children were older than 5 years and had higher levels of cow's milk–specific IgE (>85 kU/L), making it less likely that they would naturally outgrow the allergy. Significantly more children in the OIT group became fully tolerant to cow's milk after the treatment compared with those on an elimination diet (36% vs 0%). In addition, 16 of the 19 children who did not become fully tolerant were able to ingest larger amounts of cow's milk than the control group, potentially offering limited protection from accidental ingestions. Side effects in this highly allergic group were common, although only 3 of the 30 subjects on OIT were unable to complete the protocol. Nevertheless, the study showed that OIT could be efficacious in almost any type of allergic patient.

Studies to this point compared OIT with the standard of care, namely a strict elimination diet. To more rigorously define the effects of OIT, Skripak and colleagues,[29] in children with cow's milk allergy, conducted the first double-blind, placebo-controlled study of OIT. In agreement with prior studies, children receiving cow's milk OIT had a significant increase in reaction threshold compared with placebo with an average cumulative dose of 5140 mg versus 40 mg respectively. More importantly, children receiving cow's milk OIT reported symptoms with 45% of daily doses compared with only 11% reported by the placebo group. Although most of the reported symptoms with cow's milk OIT were local, about 10% of all OIT doses required treatment with an antihistamine and 0.2% (4 doses) required epinephrine compared with 1% and 0% for each treatment respectively in the placebo group. Although the question of whether the reported symptoms truly required treatment can be raised, most of the dosing in current OIT protocols is performed at home without medical supervision.

Before 2009, the literature on the treatment of peanut allergy, widely considered a more severe and lifelong food allergy, consisted mostly of sporadic case reports with larger OIT studies focused on cow's milk and egg allergy. Since then, the results of 3 independent prospective studies of OIT for peanut allergy have been published. Clark and colleagues[30] described 4 children with challenge-documented peanut allergy who underwent peanut OIT. Side effects with dosing were common but mild in nature despite the presumed increased severity of peanut allergy. All 4 children had significant increases in threshold, each ingesting between 10 and 12 peanuts (2.38–2.76 g peanut protein) during the postintervention challenge. A subsequent study by Jones and colleagues[31] not only verified these challenge results in a larger cohort but also was the first attempt to broadly define the immune changes underlying the effects of OIT. The protocol was successful because 27 of 29 children safely completed a 16-peanut (3900 mg peanut protein) food challenge. The remaining 2 children discontinued the challenge after 9 peanuts (2100 mg), considerably more than is expected in a typical accidental ingestion.

More importantly, Jones and colleagues[31] showed that underlying the clinical benefits of OIT were changes to multiple aspects of the immune system leading to the dampened allergic response. These changes included not only the decrease in allergen-specific IgE and increase in allergen-specific IgG4 previously shown by others (see **Table 1**) but also a suppression of mast cells and basophils, an increase in T_{Regs}, and a change in cytokine profile. In addition, microarray analysis of patient T cells revealed changes in several apoptotic pathways, although the significance of this result is still unknown. Blumchen and colleagues,[32] in 14 children with challenge-documented peanut allergy, showed that the increase in threshold shown by Clark and colleagues[30] and Jones and colleagues[31] persisted despite the discontinuation of OIT for 2 weeks before challenge. Cytokine analysis showed a clear decrease in T_H2 cytokines without a concomitant increase in T_H1 cytokines, arguing against OIT causing a shift in the T_H1/T_H2 skewing. Instead, a decrease in IL-2 was noted, possibly suggesting clonal anergy or deletion as a possible mechanism of OIT.

SLIT

Amidst the increased attention on OIT, some small studies investigated the potential for immunotherapy by the sublingual route. Like OIT, SLIT involves the regular administration of a small amount of allergen, but, in contrast with OIT, in which the allergen is ingested, with SLIT, it is held under the tongue for an arbitrary amount of time, typically 1 to 5 minutes. The hypothesized advantages of this modality include direct absorbance into the blood stream with avoidance of first-pass metabolism in the liver, and access to immune cells in the oral cavity such as Langerhans cells, which are believed to be protolerogenic in nature.[33] More practically, the advantages of SLIT include its ease of administration and potential for improved safety owing to the smaller doses that are allowed by its efficient absorption. One early case report by Mempel and colleagues[34] described a 29-year-old woman with 3 episodes of anaphylactic shock after kiwi ingestion who underwent successful SLIT with subsequent maintenance of tolerance for 4 months off therapy.[34,35] Enrique and colleagues[36] conducted the first double-blind, placebo-controlled study of SLIT on 29 adults with hazelnut allergy. Significant increases in threshold were achieved but, with half of the subjects diagnosed with oral allergy syndrome, its direct applicability to type 1 food allergy was not clear. Recently, the results of a double-blind, placebo-controlled study of SLIT in peanut allergic children were published by our group.[37] Children receiving 12 months of peanut SLIT therapy not only showed an increased threshold to peanut ingestion but also changes in the immune response including basophils, mast cells, peanut-specific IgE and IgG4, and cytokines. Similar to the OIT studies, this suggests not only successful desensitization but also the potential for the induction of long-term tolerance.

SAFETY

Because there are no treatments currently available for food allergy, and the risk of accidental exposure remains high, the success of these recent studies on OIT and SLIT has increased the pressure to bring these treatments to market sooner. However, there are several reasons to exercise patience. In a paper by Hofmann and colleagues[38] analyzing the safety of peanut OIT, 93% of children experienced symptoms during the initial dosing day, including 15% who required epinephrine. Subsequent home dosing was safer but 2 subjects required epinephrine for reactions. Although rare, this remains important in that, as stated previously, most doses in current OIT and SLIT protocol are administered at home without medical supervision. In a letter to the editor, Varshney and colleagues[39] described the development of symptoms during OIT with episodes of fever, during exercise, when taken on an empty stomach, and during menses in children who had previously tolerated the eliciting dose. Similar patterns of reactions have also been reported during cow's milk and egg OIT.[27] Continued study to further understand these patterns of reactions and to identify additional triggers is necessary to assure patient safety. Another reason for patience is the variable, but significant, dropout rates with current OIT protocols. The study of peanut OIT by Blumchen and colleagues[32] reported a 35% dropout rate, with children withdrawing because of adverse reactions or poor compliance. Administration of OIT can be difficult with the patient's natural aversion to the food allergen and the likelihood of reactions. With dosing recommended as daily and potentially lifelong, concerns for the efficacy and safety of OIT in noncompliant patients must be addressed. Although the ease of administration and safety profile of SLIT make it an attractive alternative to OIT, the initial change in threshold reported during peanut SLIT, although significant, remains inferior to that of peanut OIT. The clinical significance of this lower reaction threshold remains to be studied as well as the long-term risks and benefits of SLIT.

Overall, immunotherapy in the form of OIT and SLIT for food allergy has advanced significantly in recent years with more progress expected in the near future. With ample evidence of successful desensitization, ongoing studies of OIT have been focusing on blinding to more precisely describe safety and overall efficacy, as well as on immunologic parameters to predict the likelihood of long-term tolerance. OIT is also being studied in conjunction with omalizumab anti-IgE therapy (ClinicalTrials.gov #NCT00932282). Regarding SLIT, an ongoing study through the Consortium of Food Allergy Researchers (CoFAR) has been investigating the use of SLIT in adults with peanut allergy (ClinicalTrials.gov #NCT00580606). Lastly, in contrast with prior studies focused on either OIT or SLIT, investigators at Johns Hopkins University have been studying the use of both OIT and SLIT modalities in tandem for the treatment of cow's milk allergy (ClinicalTrials.gov #NCT00732654) and, more recently, for peanut allergy (ClinicalTrials.gov #NCT01084174).

SUMMARY

Food allergy is an IgE-mediated immediate-type hypersensitivity that is believed to be a result of a breakdown in the normal process of oral tolerance. Although the prevalence of food allergy continues to increase, avoidance remains the standard of care because no disease-modifying treatments are readily available. A large body of evidence has accumulated showing the successful induction of desensitization by OIT. In addition, early evidence indicates successful desensitization by SLIT. Although questions regarding the safety of the treatments and the potential for the development of long-term immunologic tolerance remain, OIT and SLIT offer some hope for the future treatment of food allergy.

ACKNOWLEDGMENTS

Dr Burks has received gifts from the Food Allergy Research Project Fund and received grant funding from the Food Allergy and Anaphylaxis Network, National Institutes of Health, and Wallace Research Foundation.

REFERENCES

1. Sampson HA. Update on food allergy. J Allergy Clin Immunol 2004;113(5): 805–19.
2. Yocum MW, Butterfield JH, Klein JS, et al. Epidemiology of anaphylaxis in Olmsted County: a population-based study. J Allergy Clin Immunol 1999;104(2 Pt 1):452–6.
3. Sampson HA. Food allergy. Part 1: immunopathogenesis and clinical disorders. J Allergy Clin Immunol 1999;103(5 Pt 1):717–28.
4. Sicherer SH, Munoz-Furlong A, Sampson HA. Prevalence of peanut and tree nut allergy in the United States determined by means of a random digit dial telephone survey: a 5-year follow-up study. J Allergy Clin Immunol 2003;112(6): 1203–7.

5. Sicherer SH, Sampson HA. Food allergy. J Allergy Clin Immunol 2010; 125(2 Suppl 2):S116–25.
6. Boyce JA, Assa'ad A, Burks AW, et al. Guidelines for the diagnosis and management of food allergy in the United States: summary of the NIAID-Sponsored Expert Panel Report. J Allergy Clin Immunol 2010;126(6):1105–18.
7. Skolnick HS, Conover-Walker MK, Koerner CB, et al. The natural history of peanut allergy. J Allergy Clin Immunol 2001;107(2):367–74.
8. de Silva IL, Mehr SS, Tey D, et al. Paediatric anaphylaxis: a 5 year retrospective review. Allergy 2008;63(8):1071–6.
9. Skripak JM, Matsui EC, Mudd K, et al. The natural history of IgE-mediated cow's milk allergy. J Allergy Clin Immunol 2007;120(5):1172–7.
10. Savage JH, Matsui EC, Skripak JM, et al. The natural history of egg allergy. J Allergy Clin Immunol 2007;120(6):1413–7.
11. Pumphrey RS, Gowland MH. Further fatal allergic reactions to food in the United Kingdom, 1999-2006. J Allergy Clin Immunol 2007;119(4):1018–9.
12. Avery NJ, King RM, Knight S, et al. Assessment of quality of life in children with peanut allergy. Pediatr Allergy Immunol 2003;14(5):378–82.
13. Cummings AJ, Knibb RC, King RM, et al. The psychosocial impact of food allergy and food hypersensitivity in children, adolescents and their families: a review. Allergy 2010;65(8):933–45.
14. Oppenheimer JJ, Nelson HS, Bock SA, et al. Treatment of peanut allergy with rush immunotherapy. J Allergy Clin Immunol 1992;90(2):256–62.
15. Nelson HS, Lahr J, Rule R, et al. Treatment of anaphylactic sensitivity to peanuts by immunotherapy with injections of aqueous peanut extract. J Allergy Clin Immunol 1997;99(6 Pt 1):744–51.
16. Burks AW, Laubach S, Jones SM. Oral tolerance, food allergy, and immunotherapy: implications for future treatment. J Allergy Clin Immunol 2008;121(6): 1344–50.
17. Chehade M, Mayer L. Oral tolerance and its relation to food hypersensitivities. J Allergy Clin Immunol 2005;115(1):3–12 [quiz: 13].
18. Kopper RA, Odum NJ, Sen M, et al. Peanut protein allergens: the effect of roasting on solubility and allergenicity. Int Arch Allergy Immunol 2005;136(1):16–22.
19. Chatila TA. Role of regulatory T cells in human diseases. J Allergy Clin Immunol 2005;116(5):949–59 [quiz: 960].
20. Levy Y, Broides A, Segal N, et al. Peanut and tree nut allergy in children: role of peanut snacks in Israel? Allergy 2003;58(11):1206–7.
21. Du Toit G, Katz Y, Sasieni P, et al. Early consumption of peanuts in infancy is associated with a low prevalence of peanut allergy. J Allergy Clin Immunol 2008; 122(5):984–91.
22. Patriarca C, Romano A, Venuti A, et al. Oral specific hyposensitization in the management of patients allergic to food. Allergol Immunopathol (Madr) 1984; 12(4):275–81.
23. Bauer A, Ekanayake Mudiyanselage S, Wigger-Alberti W, et al. Oral rush desensitization to milk. Allergy 1999;54(8):894–5.
24. Patriarca G, Buonomo A, Roncallo C, et al. Oral desensitisation in cow milk allergy: immunological findings. Int J Immunopathol Pharmacol 2002;15(1):53–8.
25. Patriarca G, Nucera E, Roncallo C, et al. Oral desensitizing treatment in food allergy: clinical and immunological results. Aliment Pharmacol Ther 2003;17(3): 459–65.
26. Buchanan AD, Green TD, Jones SM, et al. Egg oral immunotherapy in nonanaphylactic children with egg allergy. J Allergy Clin Immunol 2007;119(1):199–205.

27. Staden U, Rolinck-Werninghaus C, Brewe F, et al. Specific oral tolerance induction in food allergy in children: efficacy and clinical patterns of reaction. Allergy 2007;62(11):1261–9.

28. Longo G, Barbi E, Berti I, et al. Specific oral tolerance induction in children with very severe cow's milk-induced reactions. J Allergy Clin Immunol 2008;121(2): 343–7.

29. Skripak JM, Nash SD, Rowley H, et al. A randomized, double-blind, placebo-controlled study of milk oral immunotherapy for cow's milk allergy. J Allergy Clin Immunol 2008;122(6):1154–60.

30. Clark AT, Islam S, King Y, et al. Successful oral tolerance induction in severe peanut allergy. Allergy 2009;64(8):1218–20.

31. Jones SM, Pons L, Roberts JL, et al. Clinical efficacy and immune regulation with peanut oral immunotherapy. J Allergy Clin Immunol 2009;124(2):292–300, e291–7.

32. Blumchen K, Ulbricht H, Staden U, et al. Oral peanut immunotherapy in children with peanut anaphylaxis. J Allergy Clin Immunol 2010;126(1):83–91, e81.

33. Allam JP, Wurtzen PA, Reinartz M, et al. Phl p 5 resorption in human oral mucosa leads to dose-dependent and time-dependent allergen binding by oral mucosal Langerhans cells, attenuates their maturation, and enhances their migratory and TGF-beta1 and IL-10-producing properties. J Allergy Clin Immunol 2010;126(3): 638–45, e631.

34. Mempel M, Rakoski J, Ring J, et al. Severe anaphylaxis to kiwi fruit: Immunologic changes related to successful sublingual allergen immunotherapy. J Allergy Clin Immunol 2003;111(6):1406–9.

35. Kerzl R, Simonowa A, Ring J, et al. Life-threatening anaphylaxis to kiwi fruit: protective sublingual allergen immunotherapy effect persists even after discontinuation. J Allergy Clin Immunol 2007;119(2):507–8.

36. Enrique E, Pineda F, Malek T, et al. Sublingual immunotherapy for hazelnut food allergy: a randomized, double-blind, placebo-controlled study with a standardized hazelnut extract. J Allergy Clin Immunol 2005;116(5):1073–9.

37. Kim EH, Bird JA, Kulis M, et al. Sublingual immunotherapy for peanut allergy: clinical and immunologic evidence of desensitization. J Allergy Clin Immunol 2011; 127(3):640–6.

38. Hofmann AM, Scurlock AM, Jones SM, et al. Safety of a peanut oral immunotherapy protocol in children with peanut allergy. J Allergy Clin Immunol 2009; 124(2):286–91, e281–6.

39. Varshney P, Steele PH, Vickery BP, et al. Adverse reactions during peanut oral immunotherapy home dosing. J Allergy Clin Immunol 2009;124(6):1351–2.

40. Meglio P, Bartone E, Plantamura M, et al. A protocol for oral desensitization in children with IgE-mediated cow's milk allergy. Allergy 2004;59(9):980–7.

41. Staden U, Blumchen K, Blankstein N, et al. Rush oral immunotherapy in children with persistent cow's milk allergy. J Allergy Clin Immunol 2008;122(2):418–9.

42. Zapatero L, Alonso E, Fuentes V, et al. Oral desensitization in children with cow's milk allergy. J Investig Allergol Clin Immunol 2008;18(5):389–96.

43. Itoh N, Itagaki Y, Kurihara K. Rush specific oral tolerance induction in school-age children with severe egg allergy: one year follow up. Allergol Int 2010;59(1): 43–51.

Peptide and Recombinant Immunotherapy

Mark Larché, PhD

KEYWORDS

- Recombinant protein • Peptide • Epitope • T-cell • Regulation
- Blocking Ab

Randomized controlled clinical trials have shown that both subcutaneous allergen immunotherapy (SCIT) and sublingual allergen immunotherapy (SLIT) are clinically efficacious and disease-modifying.[1–6] SCIT has also been shown to be effective for treating allergic asthma,[7] and preventing progression of allergic rhinitis to allergic asthma.[8] However, as a result of the presence of intact B-cell epitopes, the allergenicity of treatment preparations makes treatment cumbersome because of the frequent occurrence of adverse events ranging from local reactions at the site of injection to systemic reactions that may be severe and sometimes life-threatening. Furthermore, the use of poorly defined extracts of allergen has resulted in huge variability in treatment outcomes. This variability has presented a major barrier to progress in this field through the development of molecularly characterized therapeutics that conform to modern pharmaceutical manufacturing standards and comply with regulatory requirements.

Over the past 4 decades, various technologies have been applied in an attempt to address these issues. The advent of recombinant DNA technology has enabled the molecular cloning of virtually all major allergens and has allowed the production of these molecules in recombinant form for use in both diagnosis and treatment in a "component-resolved" fashion. Recent clinical trials of recombinant allergens, described later in this article, have shown levels of efficacy comparable to existing extract-based products. Thus, a new era of allergen immunotherapy with defined products has begun. However, unmodified allergen proteins retain their allergenicity,

The author is funded by the Canada Research Chairs program, the Canadian Institutes for Health Research, AllerGen Network of Centres of Excellence, the Canadian Foundation for Innovation, the Ontario Thoracic Society, Adiga Life Sciences Inc and the McMaster University/GSK endowed Chair in Lung Immunology at St Joseph's Healthcare.

Disclosure. The author is a founder, shareholder and consultant of/to Circassia Ltd., a company developing peptide-based immunotherapy. The author is scientific founder of Adiga Life Sciences Inc, A joint venture between Circassia Ltd and McMaster University.

Department of Medicine, Firestone Institute for Respiratory Health, McMaster University, HSC 4H20, 1200 Main Street West, Hamilton, ON L8N 3Z5, Canada
E-mail address: larche@mcmaster.ca

Immunol Allergy Clin N Am 31 (2011) 377–389
doi:10.1016/j.iac.2011.03.008
0889-8561/11/$ – see front matter © 2011 Published by Elsevier Inc.

making them potentially unsafe for widespread use. Even before the advent of recombinant allergens, a variety of strategies were being developed in an attempt to reduce the allergenicity of immunotherapeutics while maintaining their ability to modify adaptive immune responses. These strategies include modification of protein surfaces with agents such as glutaraldehyde to generate "allergoids," conjugation with synthetic bacterial DNA sequences (eg, CpG motifs), mutations in native allergen amino acid sequences (to create "hypoallergens"), display of allergen fragments on the surface of virus-like particles (VLPs), and the use of multimerized allergen, fragments of allergens (polypeptides), and peptides of various lengths. Ultimately, the future of immunotherapy may lie in a combination of molecularly defined products with reduced allergenicity.

This article focuses on recent advances in the development of recombinant allergens and synthetic peptides for the treatment of allergic diseases.

RECOMBINANT ALLERGENS FOR IMMUNOTHERAPY

Reduction in the allergenicity of allergens has been achieved in a variety of ways through the use of recombinant DNA technology. Individual point mutations at sites contributing to protein folding and conformational epitopes have resulted in molecules that retain many T-cell epitopes while displaying IgE reactivity diminished by several orders of magnitude.[9–18] Alternative approaches include the generation of multiallergen hybrid molecules[19–22]; the restructuring of allergens through shuffling sequence to create a new protein with reduced IgE reactivity but intact T-cell epitopes[23,24]; the deconstruction of whole allergen sequences into polypeptide fragments[25,26]; and the identification of short synthetic peptide sequences representing T-cell epitopes.[27–31] Reassuringly, Mother Nature herself has provided a precedent in the form of the naturally occurring Bet v 1 hypoallergens Bet v 1d, Bet v 1g, and Bet v 1l,[32] which are polymorphic variants of the major birch allergen and display markedly reduced IgE reactivity.

Genes encoding the most common allergens have been cloned and expressed, allowing the production of recombinant proteins that have been used to develop diagnostic tests or IgE reactivity (in vitro) and allergen sensitivity (in vivo).[33,34] Recombinant proteins from aeroallergens have recently begun to be evaluated in the clinical setting. Results from trials of recombinants in patients allergic to grass and birch pollen have been described.

Recombinant Native Allergens

Jutel and colleagues[35] evaluated a mixture of five Timothy grass pollen allergens (Phl p1, Phl p2, Phl p5a, Phl p5b, and Phl p6) in a phase II/III trial. The study was conducted over two pollen seasons after a preseasonal up-dosing regimen followed by a maintenance dose of 40 μg of total protein. Statistically significant improvements in combined symptom and medication scores were observed after 18 months of treatment. Furthermore, significant improvements were observed in a validated rhinitis quality of life questionnaire. The allergen tolerance threshold in conjunctival provocation testing also improved although this outcome failed to achieve statistical significance. Serum allergen-specific IgG antibodies increased approximately 60-fold (IgG1) and 4000-fold (IgG4). IgG1 levels rose immediately and reached a plateau, whereas IgG4 levels increased over the course of the study. No significant changes in allergen-specific IgE concentrations were observed. Hypoallergenic variants of grass pollen allergens are currently under development for future therapy.

Pauli and colleagues[36] conducted a multicentre, randomized, double-blind, placebo-controlled trial that compared the safety and efficacy of recombinant Bet v 1a, purified natural Bet v 1, and standard birch pollen extract (compared with placebo) for immunotherapy of birch pollen–allergic individuals. Treatment was for a 2-year period with the maintenance dose of 15 ug of Bet v 1. All three treatment regimens led to highly significant decreases in daily mean rhinoconjunctivitis scores and daily mean rescue medication scores in both treatment years, despite very variable pollen seasons over the five centers.

Skin sensitivity to allergen in skin prick tests was significantly reduced in all three treatment regimens at follow-up in both years of treatment. Clinical effects were associated with marked increases in Bet v 1–specific IgG1, IgG2, and IgG4. All three treatment modalities had a comparable safety profile, with two patients in each arm experiencing serious adverse events. Most systemic events were not related to treatment, but one systemic anaphylactic reaction occurred in the purified natural Bet v 1 treatment arm. Immediate local reactions were reported in all groups, and delayed local reactions were reported in the three active treatment groups. A large number of local reactions, particularly swelling at the site of injection, were recorded in patients treated with the recombinant allergen. A total of 48 local reactions in 33 patients were recorded compared with 7 reactions to placebo, 10 reactions to nBet v 1, and 15 reactions to birch extract. No explanation for the increased incidence of local swelling reactions could be provided.[36]

Engineered Hypoallergens

Valenta and colleagues[37] provided important insight into this issue through their work with engineered hypoallergenic constructs of the major birch pollen allergen, Bet v 1. A trimeric construct of Bet v 1 and two recombinant fragments of the same molecule[38] were shown to have IgE reactivity that was several orders of magnitude lower than the native allergen. Both the trimer and the fragments induced substantially reduced skin test reactivity in birch allergic subjects.[39] When injected into rabbits, the trimer induced IgG, which blocked the binding of allergen-specific IgE to Bet v 1.[40] Recent analysis suggests that the trimer forms defined high-molecular-weight aggregates that may be responsible for its functionally reduced allergenicity.[41] Furthermore, a nasal provocation study comparing recombinant Bet v 1 with the two Bet v 1 fragments showed that in contrast to the whole allergen, the fragments did not induce an increase in allergen-specific IgE or nasal symptom scores, nor did they induce a decrease in nasal flow determined by anterior acoustic rhinometry.[42]

The two formulations (trimer and fragments) were evaluated in a phase II multicenter clinical trial. Despite difficulties with the birch pollen season (uncharacteristically low pollen counts) in one center, investigators were able to show the induction of immunologic changes consistent with a protective response to vaccination. In particular, they showed the induction of IgG subclasses (IgG1, IgG2, and IgG4; and IgA) specific for Bet v 1, which were capable of blocking basophil activation in functional in vitro assays. Furthermore, serum from subjects treated with trimer and fragments was also able to inhibit CD23-dependent facilitated allergen binding (FAB).[43] This assay assesses the ability of IgG to functionally interfere with the ability of allergen–IgE immune complexes to bind to B cells via CD23. A statistically significant reduction in FAB was observed in trimer-treated subjects, but in the fragment-treated subjects the decrease failed to achieve significance, perhaps because of the small number of subjects analyzed.

In a further study, increases in serum antibody concentrations were reflected in nasal secretions, and Bet v 1–specific IgG4 was significantly associated with reduced nasal sensitivity to Bet v 1 on nasal allergen challenge.[44] Increases in IgG antibodies specific for food allergens and associated with the birch oral allergy syndrome were also observed, likely because of cross-reactivity between allergens.[25,45] Enzyme-linked immunosorbent spot (ELISPOT) analysis of T-cell cytokine responses indicated reductions in the frequency of interleukin (IL)-5– and IL-13–secreting cells, together with the trend for reduced IL-4 and increased IL-12.[46] Furthermore, skin prick test sensitivity to birch was reduced after treatment, indicating an in vivo clinical response that could be associated with clinical efficacy.[46] However, decreases in skin test responses were observed within the fragment and trimer group but not between groups.[47] Similarly statistically significant within-group reductions were observed in nasal provocation responses before and 12 months after treatment. Again, no statistically significant differences were observed between placebo and active treatment.[47] Seasonal increases in specific IgE were significantly reduced.[25]

Based on these studies, it appears that markedly reducing the allergenicity of an allergen preparation need not necessarily reduce the ability to induce functional, allergen-specific blocking antibodies that may contribute to therapeutic efficacy. No significant differences were observed in the primary outcome (symptom and medications scores) in any of the treated groups. A post-hoc analysis of patient well-being on a 10-point visual rating scale also failed to show significant differences between the groups. A significant within-group (before treatment vs after treatment in the same individual) difference in well-being scores was observed in the trimer-treated group but not in the fragment or placebo groups.

Recently, because the two recombinant Bet v 1 fragments (described earlier) have been shown to have reduced allergenicity both in vitro and in vivo (skin prick test in allergic individuals), three recombinant hybrid proteins (Bet v 1-rs 1, Bet v 1-rs 2, and Bet v 1-mosaic) have been engineered from the primary sequence of Bet v 1 through shuffling of blocks of amino acid sequence from the native protein to create restructured Bet v 1 molecules that retain T-cell epitopes but that lack the appropriate three-dimensional structure to cross-link allergen-specific IgE on effector cells. Evaluation of IgE reactivity showed that in contrast to the native allergen, all three restructured proteins failed to bind IgE in nitrocellulose dot blot assays. The restructured proteins also showed markedly reduced ability to activate basophils (although very small numbers of individuals were analyzed), and serum from rabbits immunized with the proteins was capable of inhibiting the binding of IgE from birch-allergic subjects to native Bet v 1.[24] Thus, these novel engineered hypoallergens, which retain T-cell epitope sequences, may prove efficacious for immunotherapy of birch pollen–allergic individuals in future clinical studies.

VLPs

CpG oligodeoxynucleotides (ODN), with a structure stabilized by phosphorothioate bonds (type B CpG ODN), have a prolonged half-life, making them suitable for clinical applications. However type A CpG ODN with phosphodiester backbones induce stronger interferon (IFN)-γ responses, but are rapidly degraded. Kundig and colleagues[48] evaluated a novel delivery system consisting of VLPs derived from the bacteriophage Qβ coat protein and containing type A CpG ODN. The CpG ODN–VLP was used as an adjuvant for house dust mite immunotherapy. Based on early work showing strong immunogenicity of the construct in a murine model, a phase I clinical trial of 24 healthy volunteers was initiated to evaluate the safety and tolerability of the VLP decorated with a Der p 1 peptide known to contain B-cell epitopes. IgG and IgM antibodies directed at both the VLP and Der p 1 increased during the first month after the initial vaccination but did not appear to be boosted by subsequent administrations.

Antibody titres gradually decreased to baseline levels after 18 months. The open-label phase I/IIa clinical study reported reduced skin reactivity and conjunctival sensitivity to house dust mite in allergic subjects. Clinical changes were associated with a progressive increase in specific IgG subclasses, particularly IgG1, IgG2, and IgG4.[49]

B-Cell Epitope Vaccination

Clinically effective immunotherapy with whole allergens is associated with the induction of IgG (and to a lesser extent IgA) specific for the treatment allergen. Although no absolute correlation exists between the amount of allergen-specific IgG induced and clinical efficacy,[50] these "blocking" antibodies are widely accepted to contribute to clinical efficacy. Durham and colleagues showed the functional ability of IgG induced during immunotherapy to block the binding of IgE–allergen immune complexes to IgE Fc receptors.[51,52] Focke and colleagues[53] identified nonanaphylactic surface-exposed peptides from Bet v 1. Skin prick testing of birch pollen–allergic individuals, together with in vitro histamine release assays using basophils from these patients, showed the absence of IgE cross-linking capacity. Peptides were coupled to keyhole limpet haemocyanin (KLH), a protein to which the immune system of humans is usually naive. The resulting vaccine was used in a murine model of birch pollen allergy, and serum from immunized mice was shown to inhibit activation of rat basophil cells primed with the IgE from allergic subjects.

In more recent studies, KLH was substituted with the rhinovirus protein VP1, which was coupled to a peptide from the major grass pollen allergen Phl p1 and expressed in *Escherichia coli*. The recombinant protein did not react with IgE antibodies from grass-allergic patients and was incapable of activating IgE-primed basophils in vitro. Sera from mice and rabbits immunized with the vaccine prevented Phl p1-induced basophil activation. Sera were broadly cross-reactive with other species of grass and, in an interesting twist, IgG antibodies elicited by the vaccine inhibited the infection of cultured human epithelial cells with rhinovirus.[54] The rationale for developing vaccines based on nonallergenic B-cell epitopes is that protective IgG antibodies will be elicited without the activation of IgE-dependent allergic mechanisms. Furthermore, the use of a "carrier" molecule (to provide T-cell help) from a nonallergen molecule should avoid the induction of IgE-Independent, T-cell–dependent, late-phase reactions that have been observed in the lung and skin.[55] However, until clinical studies are performed, whether the induction of allergen-specific IgG antibodies is, in the absence of modification of the T-cell compartment and the induction of regulatory T cells, sufficient to protect from allergen challenge cannot be determined. Furthermore, the fact that activation of allergen-specific memory T cells can result in symptoms of asthma and atopic dermatitis raises the possibility that reactivation of memory T cells to a carrier molecule such as VP1 (either through immunization of a previously infected person or through infection of a previously immunized person) could lead to exacerbations of asthma.

Chimeric Fcγ-Allergen Fusion Proteins

Using a chimeric construct (GE2) of Fcγ joined to Fcε, Saxon and colleagues observed that cross-linking of high-affinity IgE receptors (FcεRI) and low-affinity IgG receptors (FcγRIIb) inhibited mast cell and basophil degranulation.[56,57] GE2 blocked allergen-dependent basophil degranulation in vitro. Furthermore, in human FcεRIα transgenic mice, GE2 inhibited Fel d 1–dependent passive cutaneous anaphylaxis in skin sensitized with human serum from cat-allergic subjects. Rhesus monkeys allergic to dust mites were refractory to allergen skin testing after treatment with GE2.[57]

The investigators went on to exploit this observation through the generation of a fusion protein consisting of Fcγ1 joined to the cat allergen Fel d 1 (GFD).[58] The rationale was that binding of the Fc portion of IgG to FcγRIIb receptors concomitantly with Fel d 1 binding to specific IgE on mast cells and basophils would lead to reduced degranulation and thus allergy symptoms. This chimeric protein was able to inhibit activation of FcϵRIα, and significantly preserve lung function and core body temperature and prevent eosinophil recruitment in a BALB/c murine model of cat allergy.[59] Degranulation of human FcϵRI-transgenic murine mast cells sensitized with human IgE specific for cat allergens was inhibited after in vivo administration of the chimeric protein. Although the construct contained Fel d 1, it did not induce mediator release, suggesting that in this form, Fel d 1 displays reduced allergenicity. Furthermore, in vitro application of the chimeric protein showed a dose-dependent inhibition of IgE-mediated histamine release from the basophils of cat allergic donors and sensitized cord blood–derived mast cells.

Further studies have shown that the chimeric protein, through coaggregation of FcϵRI and FcγRIIb, blocked degranulation and protected against allergen exposure when administered 6 hours before challenge, whereas reductions in lung, systemic, and cutaneous reactivity were apparent 2 weeks after treatment in a murine model of allergy.[60] More recently a human chimeric Fc–Fel d 1 was manufactured, and in the spring of 2011 will be undergoing a phase 0 study in which its allergenicity will be tested against equimolar amounts of Fel d 1 in graded skin testing in cat-allergic subjects, with the prediction that it will show 10-fold or less reactivity (Andrew Saxon, MD, personal communication, 2011).

T-Cell Epitope Vaccination

The first attempt to translate T-cell–directed peptide immunotherapy from murine models[56] into the clinic took the form of a vaccine comprised of two 27 amino acid polypeptides (IPC-1/IPC-2; AllervaxCat) from the major cat allergen Fel d 1. The results of four clinical trials evaluating safety and efficacy have been published to date. Cat-allergic subjects were treated with four subcutaneous injections over a 2-week period to evaluate three dose groups (7.5 μg, 75 μg, and 750 μg per injection).[61] Statistically significant improvements in lung and nasal symptom scores were reported at the highest dose. Treatment was also associated with reduced IL-4 production in peptide-specific T-cell lines derived from pre- and posttreatment blood samples and cultured in vitro.[62] Treatment with AllervaxCat was associated with reduced sensitivity to inhaled allergen challenge in a study of individuals treated with variable doses of vaccine. Improvements in allergen PD_{20} were observed in high- and medium-dose groups, although statistically all improvements occurred within-group rather than compared with placebo.[63]

Some modest efficacy was reported in a multicenter study of a regimen consisting of eight subcutaneous injections of high-dose AllervaxCat (750 μg). Although a significant improvement in pulmonary function was observed 3 weeks after therapy, this was found only in individuals with reduced baseline FEV_1.[64] Previous allergen injection immunotherapy failed in several of the subjects, and thus the study population might be considered somewhat more difficult than usual.

In a fourth study administering 250-μg weekly injections of AllervaxCat, no significant changes in outcomes were observed. Similar to other AllervaxCat studies, treatment was associated with a high incidence of adverse events related to treatment; in this case delayed symptoms of rhinitis, asthma, and pruritus.[65]

In general, adverse events occurred both acutely and up to several hours after subcutaneous injection of the vaccine. In addition to some acute IgE-mediated reactions, which occasionally required epinephrine and may have been related to the size of the peptides, most adverse events were reported in the respiratory tract and consisted of symptoms of asthma with chest tightness and shortness of breath beginning several hours (~3 hours) after dosing. Subsequently, dedicated peptide challenge studies in subjects with asthma identified major histocompatibility complex (MHC)–restricted activation of allergen-specific airway mucosal T cells as being the cause of these manifestations, in the absence of any overt signs of mast cell or basophil activation.[66] Delayed symptoms of asthma (isolated late asthmatic reactions) were reduced with successive doses of peptide, suggesting the induction of immunologic tolerance.

Over the past decade, the authors have followed up those original observations with a series of clinical studies using broader mixtures of shorter peptides from Fel d 1.[28–31,67,68] The peptides selected represent major T-cell epitopes within the protein and are spread throughout its entire sequence. In an uncontrolled, open study, one intradermal injection of a mixture of 12 peptides reduced late-phase skin reactions (LPSRs) to challenge with whole allergen. Concomitant reductions in allergen-specific proliferation and a reduction in both Th1 and Th2 cytokines were also observed.[30] Subsequently a double-blind, placebo-controlled clinical trial of the same peptide vaccine showed significant reductions in both the early-phase skin response (EPSR) and the LPSR to allergen extract challenge. Reductions in allergen-specific proliferative and cytokine responses of peripheral blood mononuclear cells (PBMC) were also observed, together with an increase in IL-10. Based on earlier observations, isolated late asthmatic reactions were expected at the peptide dose administered. However, the occurrence of these reactions was not related to the induction of allergen-specific tolerance.[31] Related mechanistic studies used PBMC isolated from subjects before and after treatment to show that proliferative and cytokine responses were reduced to peptides contained within the vaccine, but also to those that were not, indicating intramolecular tolerance (linked epitope suppression).[69]

The relationship between vaccine dose and the occurrence of isolated late asthmatic reactions was investigated in a open study in which biweekly doses of peptide were administered incrementally starting at 100 ng/mL (each peptide). In this small study, tolerance was achieved in the absence of late asthmatic reactions, suggesting that lower doses of peptide may lead to tolerance in the absence of T-effector cell activation, and further highlighting the distinct nature of the two phenomena (tolerance and isolated late asthmatic reaction).[70] The same study showed a significant reduction in airway hyperreactivity (measured by PC_{20}).[29] In contrast, no change in airway hyperresponsiveness was observed in the double-blind, placebo-controlled study described earlier.[31] However, neither study was adequately powered for this outcome, and further studies in larger groups of asthmatics are awaited to specifically address this issue.

Most recently, a seven-peptide vaccine (Toleromune Cat) has been evaluated in a phase IIa safety and tolerability study.[27] Peptide components were selected in a multistep process involving (1) direct MHC-binding assays using 10 commonly expressed MHC alleles to determine which sequences displayed promiscuous binding to MHC class II, (2) proliferation, (3) cytokine production (IFN-γ, IL-10, IL-13), and (4) histamine release assays to identify peptides with unexpected intrinsic ability to induce basophil activation. The vaccine was administered to 88 cat-allergic subjects either intradermally or subcutaneously to evaluate safety and tolerability. The dose of vaccine providing the greatest inhibition of the LPSR to allergen extract challenge was used as a secondary outcome of efficacy. Cohorts of eight cat-allergic subjects received a single injection of vaccine (n = 6) or placebo (n = 2). The vaccine was safe and well tolerated and the adverse events profile was indistinguishable from placebo. Intradermal delivery resulted in approximately 40% inhibition of the LPSR at a dose of 3 nmol of vaccine, comparable to earlier findings with a prototype vaccine.[30] Phase IIb clinical studies are currently underway to further evaluate the safety and tolerability of a vaccine and to begin to explore clinical efficacy.

Peptides have also been used in small open studies to treat bee venom allergy. The first of these studies identified immunodominant T-cell epitopes of the major bee venom allergen Api m 1[71] and used them to treat five bee venom–allergic subjects who had documented systemic allergic reactions to bee venom. Subjects received incremental doses (cumulative dose, 397.1 µg starting at 100 ng) of an equimolar mixture of peptides at weekly intervals.[72] All subjects tolerated a subcutaneous challenge with 10 µg of the major venom allergen Api m 1 after the last treatment injection, and a live bee sting challenge was subsequently tolerated by three of five subjects. Because of the small numbers of subjects and the unpredictable natural history of bee venom reactions, these results must be interpreted with caution.

In a later study, four immunodominant peptides of Api m 1 were identified using peptide–MHC binding assays to quantify the binding affinities of overlapping synthetic peptides spanning the Api m 1 sequence.[73] These peptides were subsequently evaluated in an open-label, single-blind study of subjects with mild bee venom allergy (no history of systemic reactions after bee sting).[74] The peptide vaccine was well tolerated and no treatment-related adverse events were observed. Treatment was associated with reduced proliferative and cytokine (Th1 and Th2) responses in posttreatment PBMC challenged with allergen. In agreement with findings in studies of cat peptide immunotherapy, IL-10 secretion was significantly upregulated and LPSRs to allergen were significantly reduced.

In the most recently published study, bee venom–allergic subjects were treated with three long synthetic peptides (LSP) encompassing the entire Api m 1 sequence in a RUSH desensitization protocol.[26] An incremental dosing protocol with dose escalation at 30-minute intervals and starting at 100 ng (in common with other venom studies) resulted in a cumulative dose of approximately 250 µg. Subsequently, variable maintenance injections of either 100 or 300 µg were administered at five further time points. Increased T-cell proliferation to the treatment peptides was observed, along with increases in IFN-γ and IL-10 levels, but not Th2 cytokines. Allergen-specific IgG$_4$, but not IgE, levels increased during the study. Peptide-specific IgE was induced during treatment in some subjects. No significant changes in skin reactions to intradermal allergen extract challenge were seen. No severe adverse events were reported, but two subjects experienced redness and itching of the hands.

SUMMARY

Because of the need to standardize allergen immunotherapy coupled with the desire to reduce allergic adverse events during therapy, a transition to recombinant/synthetic hypoallergenic approaches is inevitable in the near future. Mounting evidence supports the notion that effective therapy can be delivered using a limited panel of allergens or even epitopes, weakening the argument that all allergens must be present (eg, in an extract) for optimal efficacy. Moreover, standardized products will allow direct comparisons between studies and, for the first time, immunotherapy studies will be truly blinded (because of the lack of adverse events alerting study subjects and researchers to subject assignment), allowing an accurate assessment of the actual treatment effect that can be achieved with this form of intervention.

REFERENCES

1. Durham SR, Walker SM, Varga EM, et al. Long-term clinical efficacy of grass-pollen immunotherapy. N Engl J Med 1999;341(7):468–75.
2. Bousquet J, Lockey R, Malling HJ, et al. Allergen immunotherapy: therapeutic vaccines for allergic diseases. World Health Organization. American academy of Allergy, Asthma and Immunology. Ann Allergy Asthma Immunol 1998;81(5 Pt 1):401–5.
3. Calderon MA, Casale TB, Togias A, et al. Allergen-specific immunotherapy for respiratory allergies: from meta-analysis to registration and beyond. J Allergy Clin Immunol 2011;127(1):30–8.
4. Dahl R, Kapp A, Colombo G, et al. Sublingual grass allergen tablet immunotherapy provides sustained clinical benefit with progressive immunologic changes over 2 years. J Allergy Clin Immunol 2008;121(2):512–8.
5. Durham SR. SQ-standardised grass tablet sublingual immunotherapy: persistent clinical benefit and progressive immunological changes during three years treatment. Arb Paul Ehrlich Inst Bundesamt Sera Impfstoffe Frankf A M 2009;96:121–7.
6. Wilson DR, Lima MT, Durham SR. Sublingual immunotherapy for allergic rhinitis: systematic review and meta-analysis. Allergy 2005;60(1):4–12.
7. Abramson M, Puy R, Weiner J. Immunotherapy in asthma: an updated systematic review. Allergy 1999;54(10):1022–41.
8. Jacobsen L, Niggemann B, Dreborg S, et al. Specific immunotherapy has long-term preventive effect of seasonal and perennial asthma: 10-year follow-up on the PAT study. Allergy 2007;62(8):943–8.
9. Ferreira F, Rohlfs A, Hoffmann-Sommergruber K, et al. Modulation of IgE-binding properties of tree pollen allergens by site-directed mutagenesis. Adv Exp Med Biol 1996;409:127–35.
10. Okada T, Swoboda I, Bhalla PL, et al. Engineering of hypoallergenic mutants of the Brassica pollen allergen, Bra r 1, for immunotherapy. FEBS Lett 1998;434(3):255–60.
11. Swoboda I, De Weerd N, Bhalla PL, et al. Mutants of the major ryegrass pollen allergen, Lol p 5, with reduced IgE-binding capacity: candidates for grass pollen-specific immunotherapy. Eur J Immunol 2002;32(1):270–80.
12. Swoboda I, Bugajska-Schretter A, Linhart B, et al. A recombinant hypoallergenic parvalbumin mutant for immunotherapy of IgE-mediated fish allergy. J Immunol 2007;178(10):6290–6.
13. Burks AW, King N, Bannon GA. Modification of a major peanut allergen leads to loss of IgE binding. Int Arch Allergy Immunol 1999;118(2-4):313–4.
14. Rabjohn P, West CM, Connaughton C, et al. Modification of peanut allergen Ara h 3: effects on IgE binding and T cell stimulation. Int Arch Allergy Immunol 2002;128(1):15–23.
15. Stanley JS, King N, Burks AW, et al. Identification and mutational analysis of the immunodominant IgE binding epitopes of the major peanut allergen Ara h 2. Arch Biochem Biophys 1997;342(2):244–53.
16. Drew AC, Eusebius NP, Kenins L, et al. Hypoallergenic variants of the major latex allergen Hev b 6.01 retaining human T lymphocyte reactivity. J Immunol 2004;173(9):5872–9.
17. Bolhaar ST, Zuidmeer L, Ma Y, et al. A mutant of the major apple allergen, Mal d 1, demonstrating hypo-allergenicity in the target organ by double-blind placebo-controlled food challenge. Clin Exp Allergy 2005;35(12):1638–44.

18. Ferreira F, Ebner C, Kramer B, et al. Modulation of IgE reactivity of allergens by site-directed mutagenesis: potential use of hypoallergenic variants for immunotherapy. FASEB J 1998;12(2):231–42.

19. Kussebi F, Karamloo F, Rhyner C, et al. A major allergen gene-fusion protein for potential usage in allergen-specific immunotherapy. J Allergy Clin Immunol 2005; 115(2):323–9.

20. King TP, Jim SY, Monsalve RI, et al. Recombinant allergens with reduced allergenicity but retaining immunogenicity of the natural allergens: hybrids of yellow jacket and paper wasp venom allergen antigen 5s. J Immunol 2001;166(10): 6057–65.

21. Hirahara K, Tatsuta T, Takatori T, et al. Preclinical evaluation of an immunotherapeutic peptide comprising 7 T-cell determinants of Cry j 1 and Cry j 2, the major Japanese cedar pollen allergens. J Allergy Clin Immunol 2001;108(1):94–100.

22. Karamloo F, Schmid-Grendelmeier P, Kussebi F, et al. Prevention of allergy by a recombinant multi-allergen vaccine with reduced IgE binding and preserved T cell epitopes. Eur J Immunol 2005;35(11):3268–76.

23. Westritschnig K, Linhart B, Focke-Tejkl M, et al. A hypoallergenic vaccine obtained by tail-to-head restructuring of timothy grass pollen profilin, Phl p 12, for the treatment of cross-sensitization to profilin. J Immunol 2007;179(11):7624–34.

24. Campana R, Vrtala S, Maderegger B, et al. Hypoallergenic derivatives of the major birch pollen allergen Bet v 1 obtained by rational sequence reassembly. J Allergy Clin Immunol 2010;126(5):1024–31, 1031.

25. Niederberger V, Horak F, Vrtala S, et al. Vaccination with genetically engineered allergens prevents progression of allergic disease. Proc Natl Acad Sci U S A 2004;101(Suppl 2):14677–82.

26. Fellrath JM, Kettner A, Dufour N, et al. Allergen-specific T-cell tolerance induction with allergen-derived long synthetic peptides: results of a phase I trial. J Allergy Clin Immunol 2003;111(4):854–61.

27. Worm M, Lee HH, Kleine-Tebbe J, et al. Development and preliminary clinical evaluation of a peptide immunotherapy vaccine for cat allergy. J Allergy Clin Immunol 2011;127(1):89–97.

28. Alexander C, Tarzi M, Larche M, et al. The effect of Fel d 1-derived T-cell peptides on upper and lower airway outcome measurements in cat-allergic subjects. Allergy 2005;60(10):1269–74.

29. Alexander C, Ying S, Kay B, et al. Fel d 1-derived T cell peptide therapy induces recruitment of CD4CD25; CD4 interferon-gamma T helper type 1 cells to sites of allergen-induced late-phase skin reactions in cat-allergic subjects. Clin Exp Allergy 2005;35(1):52–8.

30. Oldfield WL, Kay AB, Larche M. Allergen-derived T cell peptide-induced late asthmatic reactions precede the induction of antigen-specific hyporesponsiveness in atopic allergic asthmatic subjects. J Immunol 2001;167(3):1734–9.

31. Oldfield WL, Larche M, Kay AB. Effect of T-cell peptides derived from Fel d 1 on allergic reactions and cytokine production in patients sensitive to cats: a randomised controlled trial. Lancet 2002;360(9326):47–53.

32. Arquint O, Helbling A, Crameri R, et al. Reduced in vivo allergenicity of Bet v 1d isoform, a natural component of birch pollen. J Allergy Clin Immunol 1999;104(6): 1239–43.

33. Hiller R, Laffer S, Harwanegg C, et al. Microarrayed allergen molecules: diagnostic gatekeepers for allergy treatment. FASEB J 2002;16(3):414–6.

34. Schmid-Grendelmeier P, Crameri R. Recombinant allergens for skin testing. Int Arch Allergy Immunol 2001;125(2):96–111.

35. Jutel M, Jaeger L, Suck R, et al. Allergen-specific immunotherapy with recombinant grass pollen allergens. J Allergy Clin Immunol 2005;116(3):608–13.
36. Pauli G, Larsen TH, Rak S, et al. Efficacy of recombinant birch pollen vaccine for the treatment of birch-allergic rhinoconjunctivitis. J Allergy Clin Immunol 2008; 122(5):951–60.
37. Vrtala S, Hirtenlehner K, Susani M, et al. Genetic engineering of a hypoallergenic trimer of the major birch pollen allergen Bet v 1. FASEB J 2001; 15(11):2045–7.
38. Vrtala S, Hirtenlehner K, Vangelista L, et al. Conversion of the major birch pollen allergen, Bet v 1, into two nonanaphylactic T cell epitope-containing fragments: candidates for a novel form of specific immunotherapy. J Clin Invest 1997; 99(7):1673–81.
39. Hage-Hamsten M, Kronqvist M, Zetterstrom O, et al. Skin test evaluation of genetically engineered hypoallergenic derivatives of the major birch pollen allergen, Bet v 1: results obtained with a mix of two recombinant Bet v 1 fragments and recombinant Bet v 1 trimer in a Swedish population before the birch pollen season. J Allergy Clin Immunol 1999;104(5):969–77.
40. Vrtala S, Akdis CA, Budak F, et al. T cell epitope-containing hypoallergenic recombinant fragments of the major birch pollen allergen, Bet v 1, induce blocking antibodies. J Immunol 2000;165(11):6653–9.
41. Campana R, Vrtala S, Maderegger B, et al. Altered IgE epitope presentation: a model for hypoallergenic activity revealed for Bet v. 1 trimer. Mol Immunol 2011;48(4):431–41.
42. Egger C, Horak F, Vrtala S, et al. Nasal application of rBet v 1 or non-IgE-reactive T-cell epitope-containing rBet v 1 fragments has different effects on systemic allergen-specific antibody responses. J Allergy Clin Immunol 2010;126(6): 1312–5.
43. Pree I, Shamji MH, Kimber I, et al. Inhibition of CD23-dependent facilitated allergen binding to B cells following vaccination with genetically modified hypoallergenic Bet v 1 molecules. Clin Exp Allergy 2010;40(9):1346–52.
44. Reisinger J, Horak F, Pauli G, et al. Allergen-specific nasal IgG antibodies induced by vaccination with genetically modified allergens are associated with reduced nasal allergen sensitivity. J Allergy Clin Immunol 2005;116(2): 347–54.
45. Niederberger V, Reisinger J, Valent P, et al. Vaccination with genetically modified birch pollen allergens: immune and clinical effects on oral allergy syndrome. J Allergy Clin Immunol 2007;119(4):1013–6.
46. Gafvelin G, Thunberg S, Kronqvist M, et al. Cytokine and antibody responses in birch-pollen-allergic patients treated with genetically modified derivatives of the major birch pollen allergen Bet v 1. Int Arch Allergy Immunol 2005;138(1):59–66.
47. Purohit A, Niederberger V, Kronqvist M, et al. Clinical effects of immunotherapy with genetically modified recombinant birch pollen Bet v 1 derivatives. Clin Exp Allergy 2008;38(9):1514–25.
48. Kundig TM, Senti G, Schnetzler G, et al. Der p 1 peptide on virus-like particles is safe and highly immunogenic in healthy adults. J Allergy Clin Immunol 2006; 117(6):1470–6.
49. Senti G, Johansen P, Haug S, et al. Use of A-type CpG oligodeoxynucleotides as an adjuvant in allergen-specific immunotherapy in humans: a phase I/IIa clinical trial. Clin Exp Allergy 2009;39(4):562–70.
50. Djurup R, Malling HJ. High IgG4 antibody level is associated with failure of immunotherapy with inhalant allergens. Clin Allergy 1987;17(5):459–68.

51. Wachholz PA, Soni NK, Till SJ, et al. Inhibition of allergen-IgE binding to B cells by IgG antibodies after grass pollen immunotherapy. J Allergy Clin Immunol 2003; 112(5):915–22.

52. Shamji MH, Wilcock LK, Wachholz PA, et al. The IgE-facilitated allergen binding (FAB) assay: validation of a novel flow-cytometric based method for the detection of inhibitory antibody responses. J Immunol Methods 2006;317(1–2):71–9.

53. Focke M, Linhart B, Hartl A, et al. Non-anaphylactic surface-exposed peptides of the major birch pollen allergen, Bet v 1, for preventive vaccination. Clin Exp Allergy 2004;34(10):1525–33.

54. Edlmayr J, Niespodziana K, Linhart B, et al. A combination vaccine for allergy and rhinovirus infections based on rhinovirus-derived surface protein VP1 and a nonallergenic peptide of the major timothy grass pollen allergen Phl p 1. J Immunol 2009; 182(10):6298–306.

55. Campana R, Mothes N, Rauter I, et al. Non-IgE-mediated chronic allergic skin inflammation revealed with rBet v 1 fragments. J Allergy Clin Immunol 2008; 121(2):528–30.

56. Kepley CL, Taghavi S, Mackay G, et al. Co-aggregation of FcgammaRII with FcepsilonRI on human mast cells inhibits antigen-induced secretion and involves SHIP-Grb2-Dok complexes. J Biol Chem 2004;279(34):35139–49.

57. Zhang K, Kepley CL, Terada T, et al. Inhibition of allergen-specific IgE reactivity by a human Ig Fcgamma-Fcepsilon bifunctional fusion protein. J Allergy Clin Immunol 2004;114(2):321–7.

58. Zhang K, Zhu D, Kepley C, et al. Chimeric human fcgamma-allergen fusion proteins in the prevention of allergy. Immunol Allergy Clin North Am 2007;27(1): 93–103.

59. Zhu D, Kepley CL, Zhang K, et al. A chimeric human-cat fusion protein blocks cat-induced allergy. Nat Med 2005;11(4):446–9.

60. Terada T, Zhang K, Belperio J, et al. A chimeric human-cat Fcgamma-Fel d1 fusion protein inhibits systemic, pulmonary, and cutaneous allergic reactivity to intratracheal challenge in mice sensitized to Fel d1, the major cat allergen. Clin Immunol 2006;120(1):45–56.

61. Norman PS, Ohman JL, Long AA, et al. Treatment of cat allergy with T-cell reactive peptides. Am J Respir Crit Care Med 1996;154(6 Pt 1):1623–8.

62. Marcotte GV, Braun CM, Norman PS, et al. Effects of peptide therapy on ex vivo T-cell responses. J Allergy Clin Immunol 1998;101(4 Pt 1):506–13.

63. Pene J, Desroches A, Paradis L, et al. Immunotherapy with Fel d 1 peptides decreases IL-4 release by peripheral blood T cells of patients allergic to cats. J Allergy Clin Immunol 1998;102(4 Pt 1):571–8.

64. Maguire P, Nicodemus C, Robinson D, et al. The safety and efficacy of ALLERVAX CAT in cat allergic patients. Clin Immunol 1999;93(3):222–31.

65. Simons FE, Imada M, Li Y, et al. Fel d 1 peptides: effect on skin tests and cytokine synthesis in cat-allergic human subjects. Int Immunol 1996;8(12):1937–45.

66. Haselden BM, Kay AB, Larche M. Immunoglobulin E-independent major histocompatibility complex-restricted T cell peptide epitope-induced late asthmatic reactions. J Exp Med 1999;189(12):1885–94.

67. Smith TR, Alexander C, Kay AB, et al. Cat allergen peptide immunotherapy reduces CD4 T cell responses to cat allergen but does not alter suppression by CD4 CD25 T cells: a double-blind placebo-controlled study. Allergy 2004; 59(10):1097–101.

68. Verhoef A, Alexander C, Kay AB, et al. T cell epitope immunotherapy induces a CD4(+) T cell population with regulatory activity. PLoS Med 2005;2(3):e78.

69. Campbell JD, Buckland KF, McMillan SJ, et al. Peptide immunotherapy in allergic asthma generates IL-10-dependent immunological tolerance associated with linked epitope suppression. J Exp Med 2009;206(7):1535–47.
70. Larche M. Update on the current status of peptide immunotherapy. J Allergy Clin Immunol 2007;119(4):906–9.
71. Carballido JM, Carballido-Perrig N, Kagi MK, et al. T cell epitope specificity in human allergic and nonallergic subjects to bee venom phospholipase A2. J Immunol 1993;150(8 Pt 1):3582–91.
72. Muller U, Akdis CA, Fricker M, et al. Successful immunotherapy with T-cell epitope peptides of bee venom phospholipase A2 induces specific T-cell anergy in patients allergic to bee venom. J Allergy Clin Immunol 1998;101(6 Pt 1): 747–54.
73. Texier C, Pouvelle S, Busson M, et al. HLA-DR restricted peptide candidates for bee venom immunotherapy. J Immunol 2000;164(6):3177–84.
74. Tarzi M, Klunker S, Texier C, et al. Induction of interleukin-10 and suppressor of cytokine signaling-3 gene expression following peptide immunotherapy. Clin Exp Allergy 2006;36(4):465–74.

Novel Administration Routes for Allergen-Specific Immunotherapy: A Review of Intralymphatic and Epicutaneous Allergen-Specific Immunotherapy

Seraina von Moos, Med. Pract.[a], Thomas M. Kündig, MD[b],
Gabriela Senti, MD[a],*

KEYWORDS

- Intralymphatic allergen-specific immunotherapy
- Epicutaneous allergen-specific immunotherapy
- Vaccination route • Intralymphatic vaccination
- Epicutaneous vaccination

The prevalence of allergic diseases, first described by John Bostock at the beginning of the 19th century as *catarrhus aestivus*,[1] has been continually increasing and has actually reached epidemic dimensions.[2] Initially conceived as a toxin-induced disease,[3] the pathophysiologic understanding of allergy fundamentally changed in 1986 with the discovery of immunoglobulin E (IgE).[4] However, despite such paradigm change with regard to the causative factor of allergy, treatment options have remained

This work was supported in part by the Swiss National Science Foundation (SNF), the University of Zurich, Medanz Medical GmbH (Starnberg, Germany), Allergy Innovations (Munich, Germany), MannKind Corporations (Valencia, CA, USA), and ImVisioN GmbH (Hannover, Germany).

[a] Clinical Trials Center, Center for Clinical Research, University and University Hospital Zürich, Moussonstrasse 2, 8091 Zürich, Switzerland
[b] Department of Dermatology, University Hospital Zürich, Gloriastrasse 31, 8091 Zürich, Switzerland
* Corresponding author.
E-mail address: gabriela.senti@usz.ch

unchanged for the past 100 years. Allergen-specific immunotherapy (SIT), introduced in 1911 by Leonard Noon,[3] still remains the only disease-modifying treatment option.[5,6] Strikingly, today's state of the art for SIT has not substantially changed and still consists of numerous subcutaneous injections of increasing allergen doses[7] aiming to restore normal immunity against allergens.[8] Several immunologic changes have been observed during successful SIT[6–8]: redirection of the T helper 2 (Th2)-biased allergic immune response toward a Th1-polarized response associated with reduced production of interleukin (IL)-4 and IL-5, and increased secretion of interferon gamma (IFN-γ); stimulation of allergen-specific IgG and IgA with important blocking activity and direct immune-inhibitory function; and, last but not least, generation of regulatory T cells (Tregs) producing IL-10. Yet, it is still a matter of debate which of these immunologic mechanisms is critical for symptom amelioration. Besides ongoing research on the mechanisms underlying SIT, considerable effort is currently put into the development of highly efficient and patient-convenient administration routes of SIT to facilitate its broad application. Today, only 5% of all allergic patients choose to undergo SIT,[9] even though conventional subcutaneous allergen-specific immuno-therapy (SCIT) has proven its efficacy in several randomized controlled trials.[10] The most important reasons for low treatment acceptance and poor treatment adherence[11] are the long treatment duration necessitating 50 to 80 physician-administrated injections associated with the risk of systemic allergic side effects.[11] The primary objective for the next century of SIT is therefore to increase its attractive-ness by enhancing treatment efficacy, reducing treatment duration, and offering needle-free, self-administrable treatment routes.

Recently, the development of novel "vaccine" administration routes has gained increasing interest both for vaccination against infectious disease[12] and for SIT.[13–15] The development of sublingual allergen-specific immunotherapy, harnessing the specialties of the mucosal immune system, is discussed in the article by Canonica and Passalacqua elsewhere in this issue. In this article, we discuss the rationale and the unique properties and challenges related to intralymphatic allergen-specific immunotherapy (ILIT) and epicutaneous allergen-specific immunotherapy (EPIT) while outlining the current results of preclinical and clinical trials in these fields.

DETERMINANTS OF THE IMMUNE SYSTEM'S REACTIVITY AND THE CHOICE OF THE "VACCINATION ROUTE"

For a rational choice of the vaccination route, it is essential to understand how an immune response is initiated and governed. Therefore, two basic and not mutually exclusive principles held by the two foremost immunologists of the 20th century need to be considered. First is the "geographic concept of immunogenicity," brought forward by Rolf Zinkernagel.[16,17] It is based on the observation that immune responses can be initiated only in secondary lymphoid organs (SLO), including lymph nodes, the splenic white pulp, and organized lymphoid tissue associated with mucosal organs, such as Peyer patches.[16,17] The outstanding characteristic of SLOs is their functional microarchitecture offering specialized subdivisions helping immune cells to build an efficient effector response.[18] Findings in mice that carry the alymphoplasia (aly/aly) mutation, and therefore lack functional SLOs, underscore this concept.[19] The afferent lymphatic vessel system carries the antigen from the peripheral tissue entry site to the SLOs, which is a crucial requirement for efficient induction of an immune response, as was elegantly demonstrated by skin flap experiments.[20] Lymphatic vessels originate in the peripheral tissue as blind-ended porous structures allowing entrance of cells and macromolecules up to 100 to 200 nm in size. In contrast, proximal lymphatic vessels are impermeable to molecules larger than 5 to 6 nm.[21] Depending on the antigen size, transport through the lymphatic vessel system mainly occurs as free drainage or as cell-associated transport.[21] The transporter cells are essentially tissue resident antigen-presenting cells (APCs), which, on activation by danger signals, emigrate out of the tissue by squeezing through openings between overlapping endothelial cells of lymphatic capillaries.[22] These APCs have been called the "ultimate messengers" by Polly Matzinger, who introduced the second key principle regarding initiation and governing of immune responses: *"the power of the tissue in determining the effector class."*[23] This concept is based on the observation that the first trigger for the initiation of an immune response arises in damaged peripheral tissue, which sends activation signals to educate resident APCs to induce a tissue-tailored response. Supporting such concept of APCs as "mailmen" carrying the tissue address is corroborated by the fact that dendritic cells (DCs) from different sites stimulate different types of immune responses.[24,25] Further support for the hypothesis regarding the role of tissue in tailoring the effector response arises from the observation that different tissues tend to react in a prototypical manner. The reaction pattern of the skin, or more precisely the dermis, consists of a delayed-type hypersensitivity response based on a Th1-type immune activation with secretion of interferon (IFN)-γ and IL-12, which in turn activate macrophages and induce complement-fixing antibodies (IgG2a type in mice). Conversely, the reaction pattern of mucosal sites, such as the gut, is characterized by a noninflammatory immune response characterized by local production of IgA and systemic accumulation of T cells that do not proliferate profusely or produce IFN-γ, but instead secrete IL-4, transforming growth factor β, and IL-10.[23,26]

Collectively, this indicates that besides antigen structure, dose, and time, the localization of the antigen plays a crucial role, not only for the decision as to whether to initiate an immune response, but also how to shape the response. In conclusion, direct administration of the antigen into the lymph node is likely to increase immunogenicity and to strengthen the immune response. Because the conventional way of antigen arrival via peripheral APCs, the "ultimate tissue messengers," is circumvented, presumably the response does not show a tissue-imprinted effector class direction. This implies that the choice of the peripheral antigen administration route (subcutaneously, intradermally, epicutaneously, sublingually) not only determines the magnitude of the immune response through the tissue-inherent number of APCs and the density of lymphatic capillaries, but also influences the effector class of the response through tissue-educated APCs.

INTRALYMPHATIC ALLERGEN-SPECIFIC IMMUNOTHERAPY

The long treatment duration associated with conventional SCIT likely impedes broad acceptance,[9,11] thus the attractiveness of SIT is likely to be increased by considerable reductions in treatment duration. Yet, to this purpose, treatment efficacy needs to be substantially increased. When considering the fact that only small fractions of subcutaneously injected antigen reach the draining lymph nodes,[14,27] direct intralymphatic injection of the antigen might be a promising strategy to enhance the efficacy of SIT by increasing antigen availability in the SLOs (see the geographic concept of immunogenicity).[16,17] In the following sections, we first outline the characteristic microstructure of a lymph node before summarizing results of preclinical and clinical trials testing ILIT for the treatment of IgE-mediated allergies.

Structure Impacts Function

Microarchitecture of the lymph node

The highly organized microarchitecture of SLOs is the prerequisite for the efficient induction of an immune response.[18] The close structure-function relationship has been demonstrated in mice deficient in lymphotoxinα1β2, which is crucial for the generation and maintenance of the SLOs' microarchitecture.[28] Generally, lymph nodes ore organized into 3 zones: (1) an *antigen-sampling zone* consisting of the subcapsular area and the medulla, which are rich in APCs that deliver the antigen to the T-cell and B-cell zones; (2) a *B-cell activation zone* in the cortex of the lymph node, which contains B-cell follicles; and (3) a *T-cell activation* zone in the paracortex of the lymph node. Such organization in specialized subdivisions facilitates the interaction between immune cells and antigen by juxtaposing APCs and lymphocytes in a small volume, thereby increasing the probability of encountering the cognate T cell.[18] Because an individual antigen specificity is represented by only 1 in 10^7 T cells or B cells, such concentrations of lymphocytes in the SLOs is key to the efficient induction of an immune response.[14] The end products of such interaction are high-affinity neutralizing antibodies, cytokine-producing Th cells, and cytotoxic T cells.

Challenges to intralymphatic "vaccine" administration

Although present throughout the entire human body, lymph nodes are only superficially accessible in the head-neck region and in the groin. In the groin they can be easily detected by ultrasound as hypoechoic nodules with a diameter of approximately 1.0 to 1.5 cm. Because the sensory innervation of lymph nodes is sparse, direct intralymphatic injection using a 28-gauge needle has been demonstrated to be less painful than a peripheral venous puncture.[29]

Intralymphatic Allergen-Specific Immunotherapy: A Success Story

Back to the roots of intralymphatic immunization

Intralymphatic immunization was first tested as a method to enhance immunogenicity of cancer vaccines.[30] Indeed, antitumor responses were observed to be enhanced after direct intralymphatic injection of tumor cells,[31,32] DNA plasmids,[33,34] and naked RNA[35] in preclinical as well as clinical settings. Additionally, targeted lymph node immunization has been tested as a method to develop a successful HIV vaccine using various peptides.[36,37] In all these situations, generation of strong immune responses after administration of minute antigen doses were observed to be the key characteristics of intralymphatic immunization.

Preclinical data of intralymphatic allergen-specific immunotherapy

Animal experiments demonstrated that the same observations hold true when intralymphatic immunization is used in the setting of SIT. For induction of equal humoral immune responses, allergen doses could be reduced 100 times when administered directly into the lymph node as compared with the subcutaneous route. Interestingly, intralymphatic immunization did not polarize the immune response but rather generated overall stronger Th1 and Th2 responses as measured by induction of high IgG1 and IgG2a antibodies associated with an overall increase of IL-4, IFN-γ, and IL-10 secretion. Of note, ILIT protected mice from temperature drop in an anaphylaxis challenge model, whereas SCIT did not prevent temperature drop in sensitized mice on intraperitoneal allergen challenge.[27]

Significant differences in antigen availability in the SLOs after antigen administration via the subcutaneous or intralymphatic route explain the observed efficacy results. Protein amount in the draining lymph node was demonstrated to be 100-fold higher after intralymphatic injections as compared with subcutaneous injections.[27] Confirmatory experiments in humans revealed efficient "antigen-pulsing" of lymph nodes 20 minutes after intralymphatic injections, whereas only small antigen fractions reached the lymph node 25 hours after subcutaneous injection.[14]

Clinical trials with intralymphatic allergen-specific immunotherapy
Several clinical trials testing the efficacy of ILIT for the treatment of grass pollen allergy, hymenoptera venom hypersensitivity, and cat dander allergy have provided highly promising results. For grass pollen allergy, a significant increase in allergen tolerance was observed within 4 months after administration of only 3 low-dose intralymphatic injections, whereas 1 year of continuous subcutaneous injections were necessary to obtain the same result. Overall, the cumulative allergen dose could be reduced 1000-fold. Long-term protection, decrease in allergen-specific IgE levels, and reduction in skin prick test sensitivity were similar after ILIT and conventional SCIT. Of note, ILIT proved to be safe, inducing no grade III or IV systemic allergic side effects in contrast to SCIT (ClinicalTrials.gov Identifier NCT00470457).[29] Analogous results were obtained in a multicenter trial including patients with grades III and IV bee venom allergy (Senti and colleagues, manuscript in preparation). This year, a large phase II/III trial was initiated in Denmark to assess efficacy and to optimize treatment dose of ILIT for the treatment of grass pollen allergy. First trial results are expected in 2012 (ClinicalTrials.gov Identifier NCT01166269).

Altogether, ILIT allows high therapeutic efficacy with considerably reduced treatment dose and substantially shortened treatment duration. Combined with its good safety profile, ILIT is therefore likely to increase treatment compliance and reduce socioeconomic costs.

Future directions
Anatomic targeting of antigen delivery at the site of immune initiation (ie, into the lymph node) has been demonstrated to significantly enhance immune responses. Combined with molecular targeting of antigen delivery, ILIT might have the potential to bring the ultimate goal of a single-dose allergy vaccine into reach. Molecular targeting has become possible with the engineering of so-called modular antigen transporter (MAT) allergens that precisely deliver the antigen into the major histocompatibility class II (MHC II) antigen-presentation pathway. MAT molecules consist of a *tat*-derived protein translocation domain (mediating cytoplasmic uptake) that is fused to a truncated invariant chain for targeting of the nascent MHC II molecule.[38,39] In vitro studies confirmed enhanced immunogenicity of MAT fusion allergens, which were able to induce T-cell proliferation at 100-fold lower doses compared with unmodulated recombinant allergens.[38] Additionally, MAT fusion molecules were observed to shift the immune response from a Th2 profile toward a Th1 profile in vitro[38] as well as in vivo.[40] Accordingly, MAT fusion molecules significantly enhanced efficacy of ILIT as measured by protection from anaphylactic temperature drop.[40] Accordingly, a clinical trial using IVN201 (major cat dander allergen Fel d 1 fused to MAT molecule) has recently proved to be safe and highly efficacious in alleviating clinical symptoms of cat dander allergy (Senti and colleagues, manuscript in preparation, ClinicalTrials.gov Identifier NCT00718679).

EPICUTANEOUS ALLERGEN-SPECIFIC IMMUNOTHERAPY

The need for 50 to 80 injections over 3 to 5 years is a major drawback of conventional SIT, strongly impeding its broad acceptance.[9,11] For this reason, much effort has been put into the development of needle-free and potentially self-administrable treatment routes. In light of the potent immune-surveillance function of the skin,[41,42] the good accessibility, and its proposed intrinsic Th1-type reactivity pattern[23,26] (see concept of *the power of the tissue in determining the effector class*), epicutaneous allergen-specific immunotherapy (EPIT) has the potential to emerge as a promising needle-free treatment route for IgE-mediated allergies. We first focus on the structure and immunologic function of the skin before depicting the clinical experience with EPIT.

Structure Impacts Function

The structure of the skin

Human skin is composed of 2 compartments: the epidermis and the underlying dermis.[42] The epidermis is composed of 4 strata (*stratum basale, stratum spinosum, stratum granulosum, stratum corneum*) forming altogether a protection layer that is 50 μm to 150 μm thick.[43] The physical barrier function is mainly exerted by the outermost layer, the stratum corneum, which measures 15 μm to 20 μm. It is built of cornified keratinocytes embedded in a lipid-rich matrix[42,43] that efficiently excludes molecules larger than 500 Da.[44] Interdispersed between the imbricated arrangement of keratinocytes, which are the predominant cell type of the epidermis, there are sparse specialized cells such as pigment-producing melanocytes and antigen-presenting Langerhans cells (LCs).[42] Even though accounting for only 3% to 5% of the epidermal cells, LCs cover up to 20% of the skin surface by forming a continuous network with their dendrites.[43,45] Holding, therefore, an important function as immune sentinels in first-line defense,[42] these cells are attractive vaccine targets. The nonvascularized epidermis with its "simple histology" is separated by the basement membrane from the "more complex" dermis, which harbors a great diversity of cell types as well as lymphatic and vascular conduits. Beyond fibroblasts, macrophages, and mast cells, the dermis comprises different subsets of dermal dendritic cells (DCs) as well as T cells.[42,46]

Immunologic function of the skin

The perception of the skin as a "quasi immunologic organ" dates back to 1983, when Streilein[47] introduced the concept of the skin-associated lymphoid tissue (SALT), conceived as an immunologic entity based on the interplay between keratinocytes, LCs, lymphocytes, and the skin-draining lymph nodes. Although the understanding of the immunologic functions of the skin is increasing,[41] the relative role of different DC subsets and keratinocyte-derived cytokines/chemokines, released upon infection and/or stress, in shaping adaptive immune response is not yet disentangled: are DCs the ultimate immune controllers[48] or the ultimate tissue messengers?[23] Supporting the former concept, a functional dichotomy has been observed between different skin DC subsets. Whereas epidermal LCs have been demonstrated to hold a key role in induction of CD8+ T-cell responses and in shaping a Th2-type/Treg-type response, activation of dermal DC subsets has been found to be essential for B cell class switching and induction of a Th1-type response.[49,50] In line with such observation, dermal DC subsets were observed to preferentially localize to the B-cell areas of draining lymph nodes, whereas LCs were observed to migrate to the T-cell areas.[51] Alternatively, increasing evidence supports a pivotal role of keratinocytes in governing the adaptive immune responses.[23,52] It has been proposed that epithelial cells express different molecular mediators under different conditions, thereby dictating the appropriate type of response. Hence, relatively slight stress to the epithelium, such as abrasion (without penetration), induces a predominance of thymic stromal lymphopoietin, IL-25, and IL-33, which in turn instruct noninflammatory Treg or Th2-type responses. Yet, as epithelial damage increases, expression of additional molecules, such as

IL-1α, IL-6, and tumor necrosis factor (TNF), skew the immune response toward a Th1-type response.[52] The degree of epithelial damage as the crucial event in determining the effector class response might as well explain the observed dichotomy of different DC subsets: superficial damage induces a "noninflammatory" response transmitted by LCs, whereas deeper epithelial damage induces a "proinflammatory" response that is carried by dermal DC subsets. Studies that enlighten this area would help to rationally design and target epicutaneously administered vaccines.

Challenges to epicutaneous "vaccine" administration

Even though the skin is easily accessible, simple topical application of a vaccine does not typically induce an adequate immune response because of the low permeability of the stratum corneum. Three thousand years ago, when the skin was first used as a vaccination site against smallpox, this challenge was addressed by disrupting the stratum corneum by scratching: so-called *scarification*.[12] Today, this has been replaced by tape stripping[53] and other abrasive methods[54,55] that gently remove the cornified keratinocytes without disruption of the underlying basement membrane. Recent advances in nanotechnology allow the specific targeting of APCs using microneedle arrays with defined length.[43,56] Of note, all of these methods are associated with physical irritation of keratinocytes stimulating the secretion of cytokines, which in turn activate the immune system.[52,57] Alternatively, penetration can be enhanced by skin hydration over a period of at least 4 to 10 hours[58] (ie, application of an occlusive patch leading to sweat accumulation[59,60]).

Epicutaneous Allergen-Specific Immunotherapy: In Small Steps to the New Standard of Care?

Back to the roots of "skin vaccination"

Harnessing the special properties of the skin for administration of vaccines has a long history, dating back more than 3000 years, when *variolation* was performed in China and India in an attempt to immunize against smallpox. The method of variolation was performed by scratching crusts from smallpox lesions of convalescing patients onto the skin of healthy individuals. This historical form of epicutaneous vaccination substantially reduced mortality rates of smallpox infections from 30% during natural outbreaks to less than 1%.[61] Despite such early and successful discovery of epicutaneous vaccination, this route did not attract major attention until the beginning of the 21st century, when interest in needle-free vaccination started to increase.[12,62] Encouraged by the testing of epicutaneous (transcutaneous) vaccination for various infectious diseases,[55,63,64] as well as for cancer,[65,66] epicutaneous allergen-specific immunotherapy was rediscovered.[13,53]

The role of the skin in the development of allergen-specific immunotherapy

Allergen-specific immunotherapy until recently was predominantly administered "under" the skin as "prophylactic hypodermic inoculations"[67] as described by Noon[3] and Freeman,[67] although several early attempts were made to deliver the pollen vaccination either "into" the skin or "onto" the skin to overcome the main problems associated with subcutaneous injections.

Intradermal allergen-specific immunotherapy

The first records describing administration of the "allergy vaccine" into the skin (taking advantage of the skin's specialties) date back to 1929. Soon after the introduction of SCIT by Leonard Noon,[3] the risk of suffering a "pollen shock" on subcutaneous allergen administration was recognized as a real problem.[68] Observations that such patients could be safely and successfully treated by intradermal administrations of pollen extract encouraged Phillips[69] to launch a study testing this novel route of SIT. Pollen extract was applied "into the substance of the skin, the same as an intradermal test...Such treatment was not only safe but also highly successful, leading to symptom relief in all the 29 patients after administration of less than three doses."[69]

The birth of epicutaneous allergen-specific immunotherapy

The first report on successful EPIT dates back to 1921, when an asthmatic patient experienced complete symptom relief after administration of horse hair on scarificated skin, a method called *cutiréactions répétées*.[70] More than a decade later, M. A. Ramirez readopted this method for the treatment of patients allergic to grass pollen.[71] Encouraged by these early successful reports, French allergologists substantially contributed to the revival of EPIT in the middle of the last century.[72,73] Whereas Pautrizel and colleagues[72] administered the allergen extract onto a slightly rubbed epidermis, Blamoutier and colleagues[73,74] applied the allergen drops onto heavily scarificated skin, called *méthode de quadrillage cutané*. Both observed high treatment success; however, with the method of Pautrizel and colleagues,[72] a large number of applications was necessary until symptom relief. In contrast, the method of Blamoutier and colleagues[73,74] could be performed co-seasonally, leading to symptom relief or considerable symptom amelioration after 4 treatments on average. Consistently, both reported fewer and milder allergic side effects upon EPIT than observed with SCIT.[72,73] Several clinical trials were performed in the subsequent years by Eichenberger and Storck[75] to test this type of co-seasonal desensitization. Consistently, they observed a treatment success rate of more than 80%. Generally, symptom amelioration was obtained rapidly while lasting between 3 days and 3 weeks. On average, 6 to 12 treatments were therefore required during one pollen season to be practically symptom free. Of note, treatment success rates with EPIT were higher than those observed with classical SCIT, and even patients who responded inadequately to conventional SCIT reported considerable symptom improvement under EPIT. Even though, at that time, this French *méthode de quadrillage cutané*,[73] was successfully tested from Portugal[76] to Switzerland,[75,77] it was buried in oblivion for the second half of the 20th century before its rediscovery at the beginning of the 21st century.

EPIT with tape stripping: a modification of Blamoutier and colleagues' scarification method

Based on such promising "historical" observations, we performed the first randomized placebo-controlled double-blind pilot trial to test clinical efficacy and safety of EPIT in patients allergic to grass pollen (NCT00457444). In this trial, skin scarification (before antigen administration) was replaced by the adhesive tape–stripping method. As previously demonstrated, tape stripping exerts a dual role: first, it gently removes the stratum corneum,[78] thereby facilitating penetration of the allergen into the epidermis; second, repeated tape stripping has been demonstrated to activate keratinocytes, which then secrete various proinflammatory cytokines, such as IL-1, IL-6, IL-8, TNF-α, and INF-γ, favoring maturation and emigration of DCs to the draining lymph nodes.[79,80] Following preseasonal and co-seasonal application of 12 patches in total, patients in the verum group reported a statistically and clinically significant 70% improvement of hay fever symptoms compared with 20% improvement in the placebo group. Of note, no severe systemic allergic reactions were observed, although the occurrence of a local eczematous skin reaction was frequently reported.

Encouraged by these results, a second phase I/IIa trial was initiated to find the optimal treatment dose of EPIT. A total of 132 patients were randomized to either the placebo group or to 1 of 3 verum groups, each receiving different concentration of allergen extract (Senti and colleagues manuscript in preparation, NCT00719511). To confirm efficacy and to gain insight into immunologic changes induced during EPIT, a third trial, including 98 patients, was initiated (NCT00777374). The first results are expected in 2011. Supporting our results, Agostinis and colleagues[81] recently demonstrated efficacy and safety of EPIT when used as a treatment for grass pollen allergy in children. Hay fever symptoms as well as antihistamine use were significantly reduced in the active treatment group.

EPIT with the Viaskin delivery system: the principle of the occlusive chamber

Based on observations from the atopy patch test, which is able to induce an eczematous skin reaction indicating efficient antigen penetration even on nonabraded, nonpretreated skin,[82] a French group developed EPIT using an occlusive epidermal delivery system.[59,60,83] Initially developed for diagnostic purposes (Diallertest), Viaskin technology (DBV Technologies, Paris, France) relies on the ability to deliver whole protein molecules to the skin via perspiration, generated under an occlusive chamber.[59] Whole protein, delivered via such a system, has been demonstrated to accumulate in the stratum corneum,[84] where it efficiently targets immune cells of the superficial skin layer that rapidly migrate to the draining lymph nodes.[59]

Murine studies, designed to test therapeutic efficacy of the Viaskin epidermal delivery system (EDS), demonstrated equivalence of EPIT and SCIT in preventing allergic airway reactions on inhalative allergen challenge.[59] Furthermore, EPIT using the Viaskin EDS proved to be an efficacious treatment for food allergy as measured by prevention of mast cell degranulation on oral allergen challenge in a murine model.[83] Based on such successful preclinical testing, a clinical pilot trial was launched to test clinical efficacy and safety of EPIT using the Viaskin EDS in children suffering from cow's milk allergy. After a 3-month treatment, a trend toward clinical efficacy was observed in the verum group, showing increased cumulative tolerance of milk in the provocation test. The treatment was well tolerated with no serious systemic allergic reaction; however, a significant increase of local eczematous reactions was observed.[60] Recently, phase I (NCT01170286) and phase II trials (NCT01197053) have been initiated to substantiate these findings.

Future directions

EPIT has proved its efficacy in animal and human studies. Yet, there is still potential to enhance its clinical efficacy[85] and to reduce treatment duration and the number of patch applications. Combination of allergen administration with an adjuvant, precise targeting of APCs by using microneedle arrays or encapsulation of allergen into nanoparticles or liposomes might be useful strategies to achieve such a goal.

Historically, the efficacy of SCIT has been significantly enhanced by mixing the allergen extract with the adjuvant alum.[86] Alum, however, is not very efficient on epicutaneous administration.[87] Therefore, novel adjuvants, such as cholera toxin (CT),[88] heat-labile enterotoxin from Escherichia coli (LT),[55] CpG,[87] or imidazoquinolines,[89] are currently tested as adjuvants for transcutaneous vaccination against infectious disease or cancer, respectively. CT and LT, however, which have been tested most extensively and successfully as adjuvants for transcutaneous vaccination against various infectious diseases, do not seem ideal in the setting of SIT because of their Th2 skewing potential.[43,90] Therefore, we recently tested the immune-enhancing and immune-modulatory potential of diphenylcyclopropenone when used as an adjuvant in EPIT (von Moos and colleagues, manuscript in preparation). Precise antigen delivery to the skin's APCs using microneedle arrays with defined needle length might be a promising technique to further increase treatment efficacy, as demonstrated in recent studies.[43,56] Last but not least, incorporation of antigen into elastic vesicles or nonelastic nanoparticles might open new possibilities.[43]

SUMMARY

In light of the increasing prevalence of allergic diseases,[2] which strongly contrasts the low percentage of patients choosing to undergo SCIT,[9,15] research during the next century should aim at optimization of current SIT methods to increase its attractiveness. Considering the *"geographic concept of immunogenicity"*[16,17] and the *"the power of the tissue in determining the effector class response,"*[23,26] the rational choice of the vaccination route bears the potential to substantially enhance treatment efficacy, thereby reducing treatment dose while ideally offering a needle-free and self-administrable treatment option.

We believe that allergen-specific immunotherapy, no matter whether mediated by blocking antibodies, Th1 upregulation, Th2 downregulation, or induction of Treg, can theoretically be done with one shot. In childhood diseases, one infection with the wild-type virus is sufficient to induce lifelong immunologic changes. Over the past few years, we were able to demonstrate that the immune system has evolved to optimally respond to the threat posed by live pathogens. Pathogen particles are transported into secondary lymphatic organs and internalized by professional APCs that are activated by pathogen-associated molecular patterns, which enhances innate and adaptive immunity.[21] When we mimic only one characteristic of pathogens, namely efficient drainage into lymph nodes by direct intralymphatic allergen administration, the number of allergen injections could already be reduced to 3. By combining intralymphatic antigen administration with molecular targeting of the antigen presentation pathway or the addition of pathogen-associated molecules as strong adjuvants, the vision of a single-shot allergy vaccine might become true. Even though the history of ILIT is not older than a decade,[14,29] its ability to significantly reduce treatment dose and treatment duration, as compared with conventional SCIT, has rapidly channeled the way to the first registration study initiated this year. Epicutaneous allergen-specific immunotherapy on the other hand looks back on a long history.[13] Although the first reports date back 90 years,[70] it has attracted attention only in recent years.[13,53] In contrast to ILIT, it has been developed based on empirical evidence, and the rational understanding of the immunologic processes occurring in the skin is only slowly growing. Nevertheless, there is increasing evidence for an important role of epithelial cytokines in determining the polarization of the immune response.[23,52] Several clinical trials have indeed demonstrated that EPIT has the potential to ameliorate Th2-derived

---

Box 1
Pros and cons of intralymphatic allergen-specific immunotherapy

Pros

- Reduced number of treatment applications (efficacy after 3 injections)
- Reduced treatment duration (several weeks)
- Fast symptom alleviation (within 1 month)
- Sustained treatment efficacy
- Good safety profile

Cons

- Ultrasound-guided, physician-administered, intralymphatic injections

---

Box 2
Pros and cons of epicutaneous allergen-specific immunotherapy

Pros

- Needle-free administration
- Potential self-administration
- Reduced treatment duration (1 pollen season)
- Fast symptom alleviation (co-seasonal treatment possible)
- Sustained treatment efficacy
- Good safety profile

Cons

- Local eczematous skin reaction

---

symptoms of allergic diseases[53,59,60,83]; yet, the exact immunologic mechanism underlying such immune modulation still needs to be elucidated. However, with the increasing understanding of these mechanisms and the adept use of epicutaneously active adjuvants or microneedle arrays, the efficacy of EPIT is likely to be considerably increased in the future. The outstanding characteristic of EPIT is its good safety profile, potentially based on the fact that the allergen accumulates in the nonvascularized stratum corneum, thereby preventing generalized systemic allergic reactions.

Comparing advantages and limitations of ILIT (**Box 1**) and EPIT (**Box 2**) makes it evident that the choice of either of these methods might not be a question of superiority but a matter of individual preference. Although ILIT might be the method of choice for patients seeking high treatment success within a very short time, EPIT might best be suitable for patients suffering from needle phobia and for those seeking a self-administrable treatment option. Another target population might be children, for whom injections represent a big threat leading to poor acceptance of conventional SCIT. Yet, it is especially children who benefit most from SIT,[91] as administration of SIT early in the course of allergic diseases has the potential to stop disease progression to asthma,[92] which represents a considerable health burden.[93] Such reasoning might highlight the development of a preventive patch-based allergy vaccine, accepted as part of the World Health Organization's recommended "early childhood" vaccination program, to conquer the epidemic of the 21st century.

ACKNOWLEDGMENTS

We thank the Swiss Institute of Allergy and Asthma Research (SIAF, Davos, Switzerland), Nicole Graf, and Pål Johansen for their support and helpful discussions.

REFERENCES

1. Bostock J. Of the catarrhus astivus or summer catarrh. Med Chir Trans 1828;14: 437–46.
2. Holgate ST. The epidemic of allergy and asthma. Nature 1999;402(Suppl 6760): B2–4.
3. Noon L. Prophylactic inoculation against hay fever. Lancet 1911;177(4580): 1572–3.
4. Stanworth DR. The discovery of IgE. Allergy 1993;48(2):67–71.
5. Holgate ST, Polosa R. Treatment strategies for allergy and asthma. Nat Rev Immunol 2008;8(3):218–30.

6. Larche M, Akdis CA, Valenta R. Immunological mechanisms of allergen-specific immunotherapy. Nat Rev Immunol 2006;6(10):761–71.
7. Frew AJ. Allergen immunotherapy. J Allergy Clin Immunol 2010;125(2 Suppl 2): S306–13.
8. Akdis M, Akdis CA. Therapeutic manipulation of immune tolerance in allergic disease. Nat Rev Drug Discov 2009;8(8):645–60.
9. Cox L, Calderon MA. Subcutaneous specific immunotherapy for seasonal allergic rhinitis: a review of treatment practices in the US and Europe. Curr Med Res Opin 2010;26(12):2723–33.
10. Calderon MA, Alves B, Jacobson M, et al. Allergen injection immunotherapy for seasonal allergic rhinitis. Cochrane Database Syst Rev 2007;1:CD001936.
11. Senna G, Ridolo E, Calderon M, et al. Evidence of adherence to allergen-specific immunotherapy. Curr Opin Allergy Clin Immunol 2009;9(6):544–8.
12. Mitragotri S. Immunization without needles. Nat Rev Immunol 2005;5(12):905–16.
13. Senti G, Freiburghaus AU, Kundig TM. Epicutaneous/transcutaneous allergen-specific immunotherapy: rationale and clinical trials. Curr Opin Allergy Clin Immunol 2010;10(6):582–6.
14. Senti G, Johansen P, Kundig TM. Intralymphatic immunotherapy. Curr Opin Allergy Clin Immunol 2009;9(6):537–43.
15. Cox LS, Larenas Linnemann D, Nolte H, et al. Sublingual immunotherapy: a comprehensive review. J Allergy Clin Immunol 2006;117(5):1021–35.
16. Zinkernagel RM, Ehl S, Aichele P, et al. Antigen localisation regulates immune responses in a dose- and time-dependent fashion: a geographical view of immune reactivity. Immunol Rev 1997;156:199–209.
17. Zinkernagel RM. Localization dose and time of antigens determine immune reactivity. Semin Immunol 2000;12(3):163–71 [discussion: 257–344].
18. Junt T, Scandella E, Ludewig B. Form follows function: lymphoid tissue micro-architecture in antimicrobial immune defence. Nat Rev Immunol 2008;8(10): 764–75.
19. Karrer U, Althage A, Odermatt B, et al. On the key role of secondary lymphoid organs in antiviral immune responses studied in alymphoplastic (aly/aly) and spleenless (Hox11(−)/−) mutant mice. J Exp Med 1997;185(12):2157–70.
20. Barker CF, Billingham RE. The role of afferent lymphatics in the rejection of skin homografts. J Exp Med 1968;128(1):197–221.
21. Bachmann MF, Jennings GT. Vaccine delivery: a matter of size, geometry, kinetics and molecular patterns. Nat Rev Immunol 2010;10(11):787–96.
22. Randolph GJ, Angeli V, Swartz MA. Dendritic-cell trafficking to lymph nodes through lymphatic vessels. Nat Rev Immunol 2005;5(8):617–28.
23. Matzinger P. Friendly and dangerous signals: is the tissue in control? Nat Immunol 2007;8(1):11–3.
24. Iwasaki A, Kelsall BL. Freshly isolated Peyer's patch, but not spleen, dendritic cells produce interleukin 10 and induce the differentiation of T helper type 2 cells. J Exp Med 1999;190(2):229–39.
25. Everson MP, Lemak DG, McDuffie DS, et al. Dendritic cells from Peyer's patch and spleen induce different T helper cell responses. J Interferon Cytokine Res 1998;18(2):103–15.
26. Matzinger P. The danger model: a renewed sense of self. Science 2002; 296(5566):301–5.
27. Martinez-Gomez JM, Johansen P, Erdmann I, et al. Intralymphatic injections as a new administration route for allergen-specific immunotherapy. Int Arch Allergy Immunol 2009;150(1):59–65.

28. Junt T, Tumanov AV, Harris N, et al. Expression of lymphotoxin beta governs immunity at two distinct levels. Eur J Immunol 2006;36(8):2061–75.

29. Senti G, Prinz Vavricka BM, Erdmann I, et al. Intralymphatic allergen administration renders specific immunotherapy faster and safer: a randomized controlled trial. Proc Natl Acad Sci U S A 2008;105(46):17908–12.

30. Juillard GJ, Boyer PJ. Intralymphatic immunization: current status. Eur J Cancer 1977;13(4-5):439–40.

31. Kundig TM, Bachmann MF, DiPaolo C, et al. Fibroblasts as efficient antigen-presenting cells in lymphoid organs. Science 1995;268(5215):1343–7.

32. Ochsenbein AF, Sierro S, Odermatt B, et al. Roles of tumour localization, second signals and cross priming in cytotoxic T-cell induction. Nature 2001;411(6841): 1058–64.

33. Smith KA, Tam VL, Wong RM, et al. Enhancing DNA vaccination by sequential injection of lymph nodes with plasmid vectors and peptides. Vaccine 2009; 27(19):2603–15.

34. Weber J, Boswell W, Smith J, et al. Phase 1 trial of intranodal injection of a Melan-A/MART-1 DNA plasmid vaccine in patients with stage IV melanoma. J Immunother 2008;31(2):215–23.

35. Kreiter S, Selmi A, Diken M, et al. Intranodal vaccination with naked antigen-encoding RNA elicits potent prophylactic and therapeutic antitumoral immunity. Cancer Res 2010;70(22):9031–40.

36. Lehner T, Wang YF, Cranage M, et al. Protective mucosal immunity elicited by targeted iliac lymph node immunization with a subunit SIV envelope and core vaccine in macaques. Nat Med 1996;2(7):767–75.

37. Finerty S, Stokes CR, Gruffydd-Jones TJ, et al. Targeted lymph node immunization can protect cats from a mucosal challenge with feline immunodeficiency virus. Vaccine 2001;20(1/2):49–58.

38. Crameri R, Fluckiger S, Daigle I, et al. Design, engineering and in vitro evaluation of MHC class-II targeting allergy vaccines. Allergy 2007;62(2):197–206.

39. Rhyner C, Kundig T, Akdis CA, et al. Targeting the MHC II presentation pathway in allergy vaccine development. Biochem Soc Trans 2007;35(Pt 4):833–4.

40. Martinez-Gomez JM, Johansen P, Rose H, et al. Targeting the MHC class II pathway of antigen presentation enhances immunogenicity and safety of allergen immunotherapy. Allergy 2009;64(1):172–8.

41. Kupper TS, Fuhlbrigge RC. Immune surveillance in the skin: mechanisms and clinical consequences. Nat Rev Immunol 2004;4(3):211–22.

42. Nestle FO, Di Meglio P, Qin JZ, et al. Skin immune sentinels in health and disease. Nat Rev Immunol 2009;9(10):679–91.

43. Bal SM, Ding Z, van Riet E, et al. Advances in transcutaneous vaccine delivery: Do all ways lead to Rome? J Control Release 2010;148(3):266–82.

44. Bos JD, Meinardi MM. The 500 Dalton rule for the skin penetration of chemical compounds and drugs. Exp Dermatol 2000;9(3):165–9.

45. Babiuk S, Baca-Estrada M, Babiuk LA, et al. Cutaneous vaccination: the skin as an immunologically active tissue and the challenge of antigen delivery. J Control Release 2000;66(2/3):199–214.

46. Merad M, Ginhoux F, Collin M. Origin, homeostasis and function of Langerhans cells and other langerin-expressing dendritic cells. Nat Rev Immunol 2008;8(12):935–47.

47. Streilein JW. Skin-associated lymphoid tissues (SALT): origins and functions. J Invest Dermatol 1983;80(Suppl):12s–6s.

48. Kapsenberg ML. Dendritic-cell control of pathogen-driven T-cell polarization. Nat Rev Immunol 2003;3(12):984–93.

49. Ueno H, Schmitt N, Klechevsky E, et al. Harnessing human dendritic cell subsets for medicine. Immunol Rev 2010;234(1):199–212.

50. Klechevsky E, Morita R, Liu M, et al. Functional specializations of human epidermal Langerhans cells and CD14+ dermal dendritic cells. Immunity 2008; 29(3):497–510.

51. Kissenpfennig A, Henri S, Dubois B, et al. Dynamics and function of Langerhans cells in vivo: dermal dendritic cells colonize lymph node areas distinct from slower migrating Langerhans cells. Immunity 2005;22(5):643–54.

52. Swamy M, Jamora C, Havran W, et al. Epithelial decision makers: in search of the 'epimmunome'. Nat Immunol 2010;11(8):656–65.

53. Senti G, Graf N, Haug S, et al. Epicutaneous allergen administration as a novel method of allergen-specific immunotherapy. J Allergy Clin Immunol 2009; 124(5):997–1002.

54. Frerichs DM, Ellingsworth LR, Frech SA, et al. Controlled, single-step, stratum corneum disruption as a pretreatment for immunization via a patch. Vaccine 2008;26(22):2782–7.

55. Frech SA, Dupont HL, Bourgeois AL, et al. Use of a patch containing heat-labile toxin from *Escherichia coli* against travellers' diarrhoea: a phase II, randomised, double-blind, placebo-controlled field trial. Lancet 2008;371(9629):2019–25.

56. Sullivan SP, Koutsonanos DG, Del Pilar Martin M, et al. Dissolving polymer microneedle patches for influenza vaccination. Nat Med 2010;16(8):915–20.

57. Wood LC, Jackson SM, Elias PM, et al. Cutaneous barrier perturbation stimulates cytokine production in the epidermis of mice. J Clin Invest 1992;90(2):482–7.

58. Tan G, Xu P, Lawson LB, et al. Hydration effects on skin microstructure as probed by high-resolution cryo-scanning electron microscopy and mechanistic implications to enhanced transcutaneous delivery of biomacromolecules. J Pharm Sci 2010;99(2):730–40.

59. Mondoulet L, Dioszeghy V, Ligouis M, et al. Epicutaneous immunotherapy on intact skin using a new delivery system in a murine model of allergy. Clin Exp Allergy 2010;40(4):659–67.

60. Dupont C, Kalach N, Soulaines P, et al. Cow's milk epicutaneous immunotherapy in children: a pilot trial of safety, acceptability, and impact on allergic reactivity. J Allergy Clin Immunol 2010;125(5):1165–7.

61. Eyler JM. Smallpox in history: the birth, death, and impact of a dread disease. J Lab Clin Med 2003;142(4):216–20.

62. Jodar L, Duclos P, Milstien JB, et al. Ensuring vaccine safety in immunization programmes—a WHO perspective. Vaccine 2001;19(13–14):1594–605.

63. Glenn GM, Taylor DN, Li X, et al. Transcutaneous immunization: a human vaccine delivery strategy using a patch. Nat Med 2000;6(12):1403–6.

64. Frech SA, Kenney RT, Spyr CA, et al. Improved immune responses to influenza vaccination in the elderly using an immunostimulant patch. Vaccine 2005;23(7): 946–50.

65. Stoitzner P, Sparber F, Tripp CH. Langerhans cells as targets for immunotherapy against skin cancer. Immunol Cell Biol 2010;88(4):431–7.

66. Yagi H, Hashizume H, Horibe T, et al. Induction of therapeutically relevant cytotoxic T lymphocytes in humans by percutaneous peptide immunization. Cancer Res 2006;66(20):10136–44.

67. Freeman J. Further observations on the treatment of hay fever by hypodermic inoculations of pollen vaccine. Lancet 1911;178(4594):814–7.

68. Hurwitz SH. Medicine: seasonal hay fever—some problems in treatment. Cal West Med 1930;33(1):520–1.

69. Phillips EW. Relief of hay-fever by intradermal injections of pollen extract. J Am Med Assoc 1926;86(3):182–4.
70. Vallery-Radot P, Hangenau J. Asthme d'origine équine. Essai de désensibilisation par des cutiréactions répétées. Bull Soc Méd Hôp Paris 1921;45:1251–60 [in French].
71. New York Academy of Medicine, Graduate F, Amberson JB. Diseases of the respiratory tract: Eighth Annual Graduate Fortnight of the New York Academy of Medicine. Philadelphia: W.B. Saunders; 1936. London.
72. Pautrizel R, Cabanieu G, Bricaud H, et al. Allergenic group specificity and therapeutic consequences in asthma; specific desensitization method by epicutaneous route. Sem Hop 1957;33(22):1394–403 [in French].
73. Blamoutier P, Blamoutier J, Guibert L. Treatment of pollinosis with pollen extracts by the method of cutaneous quadrille ruling. Presse Med 1959;67:2299–301 [in French].
74. Blamoutier P, Blamoutier J, Guibert L. Traitement co-saisonnier de la pollinose par l'application d'extraits de pollens sur des quadrillages cutanés: Résultats obtenus en 1959 et 1960. Revue francaise d'allergie 1961;1(2):112–20 [in French].
75. Eichenberger H, Storck H. Co-seasonal desensitization of pollinosis with the scarification-method of Blamoutier. Acta Allergol 1966;21(3):261–7.
76. Palma-Carlos AG. Traitement co-saisonnier des pollinoses au Portugal par la méthode des quadrillages cutanés. Revue Francaise d'Allergie 1967;7(2):92–5 [in French].
77. Martin-DuPan RBF, Neyroud M. Treatment of pollen allergy using the cutaneous checker square method of Blamoutier and Guilbert. Schweiz Rundsch Med Prax 1971;60(44):1469–72.
78. Dickel H, Goulioumis A, Gambichler T, et al. Standardized tape stripping: a practical and reproducible protocol to uniformly reduce the stratum corneum. Skin Pharmacol Physiol 2010;23(5):259–65.
79. Nickoloff BJ, Naidu Y. Perturbation of epidermal barrier function correlates with initiation of cytokine cascade in human skin. J Am Acad Dermatol 1994;30(4):535–46.
80. Dickel H, Gambichler T, Kamphowe J, et al. Standardized tape stripping prior to patch testing induces upregulation of Hsp90, Hsp70, IL-33, TNF-alpha and IL-8/CXCL8 mRNA: new insights into the involvement of 'alarmins'. Contact Dermatitis 2010;63(4):215–22.
81. Agostinis F, Forti S, Di Berardino F. Grass transcutaneous immunotherapy in children with seasonal rhinoconjunctivitis. Allergy 2010;65(3):410–1.
82. Turjanmaa K, Darsow U, Niggemann B, et al. EAACI/GA2LEN position paper: present status of the atopy patch test. Allergy 2006;61(12):1377–84.
83. Mondoulet L, Dioszeghy V, Vanoirbeek JA, et al. Epicutaneous immunotherapy using a new epicutaneous delivery system in mice sensitized to peanuts. Int Arch Allergy Immunol 2010;154(4):299–309.
84. Soury D, Barratt G, Ah-Leung S, et al. Skin localization of cow's milk proteins delivered by a new ready-to-use atopy patch test. Pharm Res 2005;22(9):1530–6.
85. Werfel T. Epicutaneous allergen administration: a novel approach for allergen-specific immunotherapy? J Allergy Clin Immunol 2009;124(5):1003–4.
86. Harris MC. HAY FEVER—a comparative clinical evaluation of treatment with aqueous pollen extracts, alum-precipitated pyridine pollen extracts and aqueous pollen in oil emulsions. Calif Med 1962;97(5):286–90.
87. Scharton-Kersten T, Yu J, Vassell R, et al. Transcutaneous immunization with bacterial ADP-ribosylating exotoxins, subunits, and unrelated adjuvants. Infect Immun 2000;68(9):5306–13.

88. Glenn GM, Rao M, Matyas GR, et al. Skin immunization made possible by cholera toxin. Nature 1998;391(6670):851.

89. Rechtsteiner G, Warger T, Osterloh P, et al. Cutting edge: priming of CTL by trans-cutaneous peptide immunization with imiquimod. J Immunol 2005;174(5): 2476–80.

90. Beignon AS, Briand JP, Muller S, et al. Immunization onto bare skin with synthetic peptides: immunomodulation with a CpG-containing oligodeoxynucleotide and effective priming of influenza virus-specific CD4+ T cells. Immunology 2002; 105(2):204–12.

91. Hankin CS, Cox L, Lang D, et al. Allergen immunotherapy and health care cost benefits for children with allergic rhinitis: a large-scale, retrospective, matched cohort study. Ann Allergy Asthma Immunol 2010;104(1):79–85.

92. Jacobsen L, Niggemann B, Dreborg S, et al. Specific immunotherapy has long-term preventive effect of seasonal and perennial asthma: 10-year follow-up on the PAT study. Allergy 2007;62(8):943–8.

93. Braman SS. The global burden of asthma. Chest 2006;130(Suppl 1):4S–12S.

Adjuvants and Vector Systems for Allergy Vaccines

Philippe Moingeon, PhD*, Vincent Lombardi, PhD,
Nathalie Saint-Lu, PhD, Sophie Tourdot, PhD,
Véronique Bodo, PhD, Laurent Mascarell, PhD

KEYWORDS

- Adjuvants • Allergy vaccine • Immunopotentiation
- Immunotherapy • Mucosal immunity • Vector system

Allergen-specific immunotherapy is currently the only curative treatment of type I allergies, with a unique capacity to reorient inappropriate humoral and cellular immune responses from a Th2 to a mixed Th1/T regulatory cell (Treg) pattern.[1] Following the pioneer studies by Noon and colleagues[2,3] a century ago, allergen-specific subcutaneous immunotherapy (SCIT) was established as an effective treatment of respiratory and venom allergies.[4,5] Although SCIT has been performed with soluble allergens in the United States, in most circumstances preparations combining allergen extracts with adjuvants such as aluminum hydroxide or calcium phosphate are being used in Europe.[6,7] This article reviews other adjuvants that are being investigated with the aim of reducing the number of injections needed for desensitization.

More recently, noninvasive mucosal routes of administration have been explored as an alternative to SCIT, most particularly sublingual immunotherapy (SLIT).[8] SLIT was first investigated more than 15 years ago in patients with respiratory allergies.[9–11] In this approach, the allergen extract is kept under the tongue for at least 1 to 2 minutes, to allow capture by oral dendritic cells before being swallowed. SLIT significantly reduces rhinoconjunctivitis symptoms as well as symptomatic medication uptake in patients allergic to grass, tree pollens, or house dust mites (HDM).[9–11] SLIT has mostly been conducted with allergen extracts presented as either drops or, more recently, as solid tablets. In all circumstances, high doses (usually 50–100 times the doses used for SCIT) of the allergen(s) are needed to reach clinical efficacy because SLIT is performed in the absence of any immunopotentiator.[9]

Irrespective of the route of immunization used, allergy vaccines currently available are based on either natural or modified allergen extracts, but second-generation

Research and Development, Stallergènes, 6 rue Alexis de Tocqueville, 92160 Antony, France
* Corresponding author.
E-mail address: pmoingeon@stallergenes.fr

treatments relying on recombinant proteins are being developed.[12] Given that such highly purified proteins are usually poorly immunogenic, those vaccines require new antigen presentation platforms. In this context, novel adjuvants and vector systems are needed to further improve the efficacy of subcutaneous and sublingual allergy vaccines.[13,14] Although an intrinsic adjuvant activity can be associated with the allergen itself (eg, Th2-inducing activity ascribed to Der p 1, natural adjuvants present in allergen extracts),[15–17] this review only focuses on biologic or synthetic candidate adjuvants, as well as vector systems to be used in combination with the allergen(s).

MECHANISMS OF ALLERGEN-SPECIFIC IMMUNOTHERAPY: IMPLICATIONS FOR SELECTING ADJUVANTS AND VECTOR SYSTEMS

Both SCIT and SLIT are associated with a decrease in serum allergen-specific immunoglobulin E (IgE) concomitantly with an upregulation of immunoglobulin G (IgG), most particularly IgG1 and IgG4s,[18–20] some of which may exhibit a potential blocking activity.[21,22] Such changes in the antibody balance are believed to downregulate IgE-mediated histamine release by basophils and mast cells but also to decrease IgE-mediated antigen presentation to CD4$^+$ T lymphocytes.[18–20] In a limited number of studies, an increase in allergen-specific immunoglobulin A (IgA) antibodies has also been documented in serum as well as in mucosal tissues, at least for SLIT.[23,24] Successful immunotherapy also inhibits the recruitment and activation of proinflammatory cells, such as mast cells, basophils, and eosinophils in the skin, as well as nasal or bronchial mucosae.[25–27]

In the current model of allergen-specific immunotherapy, a prominent role is attributed to CD4+ T lymphocytes in controlling the various immune effector mechanisms contributing to allergic inflammation.[18,27,28] Although allergic patients mount allergen-specific Th2 responses associated with the secretion of interleukin (IL)-4, IL-5, and IL-13 cytokines by CD4+ T cells, subcutaneous immunotherapy has been shown to redirect those allergen-specific T cell responses toward both (1) a Th1 type with an increased production of interferon-γ (IFNγ) within the blood and target organs (immunodeviation),[26,29] and (2) CD4+ Tregs capable of downregulating Th2 responses through the production of IL-10 and/or transforming growth factor β (TGFβ), or following cell-cell contact (immunosuppression).[28,30,31]

Recent studies confirmed that SLIT also induces IFNγ-producing Th1 cells as well as IL-10 or TGFβ-secreting Tregs.[27,31–34] The observed bias of the oral immune system toward tolerance induction as opposed to proinflammatory responses is explained by the peculiar tolerogenic phenotype of oral dendritic cells (DCs) observed both in murine and humans.[35–37] Specifically, 3 predominant subsets of oral DC have been described including (1) Langerhans cells found in the mucosa itself, (2) myeloid DCs along the lamina propria, and (3) plasmacytoid DCs located within subepithelial tissues.[37] All those DC subsets are prone to produce IL-10, IL-12, and possibly TGFβ in the presence of the allergen, thus supporting mixed Th1/regulatory CD4$^+$ T cell responses in draining cervical lymph nodes.[35–37] Those DCs express high levels of Toll-like receptors (TLR) such as TLR2 and TLR4, allowing modulation of the function of those cells using specific ligands.[35,37]

Based on our current understanding of immune mechanisms leading to tolerance in the course of immunotherapy, appropriate adjuvants and/or vector systems likely to enhance the efficacy of allergy vaccines include the following:

1. Synthetic or biologic adjuvants providing cosignals to immune cells, most particularly antigen-presenting cells (APCs). Such immunopotentiators should ideally reinforce allergen-specific Th1 and/or Treg responses (**Table 1**)

Table 1
Adjuvants for allergy vaccines

Immunomodulators	Comments	References
Mineral adjuvants	Aluminum hydroxide and calcium phosphate are commonly used as adjuvants in subcutaneous allergy vaccines. They work through both a depot effect (ie, slow release of the allergen, presentation as particles to target APCs) as well as an interaction with the innate immune system (eg, activation of the inflammasome)	7,13,38
Probiotics	In mice, mucosal (ie, intranasal or sublingual) administration of commensal bacteria such as *Lactococcus lactis*, *Lactobacillus plantarum* or *Bifidobacterium bifidum* together with the allergen(s) induces Th1 and/or Tregs as well as asthma improvement. Efficacious probiotics seem to interact with DCsign3 and may exhibit specific forms of teichoic acids in their wall composition, thus inducing a strong IL-10 production by immune cells. In humans, selected probiotics used as a stand-alone therapy were shown to protect children against eczema, in link with the induction of Th1 responses	39–44
Attenuated mycobacteria	In mice, heat-killed *Mycobacterium vaccae* induces Treg cells secreting IL-10 and TGFβ, conferring protection against airway inflammation. Some efficacy has also been observed in children with atopic dermatitis or asthma after intradermal administration of *M vaccae* or BCG. No synergy has been observed in humans between BCG and SLIT when using distinct administration sites	45–51
Bacterial toxins (CT, LT, CTB, LTB)	Genetically detoxified CT and LT (or B subunits without ADP-ribosyl transferase activity) retain a strong capacity to induce serum and mucosal IgA responses. The antigen/allergen can be mixed, fused, or chemically conjugated with the toxin moiety. In mice, sublingual administration of the allergen conjugated to CTB enhances tolerance induction	52,53
TLR ligands	Ligands for TLR2 (including lipopeptides, Pam3csk4), TLR4 (MPL, RC 529, OM-294-BA-MP), TLR7 (imidazoquinolines), TLR9 (CpGs) have shown some efficacy in murine models (decrease of both airway inflammation and Th2 responses, with induction of Th1 and/or Treg responses). Synthetic oligonucleotides containing CpG motifs (CpG ODN) are potent Th1 adjuvants via both the systemic and mucosal routes. Intradermal immunization with Amb a 1 fused to CpG oligonucleotides prevents allergen-induced hyperresponsiveness in mice. In humans, grass pollen allergens combined with MPL induce a strong production of specific IgG1 and IgG4 antibodies through the subcutaneous route. MPL is sometimes associated with tyrosine-absorbed glutaraldehyde modified allergen extracts. Following SLIT in grass pollen allergic patients, MPL enhanced specific IgG responses and decreased reactivity to nasal allergen challenge. A conjugate Amb a1-CpG vaccine has been tested in ragweed allergic humans through the subcutaneous route, with some level of clinical efficacy. The effect of CpG is believed to be associated with the induction of stronger Th1 responses, and possibly CD25+ Treg cells	54–63 64–68
Small synthetic molecules	In murine models, dihydroxyvitamin D_3 plus glucocorticoids, calcineurin inhibitors (cyclosporin A, FK 506), rapamycin, aspirin, and mycophenolate mofetil all enhance IL-10 production by CD4+ T cells. Dexamethasone plus dihydroxyvitamin D_3 enhance SLIT efficacy in a murine asthma model when combined with the allergen. No synergy was observed between fluticasone and SLIT in humans when using distinct administration routes	69–77

Abbreviations: BCG, bacille Calmette-Guérin; CT, cholera toxin; CTB, cholera toxin B subunit; LT, lymphotoxin; LTB, lymphotoxin subunit B; MPL, monophosphoryl lipid A; SLIT, sublingual immunotherapy.

2. Vector systems targeting the allergen to tolerogenic APCs. Specifically, mucoadhesive particulate vector systems seem well adapted to the sublingual (and other mucosal) routes where they enhance the duration of contact between the allergen(s) and the mucosa. Furthermore, presenting the allergen as a particle significantly improves the uptake by dendritic cells and macrophages with phagocytic activity (**Table 2**).

POTENTIAL ADJUVANTS AND VECTOR SYSTEMS FOR ALLERGY VACCINES
Adjuvants/Vector Systems for the Subcutaneous (and Other Parenteral) Routes

Preclinical studies

Mineral adjuvant molecules (eg, calcium phosphate or aluminum hydroxide) are well established as adjuvants for subcutaneous allergic vaccines (see **Table 1**).[7,13] Although aluminum salts activate the inflammasome and, as such, are broadly used by the vaccine industry to elicit proinflammatory responses, it is also clear that alum decreases established Th2 responses.[7] In addition to these mineral adjuvants, numerous candidate immunopotentiators have been shown in murine models to downregulate Th2 responses via parenteral routes (see **Table 1**). For example, in murine models of asthma, living or heat-killed bacteria (eg, *Lactobacillus plantarum*, *Lactococcus lactis*, *Mycobacterium vaccae*) as well as TLR ligands (eg, monophosphoryl lipid A [MPL], imidazoquinolines, CpGs) showed clear benefits when used as adjuvants.[45,54–57] The active 1,25-dihydroxy vitamin D_3 metabolite increased the effect of immunotherapy in a mouse asthma model, following induction of IL-10 and TGFβ by immune cells.[69]

Various vector systems have also been considered to target allergens to dendritic cells (see **Table 2**). For example, plasmid DNA or DNA absorbed on microparticles markedly enhance systemic and mucosal immune responses following injection.[82] In addition, fusion proteins combining the Fel d 1 allergen and the Fcγ immunoglobulin fragment have been designed. Those bifunctional molecules coengage FcεRI and FcγRII receptors, thus preventing acute reactivity to Fel d 1.[93] A recombinant fusion protein associating Bet v 1 to the bacterial S layer protein SbpA was also shown to form particles and, as a consequence, to facilitate allergen capture by APCs with subsequent induction of Th1 and Tregs.[94]

Human studies

Some new adjuvants are also being explored in humans to potentiate antigen-specific Th1 or Treg responses during SCIT (see **Table 1**). For example, the Th1 adjuvant MPL has been tested via the subcutaneous route in association with a grass pollen vaccine, with evidence for enhanced specific IgG1 and IgG4 responses leading to a potential reduction in number of preseasonal injections needed to reduce allergic symptoms.[64,65] Also, a synthetic CpG oligonucleotide (known to represent a powerful Th1 adjuvant) conjugated with purified natural Amb a 1 was shown to improve symptoms in patients with ragweed pollen allergy.[66] Administration of oral steroids (prednisone) with or without vitamin D_3 had no beneficial effect on SCIT efficacy in asthmatic children allergic to HDM.[70] In this study, a potential immunosuppressive effect of prednisone was corrected by vitamin D_3.

For vectors tested in humans via parental routes, nonreplicating viruslike particles (VLPs) generated by the spontaneous assembly of viral capsid proteins also represent an attractive alternative to express either the whole antigen/allergen, or adjuvants such as CpG oligonucleotides.[85–88] Specifically, a recombinant fusion protein associating a peptide derived from Phl p 1 with a rhinovirus-derived VP1 protein has been designed as a candidate vaccine for grass pollen allergies.[85] Association of

Table 2
Vector systems for allergy vaccines

Vectors/Delivery Systems	Comments	References
Liposomes, virosomes	Lipid-based vehicles such as liposomes can incorporate functional viral envelope proteins (leading to virosomes). Mucosal administration of such particulate antigen formulations increases specific IgG and IgA antibodies. Nasal administration of plasmid DNA complexes formulated with cationic lipids induces specific secretory IgA antibodies in the mucosa as well as serum IgG and IgA antibodies. Intranasal immunization with the antigen formulated in liposomes together with immunopotentiators (eg, LPS, MPL, or LTB) induces strong systemic and mucosal responses (with IgG and IgA in the lung and the nose).	77–79
ISCOMs	These spherical particles (30–100 nm diameter) comprise the saponin-adjuvant Quil A, cholesterol, and phospholipids mixed with the antigen. ISCOMs induce a strong systemic and mucosal Th1 adjuvant activity. ISCOM particles target both the endosomal and cytosolic compartments, thus leading to class I and class II restricted antigen presentation to T cells.	80,81
PLGA	Poly (D,L) lactic-co-glycolic acid can be used to form nanoparticles or microparticles to present the antigen/allergen, thus facilitating APC capture. Subcutaneous administration in mice of PLGA-Bet v 1 induced IgG2, Th1 and Treg responses while preventing hypersensitivity to Bet v 1	82–84
VLPs	VLPs are formed following the spontaneous assembly of capsid proteins. VLPs stimulate both humoral and cellular immune responses, leading to systemic and mucosal responses in mice and in humans. Potential VLP delivery systems include the porcine parvovirus, Norwalk virus as well as human papilloma viruses, which specifically target immature DCs. VLPs made from the $Q\beta$ phage proteins have been successfully tested in humans with mite allergies in association with the Der p 1 allergen or a CpG adjuvant	78,85–89
Carbohydrate-particles	Particles made of synthetic polymers represent a powerful means to address the antigen/allergen onto phagocytic APCs. Nanoparticles or microparticles made of maltodextrin or chitosan polymers have been shown in murine models to improve targeting of the allergen onto oral DCs and enhance tolerance induction following sublingual administration	14,23,90–92
DC targeting vectors	In mice, anti-DEC-205 antibodies coupled to ovalbumin target the antigen to DCs and induce strong specific T cell responses. Antigens coupled to kpOmpA target CD11+c mucosal (eg, nasal) DCs through Toll-like receptor 2. CyaA from *Bordetella pertussis* binds specifically to CD11b and as such has been used to target the allergen to oral DCs, thus enhancing tolerance induction via the sublingual route in a murine asthma model. STxB also targets DCs, leading to strong specific Th1 and humoral responses. Fusion proteins assembling allergens with Ig FcRs or with S layer bacterial product also enhance capture by human dendritic cells.	93–99
Plasmid DNA	Plasmid DNA has been used in preclinical models, both via parenteral and mucosal routes, alone or adsorbed on microparticles	82,100

Abbreviations: CyaA, adenylate cyclase; DC, dendritic cell; FcR, Fc fragment; ISCOMs, immunostimulating complexes; kpOmpA, outer membrane protein A from *Klebsiella pneumoniae*; LPS, lipopolysaccharide; PLGA, D,L-lactic-co-glycolic acid; STxB, shiga toxin B subunit; VLP, viruslike particle.

Fel d 1 to VLPs prevents allergenicity and enhances its capacity to elicit protective IgGs.[86] Recently, VLPs made from capsid proteins obtained from the Qβ phage coupled to a Der p 1–derived peptide were shown to be highly immunogenic in healthy volunteers,[87] with the induction of strong IgG responses after a single injection. When tested in mite allergic patients, QβG10 VLPs containing a synthetic oligonucleotide as a Th1 adjuvant significantly decreased rhinoconjunctivitis and asthma symptoms after 6 weekly injections.[88] Fusion of the Fel d 1 allergen to a modular antigen transporter (MAT) facilitates capture, processing, and efficient presentation of the allergen by APCs in association with major histocompatibility complex (MHC) class II molecules.[78] This vaccine is currently considered for clinical evaluation in humans. Other potential particulate allergen formulations that could be tested in humans include liposomes, virosomes, D,L-lactic-co-glycolic acid (PLGA), or immunostimulating complexes (ISCOMS).[80,83]

Adjuvants/Vector Systems for the Sublingual (and Other Mucosal) Route(s)

Preclinical studies

Mucosal adjuvants tested in murine models to modulate T cell polarization include bacterial toxins, such as cholera toxin (CT) and the closely related *Escherichia coli* heat-labile enterotoxin (LT), as well as their nontoxic derivatives (ie, genetically detoxified forms or B subunits without ADP-ribosyl transferase activity) (see **Table 1**). These bacterial toxins can be coadministered as a mix, conjugated or fused with soluble antigens/allergens.[52,53] Triggering TLR2 or TLR4 with either Pam3CSK4 or biologic/synthetic lipid A analogues (eg, MPL and OM-294-BA-MP), respectively, has proved effective in inducing Th1 and Treg responses via the nasal or sublingual routes.[58–61] Similarly, synthetic drugs (eg, glucocorticoids plus 1,25-dihydroxy vitamin D_3) also represent potential Treg adjuvants for sublingual immunotherapy because they are powerful inducers of IL-10 production by immune cells, such as dendritic cells and $CD4^+$ T lymphocytes.[71] Both glucocorticoids and vitamin D_3 inhibit the maturation of monocyte-derived DC, as shown by an impaired upregulation of costimulatory and MHC molecules and a diminished capacity to stimulate allogeneic T cells.[71–75] Other potential adjuvants for the sublingual (and other mucosal) routes include probiotics selected for their capacity to induce a strong IL-10 and IL-12 production by mucosal DCs. In this regard, a combination of the allergen with either *L plantarum* or *Bifidobacterium bifidum* strains enhances both allergen-specific Th1 and Treg responses as well as tolerance induction via the sublingual route.[39,71] In murine asthma models, pure Th1 adjuvants do not promote significant tolerance induction during SLIT.[39,71]

Vector systems considered for mucosal routes should protect the allergen(s) from degradation by local proteases while targeting mucosal APCs (see **Table 2**). To this end, bacterial subunits such as the outer membrane protein A from *Klebsiella pneumoniae* (OmpA) or the shiga toxin B subunit have been conjugated to antigens/allergens to target APCs (see **Table 2**).[95–97] Among those, the adenylate cyclase protein from *Bordetella pertussis* conjugated to ovalbumin (OVA) has been shown to enhance tolerance induction during SLIT in mice with OVA-induced asthma, as a consequence of a specific addressing of the allergen to oral CD11b+ tolerogenic myeloid DCs.[37,98] In addition, positively charged carbohydrate polymers have been used to generate mucoadhesive particles capable of binding efficiently to negatively charged epithelial cells, thus enhancing the duration of allergen contact with the mucosa.[23] The advantage of particulate formulations such as nanoparticles made from polymerized maltodextrin or chitosan-based microparticles is to enhance in vitro and in vivo uptake of the allergen(s) by dendritic cells, thus resulting in superior tolerance induction via the sublingual route when administered to asthmatic mice (see **Table 2**).[23,90]

Human studies

In recent years, the use of selected lactic acid bacterial strains in the prevention of allergy has also been suggested in humans (see **Table 1**). For example, oral administration of lactic acid bacteria led to reduced atopic dermatitis in children with a positive family history of type I allergy,[40] suggesting that such probiotics could also be used as adjuvants for mucosal vaccines. However, to date, no probiotics have been administered jointly with the allergen in allergic patients. The Th1 adjuvant MPL has been tested in grass pollen allergic patients through the sublingual route.[67] When used at a high dose, MPL enhanced specific IgG responses and reduced reactivity to a subsequent nasal allergen challenge (see **Table 1**). Bacille Calmette-Guérin (BCG) has also been tested in children asthmatic to mite allergens in association with SLIT, with no effect on clinical outcome.[46] One drawback in the latter study is that the adjuvant was administered via the intradermal route, whereas allergens were given sublingually. No vector systems have been tested to improve allergen delivery via the sublingual route in humans, but maltodextrin-based mucoadhesive nanoparticles have been shown to elicit strong mucosal IgA responses when administered intranasally as part of an experimental flu vaccine (see **Table 2**).

SUMMARY

A better understanding of immune mechanisms involved in the induction and maintenance of antigen-specific immune tolerance provides opportunities to design and develop appropriate adjuvants and vector systems leading to improved allergy vaccines. A guiding hypothesis in this regard is that allergy vaccines should induce both allergen-specific Th1 as well as regulatory CD4$^+$ T lymphocytes able to produce suppressive cytokines (eg, IL-10 and/or TGFβ). Identifying appropriate allergen presentation platforms could help increase the clinical efficacy of allergy vaccines and simplify immunization schemes. In addition, an expected benefit of adjuvants and vector systems modulating/targeting appropriate immune cells is to help lower the allergen dose, thus improving the safety profile. Ample evidence is now available confirming that multiple adjuvants are efficacious in murine allergy models, via both systemic and mucosal routes. Some of those adjuvants (eg, MPL, CpGs) have been shown to enhance Th1 responses in humans, but their effect on clinical efficacy remains to be firmly established. With respect to vector systems, viruslike particles represent a promising platform to present allergens and/or adjuvants to the immune system, with encouraging results obtained during SCIT of mite allergic patients. Mucoadhesive particulate vectors seem most particularly suitable to develop a new generation of safer and more efficient allergy vaccines to be administered via mucosal (ie, sublingual) routes.

REFERENCES

1. Bousquet J, Lockey R, Malling HJ. Allergen immunotherapy: therapeutic vaccines for allergic diseases. A WHO position paper. J Allergy Clin Immunol 1998;102:558–62.
2. Noon L. Prophylactic inoculation against hay fever. Lancet 1911;2:1572–3.
3. Freeman J. Further observations on the treatment of hay fever by hypodermic inoculations of pollen vaccine. Lancet 1911;2:814–7.
4. Cox L, Li JT, Nelson HS, et al. Allergen immunotherapy: a practice parameter second update. J Allergy Clin Immunol 2007;120:25–85.

5. Durham SR, Walker SM, Varga E, et al. Long term clinical efficacy of grass pollen immunotherapy. N Engl J Med 1999;341:468–75.

6. Bousquet J, Van Cauwenberge P, Khaltaev N. Allergic rhinitis and its impact on asthma. J Allergy Clin Immunol 2001;108:S147–334.

7. Wilcock LK, Francis JN, Durham SR. Aluminium hydroxide down-regulates T helper 2 responses by allergen-stimulated human peripheral blood mononuclear cells. Clin Exp Allergy 2004;34:1373–8.

8. Mascarell L, Van Overtvelt L, Moingeon P. Novel ways for immune intervention in immunotherapy: mucosal allergy vaccines. Immunol Allergy Clin North Am 2006;26:283–306.

9. Canonica GW, Bousquet J, Casale T, et al. Sub-lingual immunotherapy: World Allergy Organization Position Paper 2009. Allergy 2009;64(Suppl 91):1–59.

10. Wilson DR, Torres LI, Durham SR. Sublingual immunotherapy for allergic rhinitis. Cochrane Database Syst Rev 2003;2:CD002893.

11. Passalacqua G, Lombardi C, Troise C, et al. Sublingual immunotherapy: certainties, unmet needs and future directions. Eur Ann Allergy Clin Immunol 2009;41:163–70.

12. Valenta R, Niederberger V. Recombinant allergens for immunotherapy. J Allergy Clin Immunol 2007;119:826–30.

13. Burdin N, Guy B, Moingeon P. Immunological foundations to the quest for new vaccine adjuvants. BioDrugs 2004;18:79–93.

14. Moingeon P, de Taisne C, Almond J. Delivery technologies for human vaccines. Br Med Bull 2002;62:29–44.

15. Chapman MD, Wünschmann S, Pomés A. Protease as Th2 adjuvants. Curr Allergy Asthma Rep 2007;7:363–7.

16. Trivedi B, Valerio C, Slater JE. Endotoxin content of standardized allergen vaccines. J Allergy Clin Immunol 2003;111:777–83.

17. Barret NA, Maekawa A, Rahman OM, et al. Dectin-2 recognition of house dust mite triggers cysteinyl leukotriene generation by dendritic cells. J Immunol 2009;182:1119–28.

18. Akdis CA, Akdis M. Mechanisms of allergen-specific immunotherapy. J Allergy Clin Immunol 2011;127:18–27.

19. Durham SR, Till SJ. Immunologic changes associated with allergen immunotherapy. J Allergy Clin Immunol 1998;102:157–64.

20. Till SJ, Francis JN, Nouri-Aria K, et al. Mechanisms of immunotherapy. J Allergy Clin Immunol 2004;113:1025–34 [quiz: 35].

21. Wachholz PA, Durham SR. Induction of 'blocking' IgG antibodies during immunotherapy. Clin Exp Allergy 2003;33:1171–4.

22. van Neerven RJ, Wikborg T, Lund G, et al. Blocking antibodies induced by specific allergy vaccination prevent the activation of CD4+ T cells by inhibiting serum-IgE-facilitated allergen presentation. J Immunol 1999;163:2944–52.

23. Razafindratsita A, Saint-Lu N, Mascarell L, et al. Improvement of sublingual immunotherapy efficacy with a mucoadhesive allergen formulation. J Allergy Clin Immunol 2007;120:278–85.

24. Bahceciler NN, Arikan C, Taylor A, et al. Impact of sublingual immunotherapy on specific antibody levels in asthmatic children allergic to house dust mites. Int Arch Allergy Immunol 2005;136:287–94.

25. Durham SR, Varney VA, Gaga M, et al. Grass pollen immunotherapy decreases the number of mast cells in the skin. Clin Exp Allergy 1999;29:1490–6.

26. Durham SR, Ying S, Varney VA, et al. Grass pollen immunotherapy inhibits allergen-induced infiltration of CD4+ T lymphocytes and eosinophils in the nasal

mucosa and increases the number of cells expressing messenger RNA for interferon-gamma. J Allergy Clin Immunol 1996;97:1356–65.

27. Moingeon P, Batard T, Fadel R, et al. Immune mechanisms of allergen-specific sublingual immunotherapy. Allergy 2006;61:151–65.

28. Robinson DS, Larche M, Durham SR. Tregs and allergic disease. J Clin Invest 2004;114:1389–97.

29. Ebner C, Siemann U, Bohle B, et al. Immunological changes during specific immunotherapy of grass pollen allergy: reduced lymphoproliferative responses to allergen and shift from TH2 to TH1 in T-cell clones specific for Phl p 1, a major grass pollen allergen. Clin Exp Allergy 1997;27:1007–15.

30. Jutel M, Akdis M, Budak F, et al. IL-10 and TGF-beta cooperate in the regulatory T cell response to mucosal allergens in normal immunity and specific immunotherapy. Eur J Immunol 2003;33:1205–14.

31. Francis JN, Till SJ, Durham SR. Induction of IL-10+CD4+CD25+ T cells by grass pollen immunotherapy. J Allergy Clin Immunol 2003;111:1255–61.

32. Ciprandi G, Fenoglio D, Cirillo I, et al. Induction of interleukin 10 by sublingual immunotherapy for house dust mites: a preliminary report. Ann Allergy Asthma Immunol 2005;95:38–44.

33. Bohle B, Kinaciyan T, Gerstmayr M, et al. Sublingual immunotherapy induces IL-10-producing T regulatory cells, allergen-specific T-cell tolerance, and immune deviation. J Allergy Clin Immunol 2007;120:707–13.

34. O'Hehir RE, Gardner LM, de Leon MP, et al. House dust mite sublingual immunotherapy. The role for transforming growth factor B and functional regulatory T cells. Am J Respir Crit Care Med 2009;180:936–47.

35. Allam JP, Peng WM, Appel T, et al. Toll-like receptor 4 ligation enforces tolerogenic properties of oral mucosal Langerhans cells. J Allergy Clin Immunol 2008;121:368–74.

36. Allam JP, Novak N, Fuchs C, et al. Characterization of dendritic cells from human oral mucosa: a new Langerhans' cell type with high constitutive FcepsilonRI expression. J Allergy Clin Immunol 2003;112:141–8.

37. Mascarell L, Lombardi V, Louise A, et al. Oral dendritic cells mediate antigen-specific tolerance by stimulating Th1 and regulatory CD4+ T cells. J Allergy Clin Immunol 2008;122:603–9.

38. McKee AS, Munks MW, Marrack P. How do adjuvants work? Important considerations for new generation adjuvants. Immunity 2007;27:687–90.

39. van Overtvelt L, Moussu H, Horiot S, et al. Lactic acid bacteria as adjuvants for sublingual allergy vaccines. Vaccine 2010;28:2986–92.

40. Kalliomaki M, Salminen S, Poussa T, et al. Probiotics and prevention of atopic disease: 4-year follow-up of a randomised placebo-controlled trial. Lancet 2003;361:1869–71.

41. Grangette C, Nutten S, Palumbo E, et al. Enhanced antiinflammatory capacity of a *Lactobacillus plantarum* mutant synthesizing modified teichoic acids. Proc Natl Acad Sci U S A 2005;102:10321–6.

42. Smits HH, Engering A, van der Kleij D, et al. Selective probiotic bacteria induce IL-10-producing regulatory T cells in vitro by modulating dendritic cell function through dendritic cell-specific intercellular adhesion molecule 3-grabbing nonintegrin. J Allergy Clin Immunol 2005;115:1260–7.

43. Prescott SL, Dunstan JA, Hale J, et al. Clinical effects of probiotics are associated with increased interferon-gamma responses in very young children with atopic dermatitis. Clin Exp Allergy 2005;35:1557–64.

44. de Roock S, van Elk M, van Dijk ME, et al. Lactic acid bacteria differ in their ability to induce functional regulatory T cells in humans. Clin Exp Allergy 2010;40:103–10.

45. Zuany-Amorim C, Manlius C, Trifilieff A, et al. Long-term protective and antigen-specific effect of heat-killed *Mycobacterium vaccae* in a murine model of allergic pulmonary inflammation. J Immunol 2002;169:1492–9.

46. Arikan C, Bahceciler NN, Deniz G, et al. Bacillus Calmette-Guérin-induced interleukin-12 did not additionally improve clinical and immunologic parameters in asthmatic children treated with sublingual immunotherapy. Clin Exp Allergy 2004;34:398–405.

47. Arkwright PD, David TJ. Effect of *Mycobacterium vaccae* on atopic dermatitis in children of different ages. Br J Dermatol 2003;149:1029–34.

48. Choi IS, Koh YI. Effects of BCG revaccination on asthma. Allergy 2003;58:1114–6.

49. Townley RG, Barlan IB, Patino C, et al. The effect of BCG vaccine at birth on the development of atopy or allergic disease in young children. Ann Allergy Asthma Immunol 2004;92:350–5.

50. Smit JJ, Van Loveren H, Hoekstra MO, et al. *Mycobacterium vaccae* administration during allergen sensitization or challenge suppresses asthmatic features. Clin Exp Allergy 2003;33:1083–9.

51. Arkwright PD, David TJ. Intradermal administration of a killed *Mycobacterium vaccae* suspension (SRL 172) is associated with improvement in atopic dermatitis in children with moderate-to-severe disease. J Allergy Clin Immunol 2001; 107:531–4.

52. Freytag LC, Clements JD. Mucosal adjuvants. Vaccine 2005;23:1804–13.

53. Pizza M, Giuliani MM, Fontana MR, et al. Mucosal vaccines: non toxic derivatives of LT and CT as mucosal adjuvants. Vaccine 2001;19:2534–41.

54. Akdis CA, Kussebi F, Pulendran B, et al. Inhibition of T helper 2-type responses, IgE production and eosinophilia by synthetic lipopeptides. Eur J Immunol 2003; 33:2717–26.

55. Trujillo-Vargas CM, Mayer KD, Bickert T, et al. Vaccinations with T-helper type 1 directing adjuvants have different suppressive effects on the development of allergen-induced T-helper type 2 responses. Clin Exp Allergy 2005;35:1003–13.

56. Santeliz JV, Van Nest G, Traquina P, et al. Amb a 1-linked CpG oligodeoxynucleotides reverse established airway hyperresponsiveness in a murine model of asthma. J Allergy Clin Immunol 2002;109:455–62.

57. Johansen P, Senti G, Martinez Gomez JM, et al. Toll-like receptor ligands as adjuvants in allergen-specific immunotherapy. Clin Exp Allergy 2005;35:1591–8.

58. Patel M, Xu D, Kewin P, et al. TLR2 agonist ameliorates established allergic airway inflammation by promoting Th1 response and not via regulatory T cells. J Immunol 2005;174:7558–63.

59. Goldman M. Toll-like receptor ligands as novel pharmaceuticals for allergic disorders. Clin Exp Immunol 2007;147:208–16.

60. Lombardi V, van Overtvelt L, Horiot S, et al. The TLR2 agonist Pam3CSK4 enhances the induction of antigen-specific tolerance via the sublingual route. Clin Exp Allergy 2008;38:1819–29.

61. Mascarell L, Van Overtvelt L, Lombardi L, et al. A synthetic triacylated pseudo-dipeptide molecule promotes Th1/TReg immune responses and enhances tolerance induction via the sublingual route. Vaccine 2007;26:108–18.

62. Baldridge JR, Yorgensen Y, Ward JR, et al. Monophosphoryl lipid A enhances mucosal and systemic immunity to vaccine antigens following intranasal administration. Vaccine 2000;18:2416–25.

63. Quarcoo D, Weixler S, Joachim RA, et al. Resiquimod, a new immune response modifier from the family of imidazoquinolinamines, inhibits allergen-induced Th2 responses, airway inflammation and airway hyper-reactivity in mice. Clin Exp Allergy 2004;34:1314–20.

64. Drachenberg KJ, Wheeler AW, Stuebner P, et al. A well-tolerated grass pollen-specific allergy vaccine containing a novel adjuvant, monophosphoryl lipid A, reduces allergic symptoms after only four preseasonal injections. Allergy 2001;56:498–505.

65. Mothes N, Heinzkill M, Drachenberg KJ, et al. Allergen-specific immunotherapy with a monophosphoryl lipid A-adjuvanted vaccine: reduced seasonally boosted immunoglobulin E production and inhibition of basophil histamine release by therapy-induced blocking antibodies. Clin Exp Allergy 2003;33:1198–208.

66. Creticos PS, Schroeder JT, Hamilton RG, et al. Immunotherapy with a ragweed-toll-like receptor 9 agonist vaccine for allergic rhinitis. N Engl J Med 2006;355:1445–55.

67. Pfaar O, Barth C, Jaschke C, et al. Sublingual allergen-specific immunotherapy adjuvanted with monophosphoryl lipid A: a phase I/IIa study. Int Arch Allergy Immunol 2010;154:336–44.

68. Asai K, Foley SC, Sumi Y, et al. Amb a 1-immunostimulatory oligodeoxynucleotide conjugate immunotherapy increases CD4+CD25+ T cells in the nasal mucosa of subjects with allergic rhinitis. Allergol Int 2008;57:377–81.

69. Taher YA, van Esch BC, Hofman GA, et al. 1alpha,25-dihydroxyvitamin D3 potentiates the beneficial effects of allergen immunotherapy in a mouse model of allergic asthma: role for IL-10 and TGFβ. J Immunol 2008;180:5211–21.

70. Majak P, Rychlik B, Stelmach I. The effect of oral steroids with and without vitamin D3 on early efficacy of immunotherapy in asthmatic children. Clin Exp Allergy 2009;39:1830–41.

71. van Overtvelt L, Lombardi V, Horiot S, et al. IL-10 inducing adjuvants enhance sublingual immunotherapy efficacy. Int Arch Allergy Immunol 2008;145:152–62.

72. de Jong EC, Vieira PL, Kalinski P, et al. Corticosteroids inhibit the production of inflammatory mediators in immature monocyte-derived DC and induce the development of tolerogenic DC3. J Leukoc Biol 1999;66:201–4.

73. Penna G, Adorini L. 1 Alpha,25-dihydroxyvitamin D3 inhibits differentiation, maturation, activation, and survival of dendritic cells leading to impaired alloreactive T cell activation. J Immunol 2000;164:2405–11.

74. Piemonti L, Monti P, Allavena P, et al. Glucocorticoids affect human dendritic cell differentiation and maturation. J Immunol 1999;162:6473–81.

75. Wilckens T, De RR. Glucocorticoids and immune function: unknown dimensions and new frontiers. Immunol Today 1997;18:418–24.

76. Dao Nguyen X, Robinson DS. Fluticasone propionate increases CD4 CD25+ T regulatory cell suppression of allergen-stimulated CD4CD25 T cells by an IL-10-dependent mechanism. J Allergy Clin Immunol 2004;114:296–301.

77. de Jonge MI, Hamstra HJ, Jiskoot W, et al. Intranasal immunisation of mice with liposomes containing recombinant meningococcal OpaB and OpaJ proteins. Vaccine 2004;22:4021–8.

78. Crameri R, Kündig TM, Akdis CA. Modular antigen-translocation as a novel vaccine strategy for allergen-specific immunotherapy. Curr Opin Allergy Clin Immunol 2009;9:568–73.

79. Galvain S, André C, Vatrinet C, et al. Safety and efficacy studies of liposomes in specific immunotherapy. Curr Ther Res 1999;60:278–94.

80. Sanders MT, Brown LE, Deliyannis G, et al. ISCOM-based vaccines: the second decade. Immunol Cell Biol 2005;83:119–28.

81. Hu KF, Lovgren-Bengtsson K, Morein B. Immunostimulating complexes (ISCOMs) for nasal vaccination. Adv Drug Deliv Rev 2001;51:149–59.

82. Kim N, Kwon SS, Lee J, et al. Protective effect of the DNA vaccine encoding the major house dust mite allergens on allergic inflammation in the murine model of house dust mite allergy. Clin Mol Allergy 2006;4:1–9.

83. Schöll I, Weissenböck A, Förster-Waldl E, et al. Allergen-loaded biodegradable poly(D,L-lactic-co-glycolic) acid nanoparticles down-regulate an ongoing Th2 response in the BALB/c mouse model. Clin Exp Allergy 2004;34:315–21.

84. Jilek S, Walter E, Merkle HP, et al. Modulation of allergic responses in mice by using biodegradable poly(lactide-co-glycolide) microspheres. J Allergy Clin Immunol 2004;114:943–50.

85. Edlmayr J, Niespodziana K, Linhart B, et al. A combination vaccine for allergy and rhinovirus infections based on rhinovirus-derived surface protein VP1 and a nonallergenic peptide of the major timothy grass pollen allergen Phl p 1. J Immunol 2009;182:6298–306.

86. Schmitz N, Dietmeier K, Bauer M, et al. Displaying Fel d 1 on virus-like particles prevents reactogenicity despite greatly enhanced immunogenicity: a novel therapy for cat allergy. J Exp Med 2009;206:1941–55.

87. Kündig TM, Senti G, Schnetzler G, et al. Der p 1 peptide on virus-like particles is safe and highly immunogenic in healthy adults. J Allergy Clin Immunol 2006;117:1470–6.

88. Senti G, Johansen P, Haug S, et al. Use of A-type CpG oligodeoxynucleotides as an adjuvant in allergen-specific immunotherapy in humans: a phase I/IIa clinical trial. Clin Exp Allergy 2009;39:562–70.

89. Boisgerault F, Moron G, Leclerc C. Virus-like particles: a new family of delivery systems. Expert Rev Vaccines 2002;1:101–9.

90. Saint-Lu N, Tourdot S, Razafindrasita A, et al. Targeting the allergen to oral dendritic cells with mucoadhesive chitosan particles enhances tolerance induction. Allergy 2009;64:1003–13.

91. Gómez S, Gamazo C, San Roman B, et al. A novel nanoparticulate adjuvant for immunotherapy with Lolium perenne. J Immunol Methods 2009;348:1–8.

92. Broos S, Lundberg K, Akagi T, et al. Immunomodulatory nanoparticles as adjuvants and allergen-delivery system to human dendritic cells: implications for specific immunotherapy. Vaccine 2010;28:5075–85.

93. Terada T. New therapeutic strategies: a chimeric human-cat fusion protein inhibits allergic reactivity. Clin Exp Allergy 2006;6:96–100.

94. Gerstmayr M, Ilk N, Jahn-Schmid B, et al. Natural self-assembly of allergen-S-layer fusion proteins is no prerequisite for reduced allergenicity and T cell stimulatory capacity. Int Arch Allergy Immunol 2009;149:231–8.

95. Jeannin P, Renno T, Goetsch L, et al. OmpA targets dendritic cells, induces their maturation and delivers antigen into the MHC class I presentation pathway. Nat Immunol 2000;1:502–9.

96. Goetsch L, Gonzalez A, Plotnicky-Gilquin H, et al. Targeting of nasal mucosa-associated antigen-presenting cells in vivo with an outer membrane protein A derived from Klebsiella pneumoniae. Infect Immun 2001;69:6434–44.

97. Haicheur N, Benchetrit F, Amessou M, et al. The B subunit of Shiga toxin coupled to full-size antigenic protein elicits humoral and cell-mediated immune responses associated with a Th1-dominant polarization. Int Immunol 2003;15:1161–71.

98. El Azami El Idrissi M, Ladant D, Leclerc C. The adenylate cyclase of *Bordetella pertussis*: a vector to target antigen presenting cells. Toxicon 2002;40:1661–5.

99. Bonifaz LC, Bonnyay DP, Charalambous A, et al. In vivo targeting of antigens to maturing dendritic cells via the DEC-205 receptor improves T cell vaccination. J Exp Med 2004;199:815–24.

100. Hobson P, Barnfield C, Barnes A, et al. Mucosal immunization with DNA vaccines. Methods 2003;31:217–24.

Index

Note: Page numbers of article titles are in **boldface** type.

Immunol Allergy Clin N Am 31 (2011) 421–432
doi:10.1016/S0889-8561(11)00030-0
0889-8561/11/$ – see front matter © 2011 Elsevier Inc. All rights reserved.

immunology.theclinics.com

Erratum

Please note that in the May 2010 issue of *Immunology and Allergy Clinics of North America* (Volume 30, Issue 2), an author's last name was misspelled. The correct spelling is **M. Cavazzana-Calvo**. The article appeared on pages 237–248 and is entitled, "Gene Therapy for Primary Immunodeficiencies."

Immunol Allergy Clin N Am 31 (2011) I
doi:10.1016/j.iac.2011.03.004
0889-8561/11/$ – see front matter © 2011 Elsevier Inc. All rights reserved.

immunology.theclinics.com

Moving?

Make sure your subscription moves with you!

To notify us of your new address, find your **Clinics Account Number** (located on your mailing label above your name), and contact customer service at:

Email: journalscustomerservice-usa@elsevier.com

800-654-2452 (subscribers in the U.S. & Canada)
314-447-8871 (subscribers outside of the U.S. & Canada)

Fax number: 314-447-8029

Elsevier Health Sciences Division
Subscription Customer Service
3251 Riverport Lane
Maryland Heights, MO 63043

Printed and bound by CPI Group (UK) Ltd, Croydon, CR0 4YY

03/10/2024

01040455-0010